DAY HIKES AROUND
Orange County

GREAT HIKES

Robert Stone

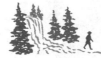

Day Hike Books, Inc.
RED LODGE, MONTANA

Published by Day Hike Books, Inc.
P.O. Box 865 · Red Lodge, Montana 59068
www.dayhikebooks.com

Distributed by National Book Network
800-243-0495 (direct order) · 800-820-2329 (fax order)

Design and maps by Paula Doherty

The author has made every attempt to provide accurate information in this book. However, trail routes and features may change— please use common sense and forethought, and be mindful of your own capabilities. Let this book guide you, but be aware that each hiker assumes responsibility for their own safety. The author and publisher do not assume any responsibility for loss, damage, or injury caused through the use of this book.

Copyright © 2017 by Day Hike Books, Inc.
2nd Edition
ISBN: 978-1-57342-074-7
eISBN: 978-1-57342-401-1

Library of Congress Control Number: 2016904465

10 9 8 7 6 5 4 3 2 1

FRONT COVER PHOTO:
Santiago Oaks Regional Park, Hike 15.
photograph courtesy of Orange County Parks: OCParks.com

BACK COVER PHOTO:
Gnarled trees along the Serrano Cow Trail in
Whiting Ranch Wilderness Park, Hike 27.
photograph courtesy of Orange County Parks: OCParks.com

Table of Contents

The Hikes

SANTA ANA MOUNTAINS

Chino Hills • Brea • Yorba Linda

Anaheim • Anaheim Hills • Orange • Tustin

Lake Forest • Foothill Ranch • Mission Viejo
Rancho Santa Margarita • Coto de Caza

Santiago Canyon Road
Silverado • Modjeska • Trabuco Canyon

Ortega Highway Corridor
to Wildomar • Murrieta • Temecula

Caspers Wilderness Park

Upper Ortega Highway
North Main Divide Road

San Mateo Canyon Wilderness

THE COASTLINE

Palos Verdes Peninsula
Torrance to Long Beach

Seal Beach to Newport Bay

Newport Bay to Dana Point

South Coast Wilderness Area:
Crystal Cove State Park
Laguna Coast Wilderness Park
Aliso and Wood Canyons Wilderness Park

Dana Point Headlands to San Mateo Point
Dana Point · San Juan Capistrano · San Clemente

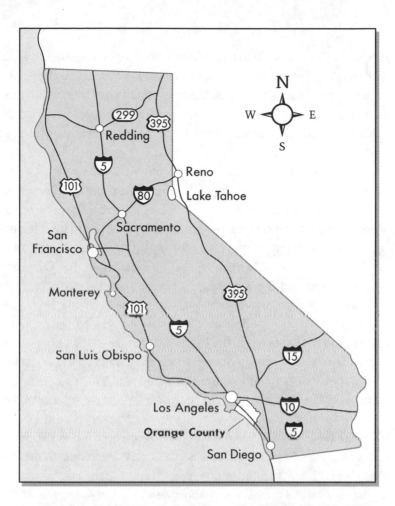

Hiking Orange County

Orange County lies along the coast in southern California between Los Angeles and San Diego. The county is framed by the Pacific Ocean on one side while the Santa Ana Mountains stretch along the entire back side of the county. The coast-to-mountain landscape creates an interesting, diverse terrain that offers many opportunities for exploration.

Despite the urban encroachment, nearly 30% of Orange County is preserved as city parklands, wilderness preserves, national forests, and state parks. Along the county's 44 miles of shoreline reside long stretches of sandy beaches, tidepools, uplifted marine terraces, eroding sandstone cliffs, promontories, peninsulas, bluffs, sheltered coves, protected wetlands, and tidal estuaries. The Cleveland National Forest and the San Mateo Canyon Wilderness cover thousands of acres of forested canyons and plateaus of the Santa Ana Range. This essential guide describes how to get to backcountry trailheads in the Santa Anas, the best trails to hike in the county's expansive parklands, and where to find access points to the coastline. Several inviting urban routes are included as well.

The hikes are divided into two sections—inland and coastal. Hikes 1—65 are located inland along the foothills and slopes of the Santa Ana Mountains. These hikes run from north to south along the range, from Chino Hills State Park to the Santa Rosa Plateau near Temecula. Hikes 66—112 are located along the coast. These hikes run from the Palos Verdes Peninsula and southward to San Clemente at the Orange—San Diego county line. In general, the coastal hikes are more urban, while the inland hikes tend to be more remote. County-wide maps on the next few pages show the overall locations of the hikes.

The Santa Ana Mountains
HIKES 1—65

Rimming the northeast side of the county are the dramatic Santa Ana Mountains, reaching over a mile high. Amongst the hills are creeks, lakes, grasslands, canyons, ridges, and hardwood forests. Protecting the open space are state and county parks, wildlife sanctuaries, wilderness areas, and the Cleveland National Forest.

The Chino Hills lie at the northern end of the Santa Anas—
Hikes 1—12. Within the expansive low-level mountains is Chino Hills
State Park, a 14,000-acre parcel of protected land. From atop the
highest summit of the park—at 1,781 feet—are 360-degree views
from the ocean to the San Gabriel Mountains. Long canyon corridors
stretch in opposite directions through the length of the park.

Moving southeast along the range, several expansive regional
parks are tucked between homes and development in the area adjacent to Anaheim Hills, Orange, and Tustin—**Hikes 13—24**. The geography largely consists of rolling, chaparral-covered slopes punctuated
with open sandstone peaks. An extensive trail system links many of
the parks, which range over hundreds of acres of open land.

The bulk of the Santa Ana range lies between the Santa Ana River
and the Ortega Highway. It remains largely undeveloped. The vehicle-
restricted Main Divide Road runs along the rugged ridgeline—from
the Ortega Highway to Highway 241—accessing the range's highest
peaks. **Hikes 25—40** are located in the area between the western foothills and the forested ridgeline. The area is characterized by
rolling hills in the lower elevations (often former ranchlands), then
merging into deep canyon corridors, dense woodlands, and rocky
sandstone summits. Many hikes here travel through stream-fed drainages to high overlooks, with views across the Orange County basin
to the ocean. Hundreds of miles of inter-connected, multi-use trails
connect the foothills to the ridgeline.

The Ortega Highway runs across the south-central end of the
Santa Anas, from San Juan Capistrano to I-15. The scenic (but some-
what treacherous) highway provides access to numerous trails into
the wilderness—**Hikes 41—60**. Caspers Wilderness Park likes in the
foothills of the highway corridor across 8,000 acres of old ranchland.
Continuing eastward, the snaking highway gains elevation as it crosses the ridge. Many backcountry trails are located along this stretch
of the highway, from hikes up to Los Pinos Peak to trails that venture
deep into the San Mateo Canyon Wilderness. The landscape features
a variety of habitats, including folded ridges covered in woodlands,
perennial streams that wind down boulder-lined creekbeds, rocky
peaks, and open slopes with the pleasant aroma of sage. The Santa

Rosa Plateau—**Hikes 61—65**—marks the southern end of the Santa Ana Mountains, where the range begins to meld into wide mesas and plateaus.

The Coastal Hikes
HIKES 66—112

The coastal hikes stretch from the Palos Verdes Peninsula (south of downtown Los Angeles) to San Mateo Point (at the Orange—San Diego county line).

Across the Orange County border at the north end is the Palos Verdes Peninsula and Long Beach—**Hikes 66—73**. This geographically interesting area includes ocean-side cliffs, beaches, coves, grassy bluffs, actively slipping landslides, and some of the best tidepools in the area. After Long Beach, the coastline turns southeast, where Orange County begins. The urban population remains dense down to Newport Bay, yet this long and wide length of sandy coastline is accessible to the public. **Hikes 74—80** offer tidal basins, beaches, and coastal bluffs, as well as piers, boardwalks, and harbor-side pathways.

Between Newport Bay and Dana Point lie three large, coastal parks that are part of the South Coast Wilderness Area. These contiguous parks comprise almost 20,000 acres of undeveloped coastal frontage in Orange County. The parks spread across numerous canyon drainages between the coast and the high inland ridges of the San Joaquin Hills. Wooded canyons, sage-covered hills, and weather-sculpted sandstone formations offer a varied landscape. **Hikes 81—100** explore the rugged upland geography along many miles of multi-use trails across this land that was formerly part of the Irvine Ranch.

The Dana Point headlands protrude into the ocean near the southern end of Orange County. The mouth of San Juan Creek, a major drainage from the Santa Ana Mountains, flows into the ocean at the point. Offshore lies a marine refuge, tidepools and a large harbor. Several pathways are located along the bluffs and shoreline—**Hikes 101—108**. Just past San Mateo Point, the vast expanse of Camp Pendleton Marine Base merges inland to the southern end of the Santa Ana Mountains.

These hikes provide an excellent cross-section of scenery and difficulty levels, ranging from coastal beach walks to steep canyon climbs with far-reaching views. Hiking times range from 30 minutes to six hours. The majority of hikes are 2–5 miles in length. Relevant maps are listed under the statistics for options to lengthen the hike. A quick glance at the hikes' statistics and summaries will allow you to choose a hike that is appropriate to your ability and intentions. The first overall map identifies the general locations of the hikes and major access roads. Several other regional maps (underlined in the table of contents), as well as maps for each hike, provide the essential details. A street guide, such as the Thomas Guide, is useful for navigating through the metropolitan areas.

A few basic necessities are recommended. Wear supportive, comfortable hiking shoes and layered clothing. Bring along plenty of water and be aware of potentially high temperatures. Bring hats, sunscreen, sunglasses, snacks, and appropriate outerwear for variable weather. Insects, including ticks, may be prolific and poison oak flourishes in many of the canyons and shady areas. Exercise caution by using insect repellent and staying on the trails. A basic first aid kit is always a good idea. Be aware that we share the land with rattlesnakes and (rarely) mountain lions.

Wildfires are common in southern California. For the latest updates on trail conditions or closures, check with the Forest Service.

Use good judgement about your capabilities—reference the hiking statistics for an approximation of difficulty—and allow extra time for exploration.

The National Forest Adventure Pass is a parking permit required by the U.S. Forest Service and issued for a fee. Adventure Passes are required in the Cleveland National Forest. The daily or annual pass can be purchased online, at any Forest Service facility, or at many local outdoor shops.

Dogs: Trail access to dogs is listed in the statistics at the top of each hike. Please note that canine companions, where allowed, must be kept on a leash of six feet or less, and clean up of dog waste is always required. Regulations may change; it is always a good idea to check with park personnel before bringing your dog.

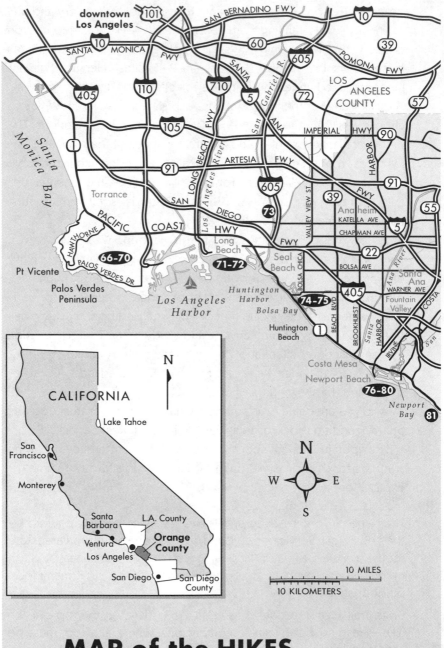

MAP of the HIKES

ORANGE COUNTY and VICINITY

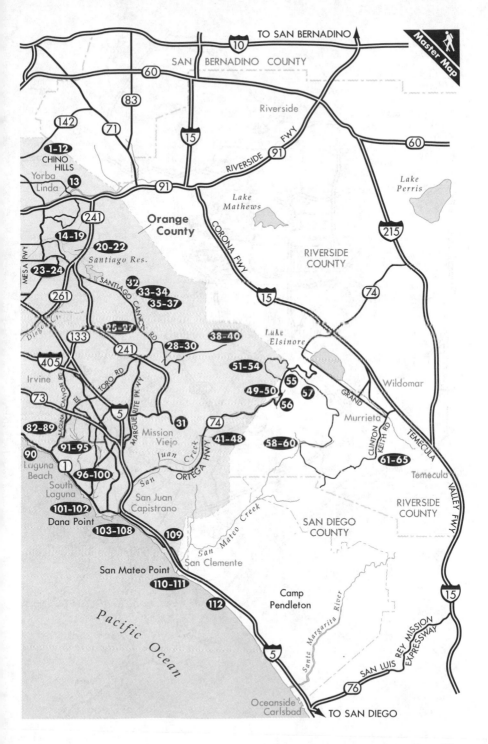

Master Map

TO SAN BERNADINO

SAN BERNADINO COUNTY

10

60

83

Riverside

142

71

15

CHINO HILLS

1-12

Yorba Linda

13

RIVERSIDE FWY

91

91

Lake Mathews

Lake Perris

Orange County

241

14-19

20-22

Santiago Res.

CORONA FWY

RIVERSIDE COUNTY

215

23-24

MESA FWY

261

SANTIAGO CANYON RD

32

33-34

35-37

74

15

25-27

Lake Elsinore

38-40

133

241

28-30

51-54

405

TORO RD

55

49-50

57

GRAND

Wildomar

Irvine

73

5

31

56

MARGUERITE PKWY

Murrieta

CLINTON KEITH RD

TEMECULA

82-89

LAGUNA CANYON RD

91-95

Mission Viejo

74

41-48

58-60

61-65

90

Laguna Beach

1

96-100

Juan Creek

ORTEGA HWY

Temecula

RIVERSIDE COUNTY

VALLEY FWY

South Laguna

San

101-102

San Juan Capistrano

San Mateo Creek

SAN DIEGO COUNTY

Dana Point

103-108

109

San Mateo Creek

15

San Mateo Point

San Clemente

110-111

112

Camp Pendleton

Santa Margarita River

Pacific Ocean

5

SAN LUIS REY MISSION EXPRESSWAY

76

Oceanside Carlsbad

TO SAN DIEGO

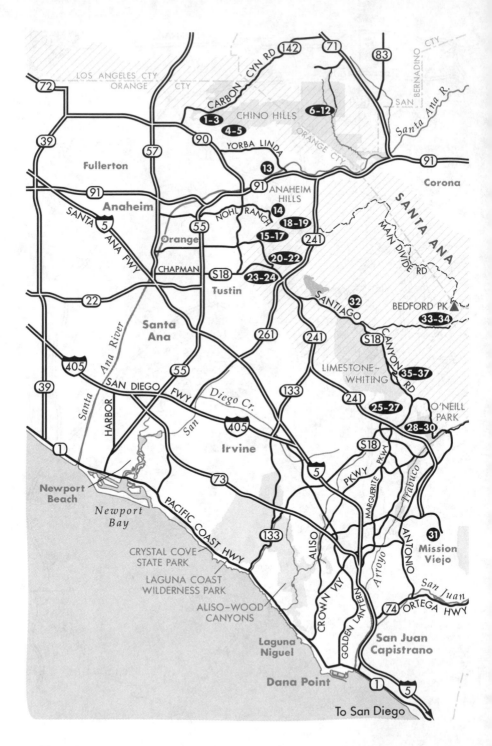

Santa Ana Mountains

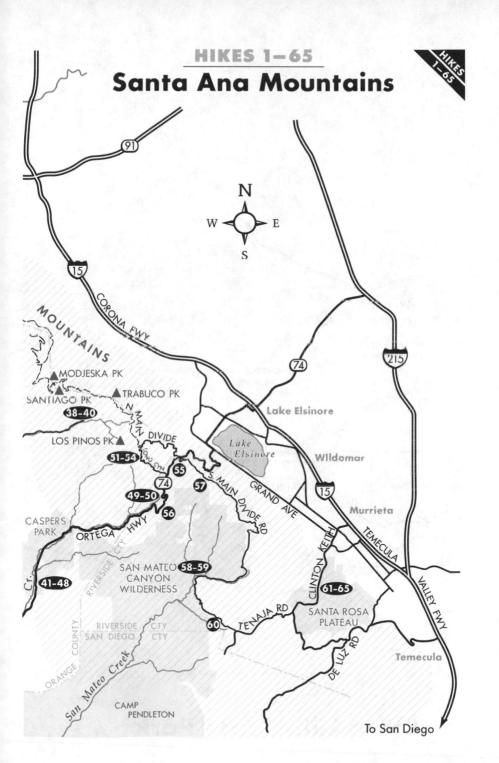

HIKES 1-65

91

N
W · E
S

15

CORONA FWY

MOUNTAINS

MODJESKA PK

SANTIAGO PK
TRABUCO PK

38-40

74

Lake Elsinore

LOS PINOS PK

N MAIN DIVIDE

51-54

Lake Elsinore

Wildomar

55

74

57

S MAIN DIVIDE RD

GRAND AVE

15

49-50

56

Murrieta

CASPERS PARK

ORTEGA HWY

RIVERSIDE CTY HWY

CLINTON KEITH

TEMECULA

41-48

Cr.

SAN MATEO CANYON WILDERNESS

58-59

61-65

VALLEY FWY

RIVERSIDE CTY
SAN DIEGO CTY

60

TENAJA RD

SANTA ROSA PLATEAU

DE LUZ RD

Temecula

ORANGE COUNTY

San Mateo Creek

CAMP PENDLETON

215

To San Diego

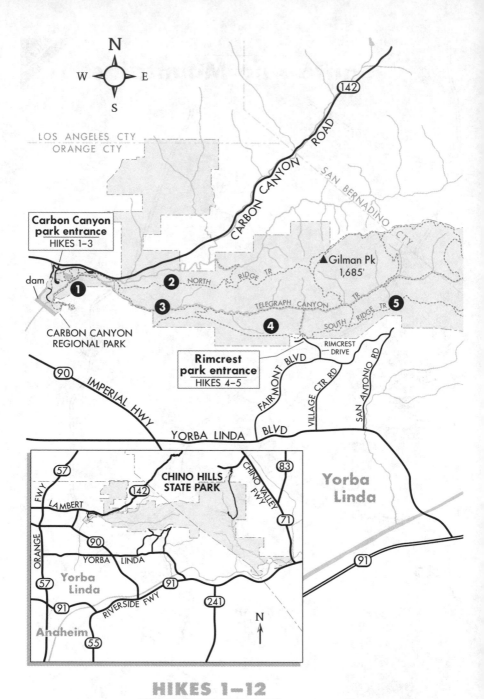

Chino Hills State Park

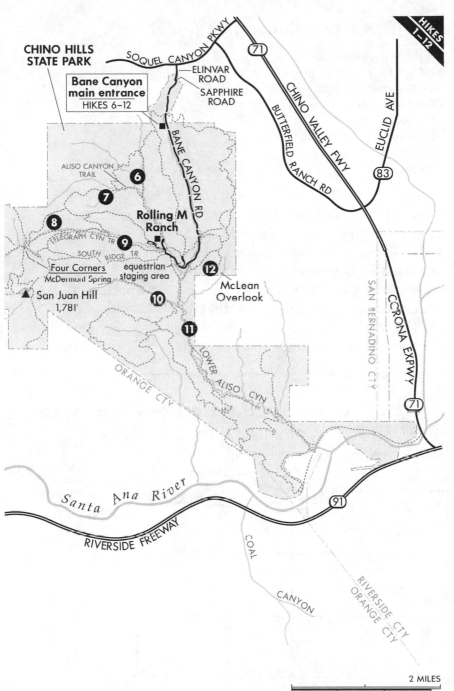

CHINO HILLS STATE PARK

SOQUEL CANYON PKWY

71

ELINVAR ROAD

Bane Canyon main entrance
HIKES 6-12

SAPPHIRE ROAD

CHINO VALLEY FWY

EUCLID AVE

BUTTERFIELD RANCH RD

BANE CANYON RD

ALISO CANYON TRAIL

6

7

83

Rolling M Ranch

8

TELEGRAPH CYN TR

9

SOUTH RIDGE TR

Four Corners
McDermont Spring

equestrian staging area

12

McLean Overlook

▲ San Juan Hill
1,781'

10

11

SAN BERNADINO CTY

CORONA EXPWY

71

ORANGE CTY

LOWER ALISO CYN

Santa Ana River

RIVERSIDE FREEWAY

91

COAL CANYON

RIVERSIDE CTY
ORANGE CTY

2 MILES

3 KILOMETERS

1. Carbon Canyon Regional Park

Hiking distance: 2.2-mile loop
Hiking time: 1 hour
Configuration: loop
Elevation gain: level
Difficulty: easy
Exposure: a mix of shade and sun
Dogs: allowed
Maps: U.S.G.S. Yorba Linda · Carbon Canyon Regional Park map

Carbon Canyon Regional Park is a 124-acre park on the rolling foothills of the Chino Hill Range in Brea. The park is situated upstream from the Carbon Canyon Dam and is adjacent to the west end of Chino Hills State Park. Appoximately half of the scenic parkland has been developed, with mowed grassland and amenities, while the other half remains natural. The wooded area includes Canary Island pines, Monterey pines, eucalyptus, pepper, walnut, willow, and sycamore trees. A magical ten-acre grove of thriving coastal redwoods was planted in 1975. With more than

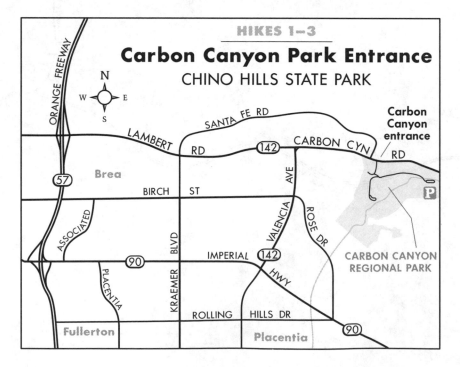

HIKES 1–3

Carbon Canyon Park Entrance
CHINO HILLS STATE PARK

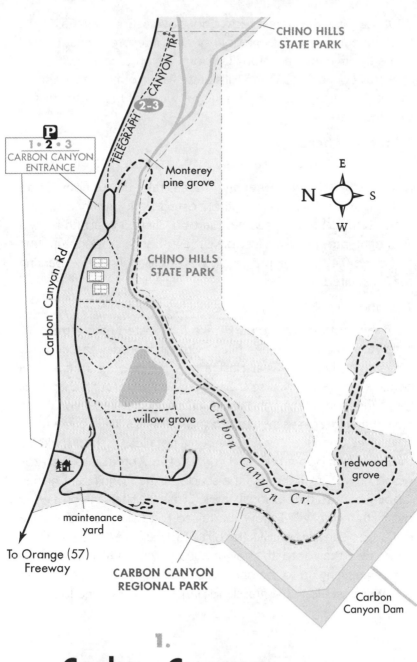

CHINO HILLS
STATE PARK

2-3

P
1 • 2 • 3
CARBON CANYON
ENTRANCE

Monterey
pine grove

E
N ◇ S
W

Carbon Canyon Rd

CHINO HILLS
STATE PARK

willow grove

Carbon Canyon Cr.

redwood
grove

maintenance
yard

To Orange (57)
Freeway

CARBON CANYON
REGIONAL PARK

Carbon
Canyon Dam

1.
Carbon Canyon
Regional Park

200 trees, it is the largest redwood grove in Southern California (and the only one in Orange County). This interpretive nature trail loops through the park along Carbon Canyon Creek.

A trail connects to Chino Hills State Park from the east end of the parking area, accessing a huge network of multi-use trails in the state park.

To the trailhead

4442 CARBON CANYON ROAD · BREA   33.922272, -117.837000

From the 57 (Orange) Freeway in Brea, take the Lambert Road exit. Drive 2.5 miles east to the posted park entrance on the right. (Lambert Road becomes Carbon Canyon Road en route.) Turn right into the park. Just past the entrance station, turn left and drive 0.4 miles to the far end of the parking lot. A parking fee is required.

The hike

From the east end of the park, take the posted nature trail into a grove of Monterey pines filled with birdhouses. Descend and curve right, heading west past a massive pepper tree with a bench at its base. Traverse the rugged terrain through chaparral. Pass a junction on the right, which crosses Carbon Canyon Creek from the wilderness sanctuary to the grassy parkland and a four-acre lake. Continue straight, walking parallel to the creekbed through a bamboo grove, and curve left 500 feet into the redwood grove. Stroll through the shade of the magnificent giants, looping back to the seasonal creek. Cross the drainage on a wide dirt path to the left. Follow the raised road along the east side of Carbon Canyon Dam. As the dirt road makes a 90-degree left bend, take the footpath straight ahead. Wind through lush foliage, zigzagging up to the park road. Veer right on the road, and follow it east along the grassland park, completing the loop. ▤

2. Gilman Peak
from North Ridge

Carbon Canyon Park Entrance

CHINO HILLS STATE PARK

Hiking distance: 7 miles round trip
Hiking time: 3.5 hours
Configuration: out-and-back
Elevation gain: 1,200 feet
Difficulty: strenuous
Exposure: mostly exposed with pockets of trees
Dogs: not allowed
Maps: U.S.G.S. Yorba Linda · Chino Hills State Park map

The Puente-Chino Hills Wildlife Corridor extends 31 miles from Whittier to the north end of the Santa Ana Mountains. Within the expansive low-level mountains is Chino Hills State Park, a 14,100-acre island of protected land surrounded by the growing urban sprawl. The elevations of the rolling hills range from 430 feet to 1,781 feet. Chaparral and woodland ecosystems, former ranch land, span across the wide open spaces and hills, providing a vital wildlife corridor. Many hiking opportunities are available across the park's 60 miles of multi-use trails (hike, biking and equestrian).

Gilman Peak is a rounded 1,685-foot peak on the western side of Chino Hills State Park. It is the second highest peak in the park, second to 1,781-foot San Juan Hill. This trail begins near the mouth of Telegraph Canyon, and follows North Ridge to the bald peak. From the open summit, the vistas extend across four counties—Los Angeles, San Bernardino, Riverside, and Orange. The views include the winter snow-capped San Gabriel Mountains in the north, the Santa Ana Mountains to the southeast, and the Orange County basin to the ocean.

This hike is an out-and-back trail to Gilman Peak along the North Ridge. Hike 3 offers a loop option, which returns to the trailhead through Telegraph Canyon.

To the trailhead

4442 CARBON CANYON ROAD · BREA   33.922272, -117.837000

From the 57 (Orange) Freeway in Brea, take the Lambert Road exit. Drive 2.5 miles east to the posted park entrance on the right. (Lambert Road becomes Carbon Canyon Road en route.) Turn right into the park. Just past the entrance station, turn left and drive 0.4 miles to the far end of the parking lot. A parking fee is required.

The hike

From the east end of the parking lot by Carbon Canyon Road, take the posted Telegraph Canyon Trail. Parallel Carbon Canyon Road several hundred yards to the Chino Hills State Park trail entrance. Enter the state park on the gravel road, and cross a bridge over a seasonal drainage to a trail gate and a junction. The right fork enters the mouth of Telegraph Canyon. Take the left fork—the North Ridge Trail. Steadily climb the north-facing slope on the dirt road while overlooking Carbon Canyon to the left. At just over one mile, cross over to the south-facing slope above Telegraph Canyon on the right. Pass a junction on the left at 1.6 miles, staying on the ridgeline. The sweeping views extend to the surrounding mountains across the three neighboring counties. Skirt the north side of Gilman Peak to a junction on the right, just shy of the post and wire fence. Curve to the right on the wide Gilman Trail, reaching the rounded 1,685-foot summit. This is the turn-around point. After enjoying the views, return along the same route. ▪

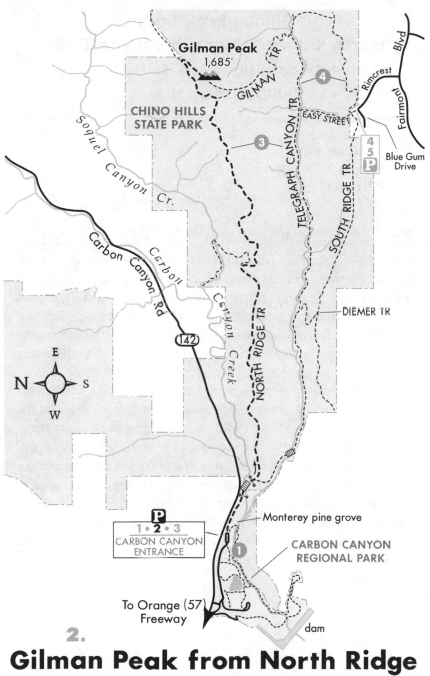

Gilman Peak
1,685'

CHINO HILLS
STATE PARK

GILMAN TR

Soquel Canyon Cr.

Carbon Canyon Rd

Carbon Canyon Creek

TELEGRAPH CANYON TR

EASY STREET

Rimcrest Blvd

Fairmont

4
5
P
Blue Gum
Drive

SOUTH RIDGE TR

DIEMER TR

NORTH RIDGE TR

142

E
N — S
W

Monterey pine grove

P
1 • 2 • 3
CARBON CANYON
ENTRANCE

CARBON CANYON
REGIONAL PARK

To Orange (57)
Freeway

dam

2.

Gilman Peak from North Ridge
CHINO HILLS STATE PARK

3. Gilman Peak Loop:
North Ridge—Telegraph Canyon Trails

Carbon Canyon Park Entrance

CHINO HILLS STATE PARK

Hiking distance: 8.2-mile loop
Hiking time: 4 hours
Configuration: loop
Elevation gain: 1,200 feet
Difficulty: strenuous
Exposure: mostly exposed ridge; partially shaded canyon
Dogs: not allowed
Maps: U.S.G.S. Yorba Linda · Chino Hills State Park map

Chino Hills State Park is located at the intersection of Orange, San Bernardino, and Riverside Counties. The diverse landscape includes open, rolling grasslands alongside stream-fed canyons with stands of oaks, sycamores, and native walnut trees. San Juan Hill (1,781 feet) and Gilman Peak (1,685 feet) are the high points of the landscape, separated by Telegraph Canyon, stretching nine miles across the parkland.

This strenuous hike loops from a high ridge to a cool canyon, offering a sampling of these ecosystems. The route begins at the state park's west end and climbs up to Gilman Peak along North Ridge. The return from the peak drops down a one-mile trail into Telegraph Canyon, then runs parallel to the wooded drainage back to the trailhead. The long canyon is the centerpiece of the park, stretching from Carbon Canyon Regional Park to Aliso Canyon by the state park headquarters (Rolling M Ranch). The canyon is a rich riparian corridor bounded by chaparral-clad hillsides.

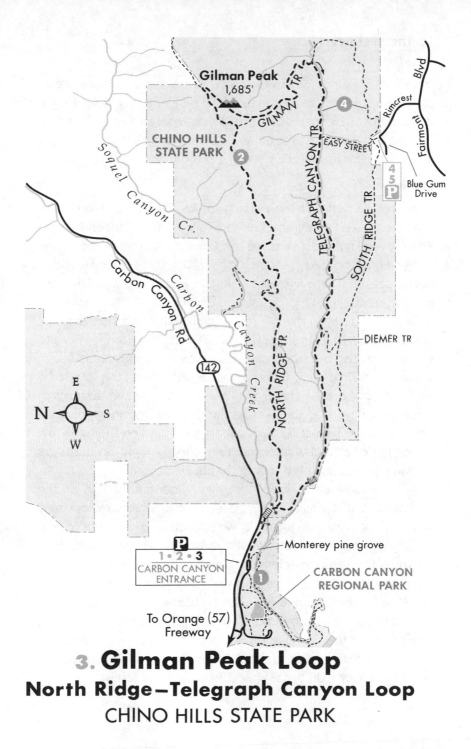

3. Gilman Peak Loop
North Ridge–Telegraph Canyon Loop
CHINO HILLS STATE PARK

To the trailhead

4442 CARBON CANYON ROAD · BREA   33.922272, -117.837000

From the 57 (Orange) Freeway in Brea, take the Lambert Road exit. Drive 2.5 miles east to the posted park entrance on the right. (Lambert Road becomes Carbon Canyon Road en route.) Turn right into the park. Just past the entrance station, turn left and drive 0.4 miles to the far end of the parking lot. A parking fee is required.

The hike

From the east end of the parking lot by Carbon Canyon Road, take the posted Telegraph Canyon Trail. Parallel Carbon Canyon Road several hundred yards to the Chino Hills State Park trail entrance. Enter the state park on the gravel road, and cross a bridge over a seasonal drainage to a trail gate and a junction. The right fork enters the mouth of Telegraph Canyon.

Begin the loop on the left fork—the North Ridge Trail. Steadily climb the north-facing slope on the dirt road, overlooking Carbon Canyon. At just over one mile, cross over to the south-facing slope above Telegraph Canyon. Pass a junction on the left at 1.6 miles, staying on the ridgeline. The sweeping views extend to the surrounding mountains across the three neighboring counties. Skirt the north side of Gilman Peak to a junction on the right, just shy of the post and wire fence. Curve to the right on the wide Gilman Trail, reaching the rounded 1,685-foot summit.

After resting and enjoying the views, continue south on the footpath (the Gilman Trail). Descend the chaparral-covered slope, and cross through an old wire fence to a knoll. Curve left, skirting around the east side of the knoll, and weave one mile down to the floor of Telegraph Canyon. Bear right on the level canyon bottom through oak and walnut woodlands beneath the 600-foot cliffs. Continue the last half of the journey down canyon, heading west to the mouth of the Telegraph Canyon. Cross a bridge over the drainage on 50 yards of paved road. Just beyond the 8-mile marker, curve right on the graveled road, completing the loop 100 yards ahead. Return to the left. ∎

4. South Ridge—Telegraph Canyon Loop
(WEST END)
Rimcrest Park Entrance

CHINO HILLS STATE PARK

Hiking distance: 5.2-mile loop
Hiking time: 2.5 hours
Configuration: loop
Elevation gain: 500 feet
Difficulty: moderate
Exposure: exposed ridge; partially shaded canyon
Dogs: not allowed
Maps: U.S.G.S. Yorba Linda · Chino Hills State Park map

South Ridge and North Ridge are long ridges that run east and west through Chino Hills State Park. Telegraph Canyon lies between the two ridges. The upper reaches of long Telegraph Canyon are located near Rolling M Ranch at the east end of the park, while the mouth of the canyon empties into Carbon Canyon Park adjacent to the west end of the state park. The chaparral slopes of the ridges frame the riparian canyon corridor.

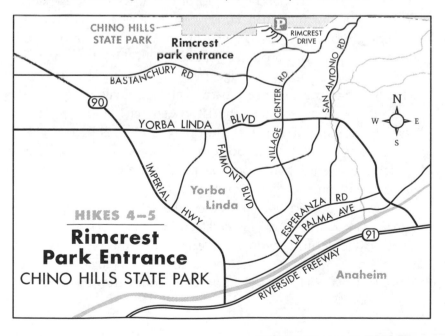

This hike starts atop South Ridge from the Rimcrest park entrance. From South Ridge, the route descends 300 feet into Telegraph Canyon. After two miles, the trail then loops back up to the ridge. The mid-length hike includes a pleasant mix of open ridge views and cool canyon vegetation.

To the trailhead

3629 RIMCREST DRIVE · YORBA LINDA   33.909025, -117.780164

From the Imperial Highway (90) in Yorba Linda, head east on Yorba Linda Boulevard. Drive 1.3 miles to Fairmont Boulevard and turn left. Continue 1.6 miles to Rimcrest Drive and turn left. Drive 0.4 miles to the end of the street at its junction with Blue Gum Drive. Park along the side of the road.

The hike

From the corner of Rimcrest Drive and Blue Gum Drive, walk up the wide, dirt path to the park entrance and trailhead on the south ridge of Telegraph Canyon. The Easy Street Trail continues straight ahead and descends 0.4 miles into Telegraph Canyon. The South Ridge Trail runs east and west (left and right).

Take the right fork and head uphill to the east, overlooking Yorba Linda and the Anaheim Hills. Meander across the long sweeping dips and rises of the rolling hills, staying atop the ridge. At one mile is a posted junction with the Little Canyon Trail on the left. The South Ridge Trail continues to San Juan Hill (Hike 5) and to the park headquarters at Aliso Canyon.

Leave the ridge and take the Little Canyon Trail on the left. Steadily descend 0.3 miles, dropping 300 feet down the north-facing slope. At the bottom of Telegraph Canyon, bear left on the Telegraph Canyon Trail, passing the Gilman Trail 100 yards ahead on the right. Continue 2 miles along the canyon floor to the posted Diemer Trail on the left, just beyond the 7-mile marker. This is the far west end of the loop. Climb 0.6 miles up the south canyon wall, returning to the west end of South Ridge. Bear left (east) and follow the undulating South Ridge Trail. Make a long, straight descent, completing the loop at the trailhead. ▦

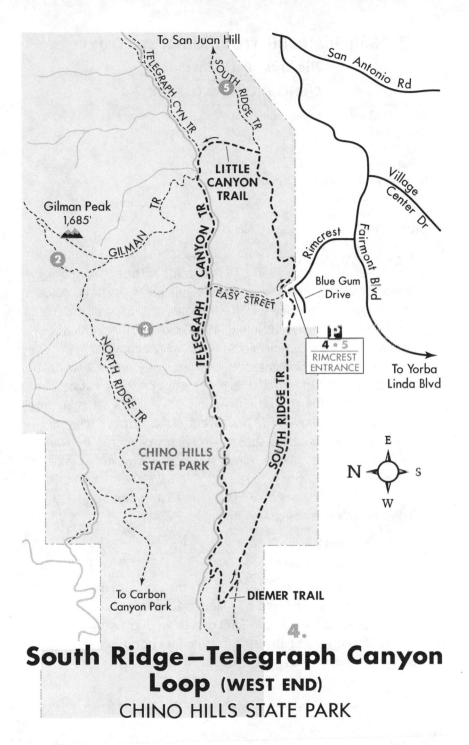

South Ridge–Telegraph Canyon
Loop (WEST END)
CHINO HILLS STATE PARK

5. San Juan Hill from Rimcrest Drive

Rimcrest Park Entrance

CHINO HILLS STATE PARK

Hiking distance: 5.6 miles round trip
Hiking time: 3 hours
Configuration: out-and-back
Elevation gain: 900 feet
Difficulty: moderate to strenuous
Exposure: exposed ridge
Dogs: not allowed
Maps: U.S.G.S. Yorba Linda and Prado Dam
Chino Hills State Park map

San Juan Hill, at an elevation of 1,781 feet, is the highest point in Chino Hills State Park. From the summit are sweeping views of the rolling landscape, which straddles three counties. The 360-degree views span from the vast Orange County plain and the ocean to the Santa Ana and San Gabriel Mountains.

San Juan Hill can be accessed from both the west and east ends of the South Ridge Trail. This hike begins on the west end of the South Ridge Trail from the Rimcrest Drive trailhead in Yorba Linda. The hike follows the exposed ridge above Telegraph Canyon. There are several short climbs and descents en route to San Juan Hill. The trail up to the summit has two approaches, which form a small loop.

San Juan Hill can be accessed from the east end of South Ridge from Rolling M Ranch (Hike 9).

To the trailhead

3629 RIMCREST DRIVE · YORBA LINDA   33.909025, -117.780164

From the Imperial Highway (90) in Yorba Linda, head east on Yorba Linda Boulevard. Drive 1.3 miles to Fairmont Boulevard and turn left. Continue 1.6 miles to Rimcrest Drive and turn left. Drive 0.4 miles to the end of the street at its junction with Blue Gum Drive. Park along the side of the road.

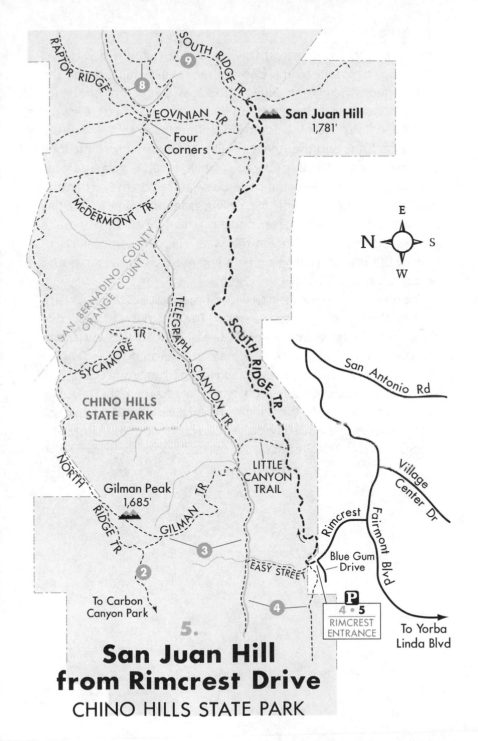

RAPTOR RIDGE

SOUTH RIDGE TR

9

8

EOVINIAN TR

San Juan Hill
1,781'

Four
Corners

McDERMONT TR

N

E

S

W

SAN BERNARDINO COUNTY
ORANGE COUNTY

TELEGRAPH CANYON TR

SOUTH RIDGE TR

TR

SYCAMORE

San Antonio Rd

CHINO HILLS
STATE PARK

Village Center Dr

NORTH RIDGE TR

GILMAN TR

Gilman Peak
1,685'

LITTLE
CANYON
TRAIL

Rimcrest

Fairmont Blvd

3

2

EASY STREET

Blue Gum
Drive

4

P
4 • 5
RIMCREST
ENTRANCE

To Carbon
Canyon Park

To Yorba
Linda Blvd

5.

San Juan Hill
from Rimcrest Drive

CHINO HILLS STATE PARK

The hike

From the corner of Rimcrest Drive and Blue Gum Drive, walk up the wide, dirt path to the park entrance and trailhead on the south ridge of Telegraph Canyon. The Easy Street Trail continues straight ahead and descends 0.4 miles into Telegraph Canyon. Take the right fork on the South Ridge Trail. Head east, overlooking Yorba Linda and the Anaheim Hills. Meander across the long sweeping dips and rises of the rolling hills, steadily gaining elevation atop the ridge. Pass the Little Canyon Trail on the left at one mile (Hike 4). Continue on the rolling ridge, passing a few unmarked neighborhood access paths on the right and utility roads on the left. As you approach the west flank of San Juan Hill, a narrow but distinct path veers right and ascends the summit—the return route.

For now, stay on the main trail (the fire road), skirting the north face of the hill to a posted junction. The South Ridge Trail continues east to the Rolling M Ranch, the park headquarters. Curve sharply to the right on the San Juan Trail, and continue 0.1 mile towards the summit by power poles. Just before reaching the utility poles, a narrow side path curves off to the right. Take this east-west footpath to the summit and a four-foot survey marker. After savoring the 360-degree vistas, return on the footpath to the South Ridge Trail. Retrace your steps back to the trailhead. ▪

6. Upper Aliso Canyon
Bane Canyon (main) Entrance
CHINO HILLS STATE PARK

Hiking distance: 2.8 miles round trip
Hiking time: 1.5 hours
Configuration: lollipop loop
Elevation gain: 300 feet
Difficulty: easy
Exposure: exposed with pockets of trees
Dogs: not allowed
Maps: U.S.G.S. Prado Dam · Chino Hills State Park map

Upper Aliso Canyon is an isolated, stream-fed canyon tucked between Bane Canyon and Telegraph Canyon at the northeast corner of Chino Hills State Park. The canyon has retained its natural undisturbed character. The trail gently climbs through the canyon from Rolling M Ranch (the park headquarters) at the end

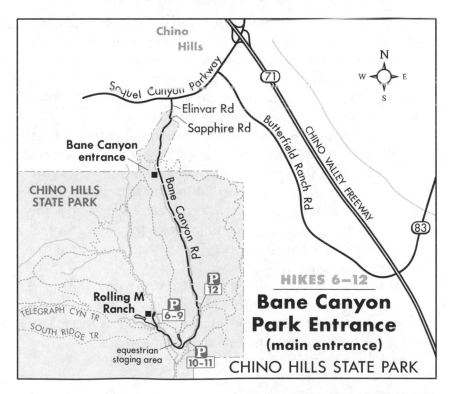

HIKES 6–12

**Bane Canyon
Park Entrance**

(main entrance)

CHINO HILLS STATE PARK

of the main entrance road. The diverse route weaves through the pristine creek bottom, crosses rounded grassy slopes overlooking the eastern portion of the park, and returns down a riparian ravine with oak and sycamore trees.

To the trailhead

4721 SAPPHIRE ROAD · CHINO HILLS 33.923644, -117.705867

From the Riverside (91) Freeway in Corona, take the Corona Expressway (71) north for 7 miles to the Soquel Canyon Parkway exit. (En route, the Corona Expressway becomes the Chino Valley Freeway.) Turn left and drive 1.2 miles to Elinvar Road. Turn left and continue 0.2 miles to Sapphire Road. Turn left and immediately turn right on the posted state park road—Bane Canyon Road. Follow the unpaved road 3.3 miles to the parking lot at the end of the road. (The first 2.3 miles are gravel and the last mile is paved.) An entrance fee is required.

The hike

From the far end of the parking lot, where the pavement ends, take the posted trail past the windmill. Follow the west bank of Aliso Creek, lined with sycamore and willow trees. Wind up the canyon bottom through grassy, rolling hills dotted with oaks. Climb gently out of the canyon to a posted footpath on the right under the towering power poles—the return route.

Begin the loop straight ahead on the main trail (left). Continue to a Y-fork. The left fork leads to Raptor Ridge and Four Corners. Veer to the right, staying on the Upper Aliso Canyon Trail. Weave up the hillside to the north, overlooking the folded hills of the state park. Top the crest and descend, zigzagging across the upper canyon while overlooking the drainage to the east that is filled with oaks and sycamores. The road portion of the trail ends by a power pole.

Take the posted footpath on the left, dropping into the drainage to a T-junction. The left fork heads north, up the canyon to Bane Ridge near the park entrance. Take the right fork and follow the single-track trail downstream through a lush drainage. Cross a footbridge, completing the loop. Return to the left. ▪

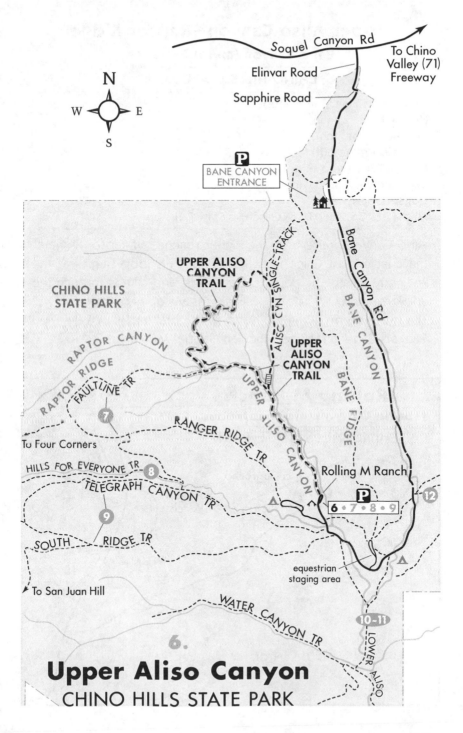

Soquel Canyon Rd

To Chino
Valley (71)
Freeway

Elinvar Road

Sapphire Road

N
W · E
S

P
BANE CANYON
ENTRANCE

Bane Canyon Rd

UPPER ALISO
CANYON
TRAIL

ALISO CYN SINGLE-TRACK

CHINO HILLS
STATE PARK

BANE CANYON

UPPER
ALISO
CANYON
TRAIL

RAPTOR CANYON

BANE RIDGE

RAPTOR RIDGE

FAULTLINE TR

UPPER ALISO CANYON

7

RANGER RIDGE TR

To Four Corners

Rolling M Ranch

HILLS FOR EVERYONE TR **8**

P
6 · 7 · 8 · 9

12

TELEGRAPH CANYON TR

9

SOUTH RIDGE TR

equestrian
staging area

To San Juan Hill

WATER CANYON TR

10-11

LOWER ALISO

6.

Upper Aliso Canyon
CHINO HILLS STATE PARK

39

7. Upper Aliso Canyon—Raptor Ridge
Bane Canyon (main) Entrance
CHINO HILLS STATE PARK

Hiking distance: 4-mile loop
Hiking time: 2 hours
Configuration: loop
Elevation gain: 600 feet
Difficulty: easy to moderate
Exposure: exposed with pockets of trees
Dogs: not allowed
Maps: U.S.G.S. Prado Dam · Chino Hills State Park map

Aliso Canyon drains from the higher reaches of Raptor Ridge at the east end of Chino Hills State Park. This loop begins at the Rolling M Ranch, the park headquarters, and climbs through the upper canyon towards the rolling, grassy slopes of Raptor Ridge. The loop returns along the ridge, with great views of Telegraph Canyon, San Juan Hill, and the San Gabriel Mountains.

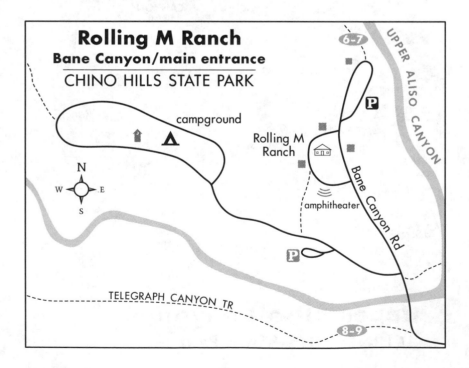

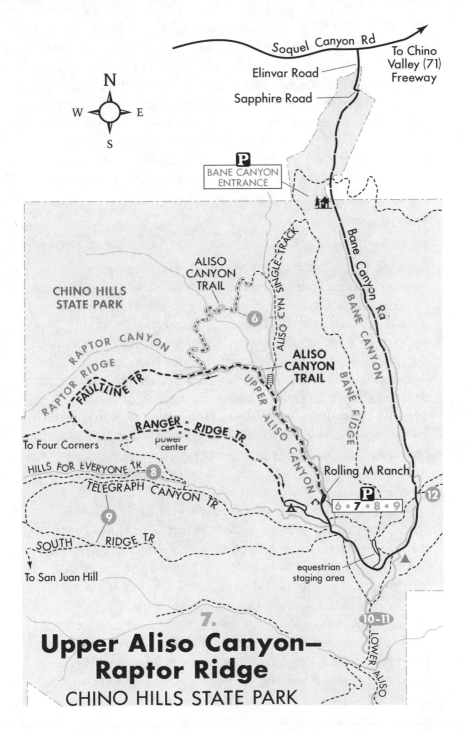

To Chino
Valley (71)
Freeway

Soquel Canyon Rd

Elinvar Road

Sapphire Road

P
BANE CANYON
ENTRANCE

N
W · E
S

CHINO HILLS
STATE PARK

ALISO
CANYON
TRAIL

ALISO CYN SINGLE-TRACK

Bane Canyon Rd

BANE CANYON

BANE CANYON

6

**ALISO
CANYON
TRAIL**

UPPER ALISO

RAPTOR CANYON

RAPTOR RIDGE

FAULTLINE TR

BANE RIDGE

RANGER RIDGE TR

power center

To Four Corners

Rolling M Ranch

P
6 · **7** · 8 · 9

12

HILLS FOR EVERYONE TK

8

TELEGRAPH CANYON TR

UPPER ALISO CANYON

9

SOUTH RIDGE TR

To San Juan Hill

equestrian
staging area

10-11

LOWER ALISO

7.
Upper Aliso Canyon–
Raptor Ridge
CHINO HILLS STATE PARK

To the trailhead

From the Riverside (91) Freeway in Corona, take the Corona Expressway (71) north for 7 miles to the Soquel Canyon Parkway exit. (En route, the Corona Expressway becomes the Chino Valley Freeway.) Turn left and drive 1.2 miles to Elinvar Road. Turn left and continue 0.2 miles to Sapphire Road. Turn left and immediately turn right on the posted state park road—Bane Canyon Road. Follow the unpaved road 3.3 miles to the parking lot at the end of the road. (The first 2.3 miles are gravel and the last mile is paved.) An entrance fee is required.

The hike

4721 SAPPHIRE ROAD · CHINO HILLS   33.923644, -117.705867

From the far end of the parking lot, where the pavement ends, take the posted trail past the windmill. Follow the west bank of Aliso Creek, lined with sycamore and willow trees. Wind up the canyon bottom through grassy, rolling hills dotted with oaks. Climb gently out of the canyon, passing a posted footpath on the right under towering power poles. Continue to a Y-fork. The right fork zigzags up Upper Aliso Canyon (Hike 6). Take the left fork toward Raptor Ridge, climbing to the end of the road/trail. Continue straight on the posted single-track footpath, climbing the spine of the hill to the top of Raptor Ridge. The footpath (Faultline Trail) ends at a T-junction. To the right leads to Telegraph Canyon at Four Corners (a picnic area and overlook at a trail junction).

Bear left, enjoying the spectacular vistas of San Juan Hill and South Ridge to the southeast and the San Gabriel Mountains to the northwest. Follow the sinuous ridge east to a distinct junction by power lines. The right fork weaves down the hillside to Telegraph Canyon at the Hills For Everyone Trail (Hike 8). Stay on the hilly ridge to a power center atop the knoll. Take the Ranger Ridge Trail, a footpath on the right (southeast) edge of the knoll. Head east to the end of the upper ridge, and follow the ridge downhill into a meadow. Curve around the backside of the Rolling M Ranch buildings to the campground and park road. Return to the parking area towards the left. ■

8. Hills For Everyone—
Four Corners—Telegraph Canyon Loop

Bane Canyon (main) Entrance

CHINO HILLS STATE PARK

Hiking distance: 5-miles round trip
Hiking time: 2.5 hours
Configuration: lollipop loop
Elevation gain: 600 feet
Difficulty: easy to moderate
Exposure: mix of sun and shade
Dogs: not allowed
Maps: U.S.G.S. Prado Dam · Chino Hills State Park map

The Hills For Everyone Trail is a hiking only footpath at the east end of Chino Hills State Park. The path follows a seasonal tributary of Aliso Creek through a small draw near the head of Telegraph Canyon. The lush riparian corridor is filled with groves of oak, sycamore, and walnut trees, with an understory of ferns, berry vines, and watercress. For hundreds of years, the drainage attracted the Gabrieleno Indians for hunting and food gathering. The 1.3-mile meandering footpath has interpretive panels that describe Gabrieleno Indian life, wildlife, and surrounding vegetation. At the west end of the loop is a picnic area and great views at Four Corners (a major trail junction). The trail descends back to the trailhead on the multi-use Telegraph Canyon Trail.

To the trailhead

4721 SAPPHIRE ROAD · CHINO HILLS   33.923644, -117.705867

From the Riverside (91) Freeway in Corona, take the Corona Expressway (71) north for 7 miles to the Soquel Canyon Parkway exit. (En route, the Corona Expressway becomes the Chino Valley Freeway.) Turn left and drive 1.2 miles to Elinvar Road. Turn left and continue 0.2 miles to Sapphire Road. Turn left and immediately turn right on the posted state park road—Bane Canyon Road. Follow the unpaved road 3.3 miles to the parking lot at the end of the road. (The first 2.2 miles are gravel and the last mile is paved.) An entrance fee is required.

The hike

Walk 260 yards back down the park road to the bottom of the hill and the posted Telegraph Canyon Trail on the right. Head up the dirt road on the south wall of Telegraph Canyon. At one mile is a posted junction. The Telegraph Canyon Trail continues west to the South Ridge Trail—the return route.

Bear right to start the loop. Walk a few feet to another junction. The main trail continues up to Raptor Ridge (Hike 7). Bear left on the posted Hills For Everyone Nature Trail. The footpath follows the edge of the serpentine drainage lined with oak groves and scattered sycamores. Cross a wooden footbridge over the drainage, and wind through the narrow, shaded canyon. Near the head of the canyon, cross a footbridge to the north side of the seasonal stream. The trail ends at a junction with the Telegraph Canyon Trail on a saddle, 20 yards east of a picnic area at Four Corners (McDermont Spring).

From Four Corners, trails lead south on the Eovinian Delight Trail to South Ridge, northeast to Raptor Ridge, and west into Telegraph Canyon. For this hike, head east on the Telegraph Canyon Trail, meandering through the rolling, grassy hills dotted with oaks. Top the crest to great views, then descend to a Y-fork. The right fork leads to the South Ridge Trail. Bear left, staying on the Telegraph Canyon Trail. Curve right near a power pole and descend, completing the loop. Retrace your steps back on the Telegraph Canyon Trail. ∎

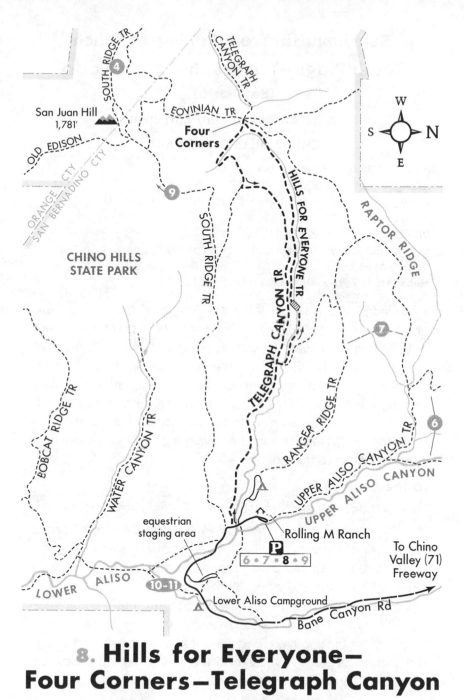

8. Hills for Everyone–
Four Corners–Telegraph Canyon
CHINO HILLS STATE PARK

9. San Juan Hill from Rolling M Ranch

South Ridge—Telegraph Canyon Loop

(EAST END)

Bane Canyon (main) Entrance

CHINO HILLS STATE PARK

Hiking distance: 7.5-miles round trip
Hiking time: 4 hours
Configuration: loop with out-and-back trail to San Juan Hill
Elevation gain: 1,100 feet
Difficulty: moderate to strenuous
Exposure: mostly exposed with pockets of trees in canyon
Dogs: not allowed
Maps: U.S.G.S. Prado Dam · Chino Hills State Park map

South Ridge spans almost the entire length of Chino Hills State Park. Near its center is San Juan Hill, the highest point in the park at 1,781 feet. San Juan Hill can be accessed from the west at Rimcrest Drive (Hike 5) or from the east from Rolling M Ranch—this hike. The moderately strenuous route begins at Upper Aliso Canyon, travels through Telegraph Canyon Trail en route to San Juan Hill, then makes a return loop back down the South Ridge Trail. From atop the summit are sweeping, 360-degree views from the ocean to the mountains.

To the trailhead

4721 SAPPHIRE ROAD · CHINO HILLS   33.923644, -117.705867

From the Riverside (91) Freeway in Corona, take the Corona Expressway (71) north 7 miles to the Soquel Canyon Parkway exit. (En route, the Corona Expressway becomes the Chino Valley Freeway.) Turn left and drive 1.2 miles to Elinvar Road. Turn left and continue 0.2 miles to Sapphire Road. Turn left and immediately turn right on the posted state park road—Bane Canyon Road. Follow the unpaved road 3.3 miles to the parking lot at the end of the road. (The first 2.2 miles are gravel and the last mile is paved.) An entrance fee is required.

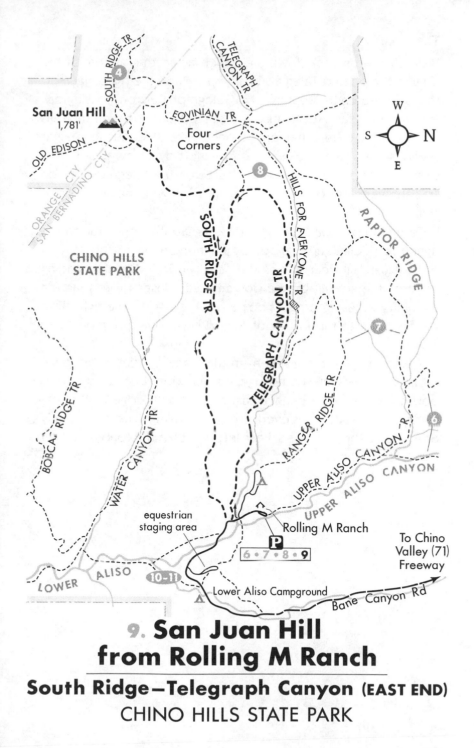

9. San Juan Hill from Rolling M Ranch

South Ridge–Telegraph Canyon (EAST END)

CHINO HILLS STATE PARK

The hike

Walk 260 yards back down the park road to the bottom of the hill and the posted Telegraph Canyon Trail on the right. Head up the dirt road on the south wall of Telegraph Canyon, passing oak and walnut trees. At one mile is a posted junction with the Hills For Everyone Nature Trail on the right (Hike 8). Continue straight ahead, slowly gaining elevation. Curve left by a power pole to a posted junction, just beyond 2 miles. Leave the Telegraph Canyon Trail and veer left, descending to a junction with the South Ridge Trail.

To head up to San Juan Hill, take the South Ridge Trail to the right (west). Climb up to a posted junction on the northeast flank of San Juan Hill. Bear left on the San Juan Trail 0.1 mile, heading towards the summit by the power poles. Just before reaching the utility poles, a narrow side path curves off to the right. Take this footpath to the 1,781-foot summit by a four-foot monument marker.

After enjoying the vistas from the highest point in the park, return to the lower South Ridge Trail junction (back to the loop portion of the hike). Continue east on the South Ridge Trail, crossing the open, rolling hills overlooking the Rolling M Ranch. Steadily descend to the park road. Bear left and take the road a quarter mile back to the parking lot. ▨

10. Water Canyon
Bane Canyon (main) Entrance
CHINO HILLS STATE PARK

Hiking distance: 3.5 miles round trip
Hiking time: 2 hours
Configuration: out-and-back
Elevation gain: 200 feet
Difficulty: easy
Exposure: mix of sun and shade
Dogs: not allowed
Maps: U.S.G.S. Prado Dam · Chino Hills State Park map

Water Canyon is one of the prettiest canyons in Chino Hills State Park. The steep-walled canyon, located in the southeast arm of the park, winds through a riparian woodland lush with willow, sycamore, oak, and native walnut trees. The hiking-only trail follows the north grassland slope near the shady canyon bottom, heading upstream through the narrow, pristine canyon.

To the trailhead

4721 SAPPHIRE ROAD · CHINO HILLS   33.919909, –117.699421

From the Riverside (91) Freeway in Corona, take the Corona Expressway (71) north 7 miles to the Soquel Canyon Parkway exit. (En route, the Corona Expressway becomes the Chino Valley Freeway.) Turn left and drive 1.2 miles to Elinvar Road. Turn left and continue 0.2 miles to Sapphire Road. Turn left and immediately turn right on the posted state park road—Bane Canyon Road. Follow the unpaved road 2.6 miles to the posted Lower Aliso Campground on the left. Parking spaces are on the right side of the road before the campground turnoff. If full, continue 0.2 miles to the equestrian staging area parking area on the right. An entrance fee is required.

The hike

From the campground entrance, walk 0.1 mile down the campground road to the gated trailhead on the right. Stroll south through the open, rolling grasslands along the seasonal stream lined with sycamores, willows, and oaks. At 0.6 miles, cross a wooden bridge over Aliso Creek to a T-junction. The Lower Aliso Canyon Trail stays left (Hike 11).

Bear right on the Scully Ridge Trail. Continue 100 yards to the posted Water Canyon Trail on the right. Take the grassy footpath to the right. Walk through the tall riparian vegetation, willows, and oaks. Cross a wooden bridge over the stream, and continue up the green canyon corridor, passing a dense grove of prickly pear cactus. The trail fades just past a drainage split by a distinct singular palm tree. Return along the same route. ■

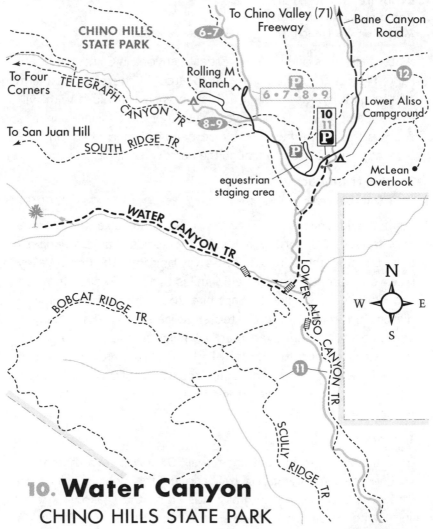

10. **Water Canyon**
CHINO HILLS STATE PARK

11. Scully Ridge— Lower Aliso Canyon

Bane Canyon (main) Entrance

CHINO HILLS STATE PARK

Hiking distance: 6-mile loop
Hiking time: 3 hours
Configuration: loop
Elevation gain: 400 feet
Difficulty: moderate
Exposure: mostly exposed
Dogs: not allowed
Maps: U.S.G.S. Prado Dam · Chino Hills State Park map

Scully Ridge stretches through the southeast corner of Chino Hills State Park. This long loop hike begins in Bane Canyon from the main entrance road and climbs up to undulating Scully Ridge. There are 360-degree views of the rolling hillsides from atop the open ridge. The route then drops down into Lower Aliso Canyon, following the seasonal stream through a wide, flat valley bottom.

To the trailhead

4721 SAPPHIRE ROAD · CHINO HILLS   33.919909, –117.699421

From the Riverside (91) Freeway in Corona, take the Corona Expressway (71) north for 7 miles to the Soquel Canyon Parkway exit. (En route, the Corona Expressway becomes the Chino Valley Freeway.) Turn left and drive 1.2 miles to Elinvar Road. Turn left and continue 0.2 miles to Sapphire Road. Turn left and immediately turn right on the posted state park road—Bane Canyon Road. Follow the unpaved road 2.6 miles to the posted Lower Aliso Campground on the left. Parking spaces are on the right side of the road before the campground turnoff. If full, continue 0.2 miles to the equestrian staging area parking area on the right. An entrance fee is required.

The hike

From the campground entrance, walk 0.1 mile down the campground road to the gated trailhead on the right. Stroll south through the open, rolling grasslands along the seasonal stream lined with sycamores, willows, and oaks. At 0.6 miles, cross a wooden bridge over Aliso Creek to a T-junction. The Lower Aliso Canyon Trail stays left.

Bear right and begin the loop on the Scully Ridge Trail. Pass the Water Canyon Trail 100 yards ahead on a horseshoe left bend (Hike 10). Steadily climb the hillside, passing the Bobcat Ridge Trail on the right. The serpentine Scully Ridge Trail follows the contours of the hillside along the west ridge of Aliso Canyon. Top the crest to 360-degree vistas of the surrounding mountains. Descend and cross a narrow ridge between Brush Canyon and Lower Aliso Canyon. Curve right and weave along the ridge to a posted Y-fork at 2.7 miles. Leave Scully Ridge and curve left on the Brush Canyon Trail. Zigzag downhill one mile on an easy grade along five switchbacks to the bottom of the wide Lower Aliso Canyon.

Bear left and meander gently upstream along the canyon floor, crossing two wooden footbridges over Aliso Creek. After the second bridge, complete the loop in about 200 yards. Return to the right along the same trail. ■

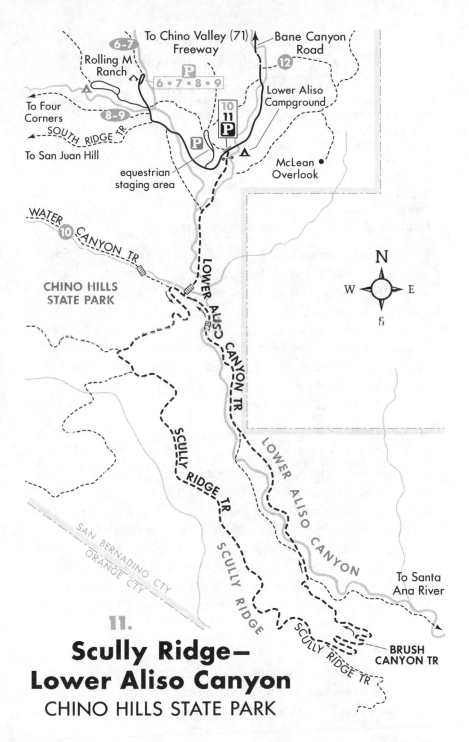

To Chino Valley (71)
Freeway

Bane Canyon
Road

Rolling M
Ranch

6·7·8·9

To Four
Corners

Lower Aliso
Campground

SOUTH RIDGE TR

To San Juan Hill

equestrian
staging area

McLean
Overlook

WATER

CANYON TR

CHINO HILLS
STATE PARK

LOWER ALISO CANYON TR

SCULLY RIDGE TR

LOWER ALISO CANYON

SAN BERNADINO CTY

ORANGE CTY

SCULLY RIDGE

SCULLY RIDGE TR

To Santa
Ana River

BRUSH
CANYON TR

N
W E
S

11.

Scully Ridge–
Lower Aliso Canyon
CHINO HILLS STATE PARK

12. McLean Overlook

Bane Canyon (main) Entrance

CHINO HILLS STATE PARK

Hiking distance: 2.4 miles round trip
Hiking time: 1 hour
Configuration: out-and-back
Elevation gain: 200 feet
Difficulty: easy
Exposure: open hilltop
Dogs: not allowed
Maps: U.S.G.S. Prado Dam · Chino Hills State Park map

The McLean Overlook is a 940-foot knoll with commanding vistas across Chino Hills State Park. From the summit are views across the rolling grasslands and canyons, including Upper and Lower Aliso Canyon, Bane Canyon, Telegraph Canyon, San Juan Hill, the Rolling M Ranch, the San Gabriel Mountains, and the Santa Ana Mountains. The McLean Overlook Trail, a 1.2-mile mile dirt road, begins where Bane Canyon and Slaughter Canyon merge at the east end of the state park. The little-used trail offers solitude and quiet contemplation from the overlook.

To the trailhead

4721 SAPPHIRE ROAD · CHINO HILLS   33.924565, -117.697265

From the Riverside (91) Freeway in Corona, take the Corona Expressway (71) north for 7 miles to the Soquel Canyon Parkway exit. (En route, the Corona Expressway becomes the Chino Valley Freeway.) Turn left and drive 1.2 miles to Elinvar Road. Turn left and continue 0.2 miles to Sapphire Road. Turn left and immediately turn right on the posted state park road—Bane Canyon Road. Follow the unpaved road 2.3 miles to the scenic overlook sign on the left. Park in small pullouts on the sides of the road. An entrance fee is required.

The hike

Two trails lead from the trailhead. The Slaughter Canyon Trail (a footpath) veers off to the left and heads northeast. Take the wide main route—an old dirt road—passing the scenic overlook sign. Walk past the trail gate, and steadily climb up the hillside on the south edge of Slaughter Canyon. Curve clockwise around the hillside. At just over a half mile, as the trail levels out, a footpath on the right descends to the campground. Stay on the main trail at a near-level grade to a large flat clearing. Climb the wood steps and continue 20 yards to the McLean Overlook, a knoll with a bench and 360-degree panoramas. ■

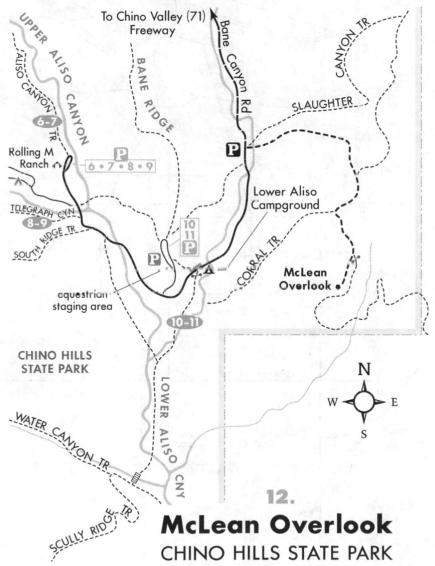

12.
McLean Overlook
CHINO HILLS STATE PARK

Anaheim Hills
Orange • North Tustin

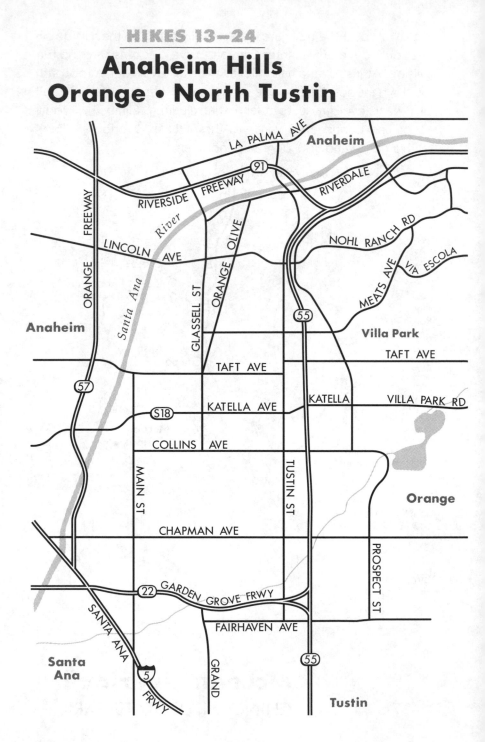

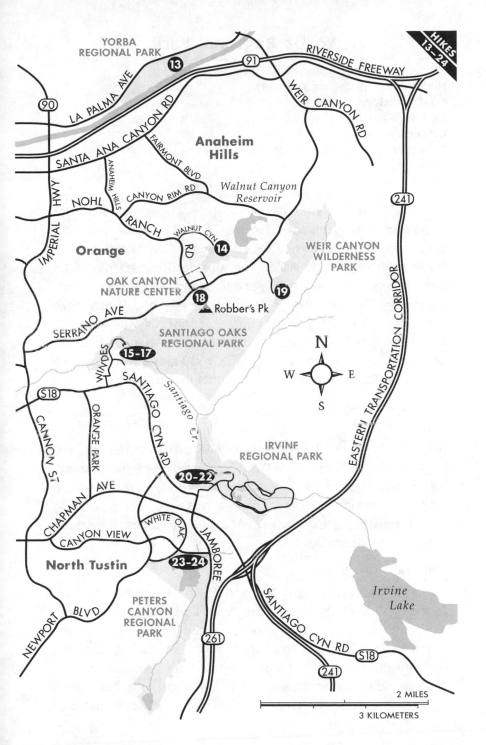

YORBA
REGIONAL PARK

13

RIVERSIDE FREEWAY

LA PALMA AVE

WEIR CANYON RD

91

90

SANTA ANA CANYON RD

FAIRMONT BLVD

**Anaheim
Hills**

*Walnut Canyon
Reservoir*

IMPERIAL HWY

NOHL

ANAHEIM HILLS

CANYON RIM RD

RANCH

WALNUT CYN RD

14

Orange

241

WEIR CANYON
WILDERNESS
PARK

OAK CANYON
NATURE CENTER

18

19

🔺 Robber's Pk

SERRANO AVE

SANTIAGO OAKS
REGIONAL PARK

N

WINDES

15-17

W ⟡ E

S

S18

SANTIAGO CYN RD

Santiago Cr.

CANNON ST

ORANGE PARK AVE

IRVINE
REGIONAL PARK

EASTERN TRANSPORTATION CORRIDOR

20-22

CHAPMAN AVE

WHITE OAK

JAMBOREE

CANYON VIEW

*Irvine
Lake*

North Tustin

23-24

NEWPORT BLVD

PETERS
CANYON
REGIONAL
PARK

SANTIAGO CYN RD

261

S18

241

2 MILES

3 KILOMETERS

57

13. Yorba Regional Park

Hiking distance: 0.5 miles to 2.5-mile multi-loop
Hiking time: 15 minutes to 2 hours
Configuration: multiple loops
Elevation gain: level
Difficulty: easy
Exposure: grassy parkland with shady groves of trees
Dogs: allowed
Maps: U.S.G.S. Orange · Yorba Regional Park map

Yorba Regional Park stretches along the north side of the Santa Ana River in Anaheim for 1.5 miles. The picturesque 166-acre park, once part of Bernardo Yorba's expansive cattle ranch, is framed by the rolling hills of Yorba Linda. The park has three lakes, grassy meadows, picnic shelters, and natural trails winding through the parkland. Trails circle the lake and footbridges cross the stream. The trail system also connects with the Santa Ana River Trail, a 24-mile paved path that crosses the length of Orange County from Yorba Linda, by Weir Canyon Road, to Huntington Beach, where the river meets the sea.

To the trailhead

7600 EAST LA PALMA AVE · ANAHEIM   33.871473, -117.763508

From the 91 (Riverside) Freeway in Anaheim, take the Imperial Highway (90) exit, and drive 0.4 miles north to La Palma Avenue. Turn right and drive 1.8 miles to the main park entrance on the right. Turn right into the park. Turn right again and park in Lot 6 on the left near the lake (or wherever a parking space is available). A parking fee is required.

The hike

Cross the grassy picnic area to the path on the edge of the lake. To the right, the path follows the north side of the lake (the return route). Continue straight and cross the bridge over the lake channel to a T-junction. The path follows the south end of the park in both directions. To the right, the trail weaves through pines, willows, sycamores, and cottonwoods. Side paths lead to the shoreline of the lakes and fishing decks. Running parallel

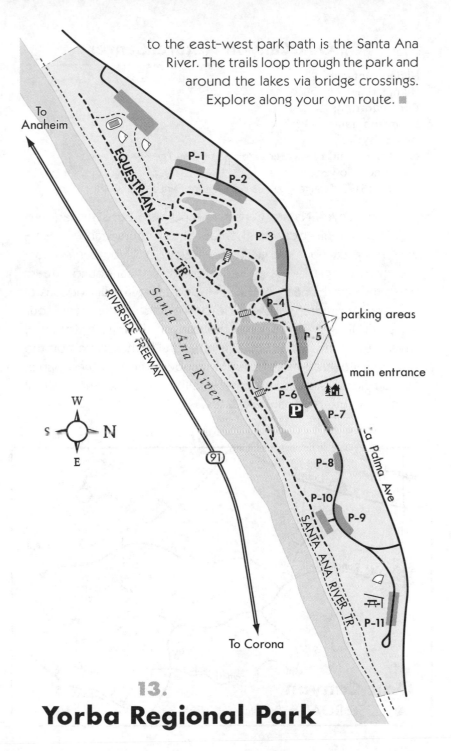

to the east-west park path is the Santa Ana
River. The trails loop through the park and
around the lakes via bridge crossings.
Explore along your own route. ■

To
Anaheim

EQUESTRIAN

TR.

RIVERSIDE FREEWAY

Santa Ana River

P-1
P-2
P-3
P-4
P-5
P-6
P
P-7
P-8
P-10
P-9
P-11

parking areas

main entrance

La Palma Ave

SANTA ANA RIVER TR.

W
S —◇— N
E

91

To Corona

13.
Yorba Regional Park

14. Oak Canyon Nature Center

Hiking distance: 2.5-mile loop
Hiking time: 1.5 hours
Configuration: loop
Elevation gain: 300 feet
Difficulty: easy
Exposure: a mix of sage-covered hillside and oak woodlands
Dogs: not allowed
Maps: U.S.G.S. Orange · Oak Canyon Nature Center Trail Guide

The Oak Canyon Nature Center is a 60-acre oasis tucked into the Anaheim Hills between homes, a golf course, and a reservoir. Three canyons merge in this tree-filled suburban wilderness, providing a sense of remoteness. A year-round stream flows through the heart of the secluded sanctuary under coastal live oak, sycamore, willow, elderberry, and walnut trees. Four miles of hiking trails connect the canyon walls with the lush, stream-fed canyon bottom. This hike circles the canyon on the chaparral-covered hillsides and meanders through the riparian canyon floor. The nature center facility has a museum, natural history exhibits, and nature classes.

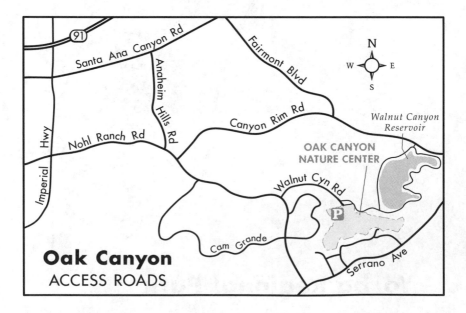

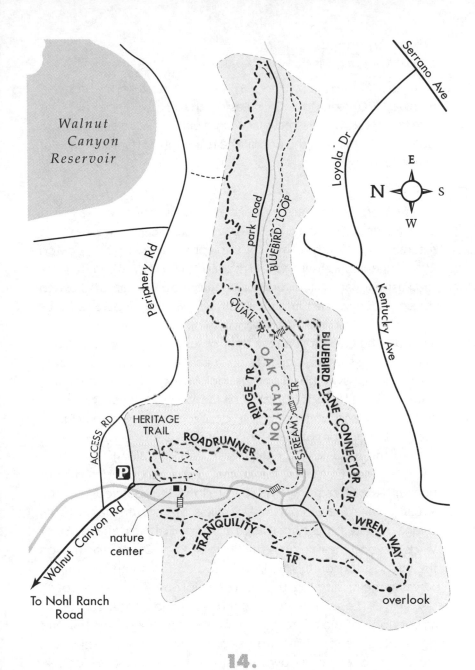

14.
Oak Canyon
Nature Center

To the trailhead

From the 91 (Riverside) Freeway in Anaheim, take the Imperial Highway (90) exit. Drive 0.7 miles south to Nohl Ranch Road and turn left. Head 1.7 miles east to Walnut Canyon Road and turn left. Continue 0.5 miles to the end of the road. Turn left into the nature center parking lot.

The hike

Cross the access road to the Oak Canyon Nature Center. Head left on the signed Heritage Trail, a paved, handicapped-accessible nature loop. Gently climb to the upper level to the posted Roadrunner Ridge Trail on the right. Take the dirt path and traverse the east canyon wall, overlooking a lush, bowl-shaped draw to the south. Curve east into Oak Canyon, passing sandstone caves on the left. Wind along the contours of the northern cliffs to a junction. The Quail Trail on the right descends to the floor of Oak Canyon for a shorter loop. Continue east and ascend the hillside on a series of switchbacks to just below the ridge. A connector path on the left leads 30 yards to the Walnut Canyon Reservoir. At the east end of the canyon, descend to the unpaved park road at the bottom of Oak Canyon at the park boundary.

Take the road to the right (west), walking along the stream under a canopy of oaks. The stream crosses the road at a junction with the Stream Trail. The road follows the south edge of the stream, while the Stream Trail parallels the north side. A footbridge reunites the two routes a short distance ahead. Sixty yards beyond their union is the Bluebird Lane Connector Trail on the left. Go left on this trail, and head up the south canyon hill. Traverse the hillside to a trail split. Stay left on Wren Way through oak groves. Loop around the southwest end of the canyon to an overlook of the entire canyon. Follow the Tranquility Trail and descend steps to a T-junction. Bear left to a bridge behind the nature center and cross over the stream, completing the loop. ■

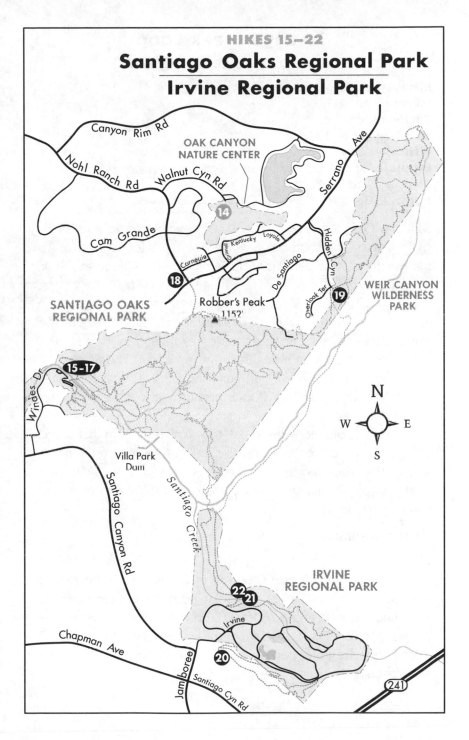

Santiago Oaks Regional Park
Irvine Regional Park

Canyon Rim Rd

OAK CANYON
NATURE CENTER

Nohl Ranch Rd

Walnut Cyn Rd

Serrano Ave

Cam Grande

14

Kentucky

Loyola

Hidden Cyn

Grijalwa

Carnegie

De Santiago

18

Overlook Ter

19

WEIR CANYON
WILDERNESS
PARK

SANTIAGO OAKS
REGIONAL PARK

Robber's Peak
1152'

15-17

Windes Dr

N

W   E

S

Villa Park
Dam

Santiago Creek

Santiago Canyon Rd

IRVINE
REGIONAL PARK

22 21

Chapman Ave

Jamboree

20

Irvine

Santiago Cyn Rd

241

15. Santiago Creek Loop
SANTIAGO OAKS REGIONAL PARK

Hiking distance: 2.5-mile loop
Hiking time: 1.25 hours
Configuration: loop
Elevation gain: 100 feet
Difficulty: easy
Exposure: open foothills with riparian corridor along creek
Dogs: allowed
Maps: U.S.G.S. Orange · Santiago Oaks Regional Park map

Santiago Oaks Regional Park is a 1,269-acre reserve in the city of Orange on the south edge of Anaheim Hills (cover photo). To the northeast, the park borders Weir Canyon Wilderness Park. An extensive trail system offers many miles of trails for hikers, bikers, and equestrians. Santiago Creek, the main tributary of the Santa Ana River, runs through the lower end of the park at the main trailhead. This section of the creek meanders through the center of the park and was a Native American village site for thousands of years. In 1879, a small clay dam was built for irrigation. It was destroyed by floods and rebuilt in 1892 with river rock and cement.

This hike strolls along the creek to the historic dam that spans 110 feet. The trail continues up the rolling foothills on the north side of the creek and through an old nursery of ornamental and exotic trees. The nursery was planted in 1955 by former land owner Harry Rinker.

To the trailhead

2145 WINDES DRIVE · ORANGE   33.821403, -117.775414

From the 55 (Costa Mesa) Freeway in Orange, take the Katella Avenue exit. Drive 3.1 miles east to Windes Drive (one mile east of Cannon Street) and turn left. (En route, Katella Avenue becomes Villa Park Road and Santiago Canyon Road.) Continue 0.7 miles into the regional park. Park in the lot on the right. A parking fee is required.

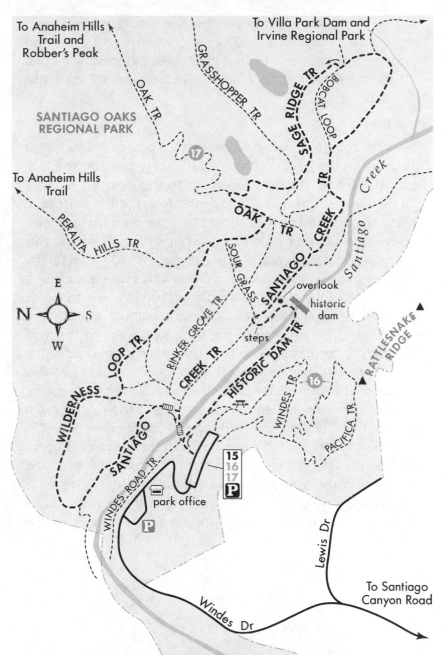

To Anaheim Hills
Trail and
Robber's Peak

To Villa Park Dam and
Irvine Regional Park

GRASSHOPPER TR

SAGE RIDGE TR

BOBCAT LOOP

OAK TR

SANTIAGO OAKS
REGIONAL PARK

17

To Anaheim Hills
Trail

PERALTA HILLS TR

OAK TR

SANTIAGO CREEK TR

Santiago Creek

E
N ✦ S
W

SOUR GRASS

RINKER GROVE TR

SANTIAGO

overlook

historic
dam

steps

RATTLESNAKE RIDGE

WILDERNESS LOOP TR

CREEK TR

HISTORIC DAM TR

WINDES TR

16

PACIFICA TR

SANTIAGO

WINDES ROAD TR

15
16
17
P

park office

P

Lewis Dr

To Santiago
Canyon Road

Windes Dr

15. Santiago Creek Loop
SANTIAGO OAKS REGIONAL PARK

From the 91 (Riverside) Freeway in Anaheim, take the Imperial Highway (90) exit, and drive 3.2 miles south to Santiago Canyon Road. (En route, Imperial Highway becomes Cannon Street.) Turn left and drive one mile to Windes Drive. Continue 0.7 miles into the regional park.

The hike

Cross the road from the park office to a posted Y-fork. Begin the loop on the Historic Dam Trail to the right, soon reaching another junction. The right fork leads to the Windes Trail (Hike 16). Stay left up the south side of the forested canyon. Curve left to the dam and pool bordered by a sedimentary rock wall. Follow the footpath through a tunnel of lush vegetation and willow trees. Cross the seasonal drainage, and climb 37 wood steps to a T-junction with the Santiago Creek Trail. Bear right, passing an overlook of the 19-foot-high dam and an information board at a junction with the Oak Trail. Continue straight to a Y-fork with the Bobcat Loop and stay to the right. Pass a trail on the right that leads to the massive Villa Park Dam, sitting at the head of the canyon. The main path joins the Bobcat Loop.

Veer right onto the Sage Ridge Trail. Traverse the south-facing slope, overlooking the Santiago Creek Canyon to a junction with the Oak Trail. The right fork leads up to Robber's Peak (Hike 17). Bear left and descend to a junction with the Wilderness Loop. Head to the right 0.9 miles, passing the Sour Grass Trail to the northwest corner of the county park. Curve left, looping onto the Santiago Creek Trail. Stay to the right at the next two junctions, and cross a bridge over Santiago Creek, completing the loop. ▥

16. Windes—Pacifica Loops
to Rattlesnake Ridge
SANTIAGO OAKS REGIONAL PARK

Hiking distance: 0.7-mile double loop
Hiking time: 45 minutes
Configuration: double loop
Elevation gain: 250 feet
Difficulty: easy
Exposure: mostly exposed slopes with riparian vegetation along creek
Dogs: allowed
Maps: U.S.G.S. Orange · Santiago Oaks Regional Park map

In the early 1930s, George Lemke and William Windes grew Valencia oranges for Sunkist on this site in Santiago Oaks Regional Park. On the south side of Santiago Creek, six acres of the 26-acre original orange grove still produce fruit. Adjacent to the grove is the Windes/Blome ranch house, built in 1938. It is currently the ranger office and nature center with exhibits, programs, and a picnic area.

The Windes Nature Trail is an interpretive trail that begins by the nature center. It climbs the steep slopes and connects with the Pacifica Trail to the 770-foot north summit of Rattlesnake Ridge. The views from the ridge span to Robber's Peak, overlooking the park's trail system.

To the trailhead

2145 WINDES DRIVE · ORANGE   33.821403, -117.775414

From the 55 (Costa Mesa) Freeway in Orange, take the Katella Avenue exit. Drive 3.1 miles east to Windes Drive (one mile east of Cannon Street) and turn left. (En route, Katella Avenue becomes Santiago Canyon Road.) Continue 0.7 miles into the regional park. Park in the lot on the right. A parking fee is required.

From the 91 (Riverside) Freeway in Anaheim, take the Imperial Highway (90) exit, and drive 3.2 miles south to Santiago Canyon Road. (En route, Imperial Highway becomes Cannon Street.) Turn left and drive one mile to Windes Drive. Continue 0.7 miles into the regional park.

The hike

From the far east end of the parking lot, take the paved rock path. Pass the picnic area to the posted Windes Nature Trail. Bear left and traverse the north-facing slope, passing conglomerate rock formations and caves. Climb the steps while overlooking Santiago Canyon and the lush riparian vegetation along the creek. Continue climbing on the hillside ledge, and loop back to the west. Drop down to a junction with the Pacifica Trail, a 0.4-mile loop on the upper slope.

Bear left 20 yards to a junction. Begin the second loop on the right fork through oak, bay, and eucalyptus trees. Steadily climb on three switchbacks to Rattlesnake Ridge and an overlook with a bench. The vistas extend across Orange County to the ocean. Follow the ridge southeast to the north summit, with vistas of the park's trail system, the historic dam, and Robber's Peak. Zigzag down the hillside, completing the upper loop. Return to the lower loop and stay left, weaving down the hillside to the paved rock path. ■

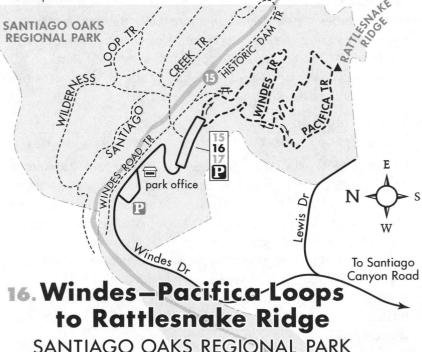

16. Windes–Pacifica Loops to Rattlesnake Ridge

SANTIAGO OAKS REGIONAL PARK

17. Robber's Peak
from Santiago Creek

SANTIAGO OAKS REGIONAL PARK

Hiking distance: 3 miles round trip
Hiking time: 1.5 hours
Configuration: out-and-back
Elevation gain: 700 feet
Difficulty: moderate
Exposure: exposed chaparral-covered slopes
Dogs: allowed
Maps: U.S.G.S. Orange · Santiago Oaks Regional Park map

Robber's Peak is a 1,152-foot sandstone peak in the Anaheim Hills, geographically known as the Peralta Hills. From the peak are 360-degree sweeping vistas of Santiago Oaks Regional Park, Oak Canyon, Weir Canyon Wilderness Park, the Chino Hills, the Santa Ana Mountains, and the Orange County basin.

Robber's Peak can be accessed from the east or west. This hike begins from the west at the trailhead hub in Santiago Oaks Regional Park. The hike follows a riparian oak woodland along the banks of Santiago Creek, then climbs the chaparral-covered rolling hills up to the peak.

To the trailhead

2145 WINDES DRIVE · ORANGE   33.821403, -117.775414

From the 55 (Costa Mesa) Freeway in Orange, take the Katella Avenue exit. Drive 3.1 miles east to Windes Drive (1 mile east of Cannon Street) and turn left. (Katella Avenue becomes Santiago Canyon Road en route.) Continue 0.7 miles into the regional park. Park in the lot on the right. A parking fee is required.

From the 91 (Riverside) Freeway in Anaheim, take the Imperial Highway (90) exit, and drive 3.2 miles south to Santiago Canyon Road. (Imperial Highway becomes Cannon Street en route.) Turn left and drive 1 mile to Windes Drive. Continue 0.7 miles into the regional park.

The hike

Cross the road from the park office to a posted Y-fork. Veer left on the Santiago Creek Trail, and follow the north side of the creek through an oak grove to a posted junction by a trail kiosk. Bear left on the Oak Trail, and head up the slope. Pass a series of connecting paths. After the Sage Ridge Trail, the path gets steeper, climbing the spine of the hill. To the left are eroded sandstone outcrops with caves. Pass through two trail gates, leaving the regional park. Beyond the second gate, the trail becomes the Anaheim Hills Trail. Curve left to an overlook, with views from the metropolis to the sea. The Peralta Hills Trail merges from the left. Continue under the power lines to a kiosk and a connector trail from Serrano Avenue by the Anaheim Hills Elementary School. Robber's Peak is the prominent formation with the large sandstone outcroppings atop the summit. At the base of Robber's Peak, the Anaheim Hills Trail curves right along a fenceline.

To ascend the peak, stay left and walk through the gate. A short distance ahead, a distinct footpath angles right and ascends the hill to the peak. At the summit, the path merges with a trail ascending from the east. After savoring the views, return along the same trail.

To extend the hike an additional 3.5 miles, continue with Hike 18 from the base of Robber's Peak. ■

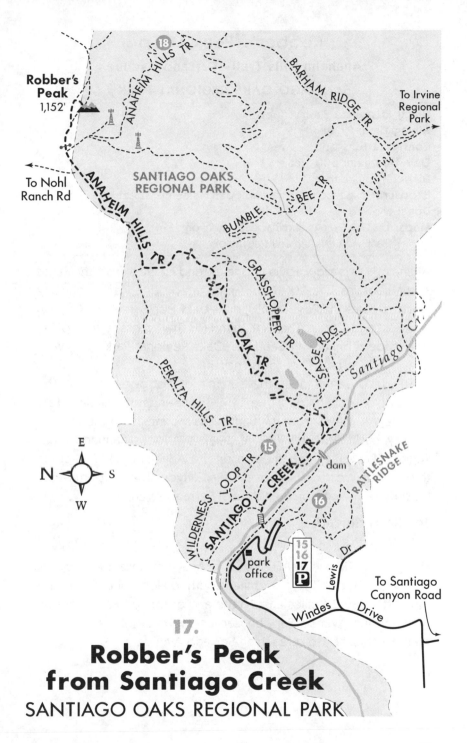

Robber's Peak
1,152'

To Nohl
Ranch Rd

To Irvine
Regional
Park

SANTIAGO OAKS
REGIONAL PARK

ANAHEIM HILLS TR

BARHAM RIDGE TR

ANAHEIM HILLS TR

BUMBLE

BEE TR

GRASSHOPPER TR

OAK TR

SAGE RDG

Santiago Cr.

PERALTA HILLS TR

WILDERNESS LOOP TR

SANTIAGO CREEK TR

dam

RATTLESNAKE RIDGE

park
office

Lewis Dr

To Santiago
Canyon Road

Windes Drive

N E S W

15

16

18

15
16
17
P

17.
Robber's Peak
from Santiago Creek
SANTIAGO OAKS REGIONAL PARK

18. Robber's Peak Loop
Anaheim Hills Trail—Serrano Avenue
SANTIAGO OAKS REGIONAL PARK

Hiking distance: 3.8-mile loop
Hiking time: 2 hours
Configuration: loop
Elevation gain: 600 feet
Difficulty: moderate
Exposure: exposed ridgeline and open residential street
Dogs: allowed
Maps: U.S.G.S. Orange and Black Star Canyon
Santiago Oaks Regional Park map

Anaheim Hills is a low, rolling ridge extending west from the Santa Ana Mountains. The 1,000-foot elongated ridge, geographically referred to as the Peralta Hills, rises between Santa Ana Canyon and Santiago Creek. The Anaheim Hills Trail crosses the rolling landscape, connecting Santiago Oaks Regional Park with Weir Canyon Wilderness Park to the north.

This hike begins near the summit of Robber's Peak at the end of Nohl Ranch Road. The 1,152-foot sandstone peak offers 360-degree views from the Santa Ana Mountains to the Orange County basin. The trail to the peak overlooks Santiago Oaks Regional Park, then heads north on the Anaheim Hills Trail along the sinuous west cliffs above Weir Canyon. The route makes a loop by returning along residential Serrano Avenue.

To the trailhead

6494 SERRANO AVE · ANAHEIM   33.830906, –117.760683

From the 91 (Riverside) Freeway in Anaheim, take the Imperial Highway (90) exit. Drive 0.7 miles south to Nohl Ranch Road and turn left. Head 2.4 miles east to the end of the road at a junction with Serrano Avenue. Park on Carnegie Avenue, the side street on the left just before reaching Serrano Avenue.

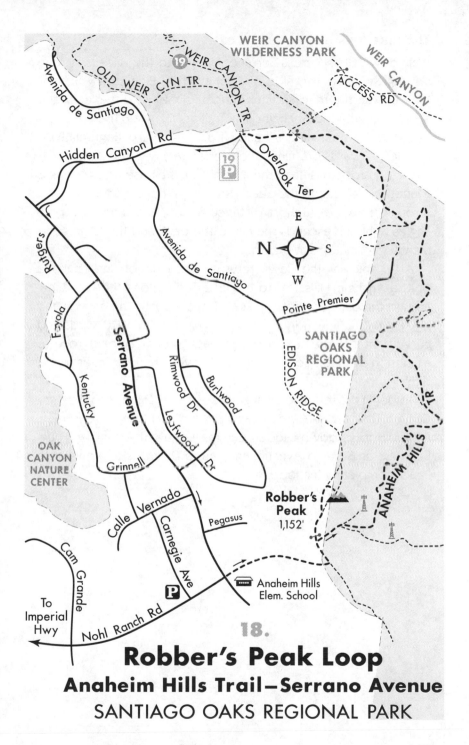

18.
Robber's Peak Loop
Anaheim Hills Trail—Serrano Avenue
SANTIAGO OAKS REGIONAL PARK

The hike

Walk downhill and cross Serrano Avenue to the wide dirt road skirting the left (east) side of Anaheim Hills Elementary School. Walk up the fire road and curve right, climbing to the kiosk and T-junction with the Anaheim Hills Trail at 0.2 miles. The right fork descends to the main trailhead of Santiago Oaks Regional Park. Bear left towards prominent Robber's Peak, with the large sandstone outcroppings atop the summit. At the base of the peak is a junction. To ascend the peak, detour on the left fork and walk through the gate. A short distance ahead, a distinct footpath angles right and ascends the hill to the peak and the large sedimentary formations at the apex.

After enjoying the views, return to the junction and continue on the Anaheim Hills Trail to the left. Curve along the fenceline, around the base of Robber's Peak. Descend into the canyon and zigzag to the next ridge. At the ridge, bear left 100 yards and curve right into the next drainage. Pass through an oak grove to a junction by metal posts. The Weir Canyon Trail continues to the right.

To begin the return loop, take the left fork 0.1 mile to the Weir Canyon Trailhead at Hidden Canyon Road and Overlook Terrace. Walk 0.5 miles down Hidden Canyon Road to Serrano Avenue. Bear left on Serrano Avenue, and return 0.9 miles to Nohl Ranch Road, completing the loop. ■

19. Weir Canyon Loop

WEIR CANYON WILDERNESS PARK

Hiking distance: 3.8-mile loop
Hiking time: 2 hours
Configuration: loop
Elevation gain: 300 feet
Difficulty: moderate
Exposure: exposed ridgeline
Dogs: allowed
Maps: U.S.G.S. Black Star Canyon

Bordered by encroaching development, Weir Canyon Wilderness Park is an expansive protected area in the Anaheim (Peralta) Hills. The parkland borders Santiago Oaks Regional Park to its south end (which has since incorporated the Weir Canyon lands). The rolling Anaheim Hills, a westward extension of the Santa Ana Mountains, offers an easy escape from the urban sprawl.

The Weir Canyon Loop weaves in and out of small side canyons high on the west wall of Weir Canyon. The westward views overlook the Orange County basin while the eastward views highlight the undeveloped foothills and canyon landscape, stretching to the peaks of the Santa Ana Mountains.

To the trailhead

SOUTH HIDDEN CANYON ROAD · ANAHEIM   33.830480, -117.744387

From the 91 (Riverside) Freeway in Anaheim, take the Weir Canyon Road exit. Drive 0.7 miles south to Serrano Avenue and turn right. Continue 2 miles to Hidden Canyon Road and turn left. Drive 0.5 miles to the end of the road at the junction with Overlook Terrace. Park alongside the curb on Hidden Canyon Road.

The hike

Walk to the trailhead, directly across the road from the end of Hidden Canyon Road. Take the wide dirt path 0.1 mile to a junction. The right fork passes metal posts on the Anaheim Hills Trail (Hike 18). Curve left 70 yards to a gate. Take the posted Weir Canyon Trail to the left, parallel to the barbed wire fence. Pass cavernous sandstone outcroppings on the left while overlooking

Weir Canyon on the right. Follow the west canyon wall along several dips and rises, curving in and out of small ravines and drainages. The serpentine path slowly descends into the canyon, passing beneath a white sandstone wall on the left. As you near the residential area atop the canyon, curve left and head uphill, parallel to the homes.

Near the upper reaches of Weir Canyon, curve left and begin the return of the loop. Pass an enormous water tank and follow the ridge south, overlooking Walnut Canyon Reservoir and Oak Canyon (Hike 14). The vistas extend across Orange County, from the Chino Hills to the ocean. Drop down to the Avenida de Santiago cul-de-sac. Walk 0.35 miles down the street to Hidden Canyon Road, and complete the loop 0.2 miles to the left. ▪

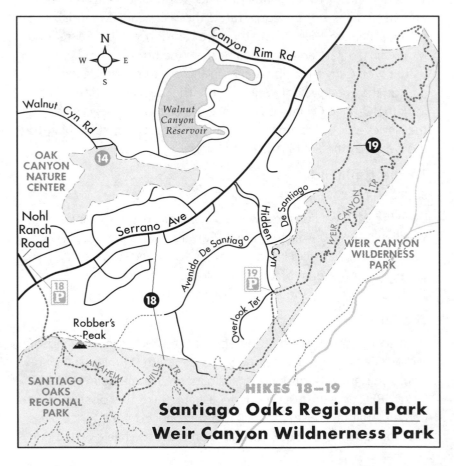

HIKES 18–19

Santiago Oaks Regional Park
Weir Canyon Wildnerness Park

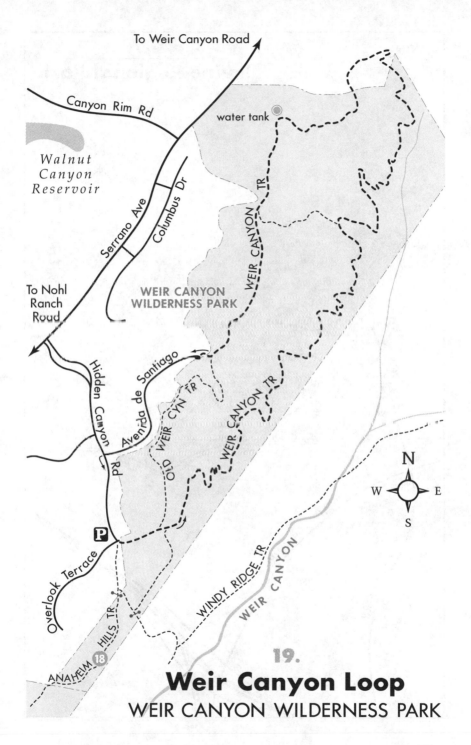

To Weir Canyon Road

Canyon Rim Rd

water tank

Walnut Canyon Reservoir

Serrano Ave

Columbus Dr

WEIR CANYON TR

WEIR CANYON WILDERNESS PARK

To Nohl Ranch Road

Hidden Canyon Rd

Avenida de Santiago

OLD WEIR CYN TR

WEIR CANYON TR

N
W · E
S

P

Overlook Terrace

ANAHEIM HILLS TR

WINDY RIDGE TR

WEIR CANYON

WEIR CANYON

18

19.

Weir Canyon Loop
WEIR CANYON WILDERNESS PARK

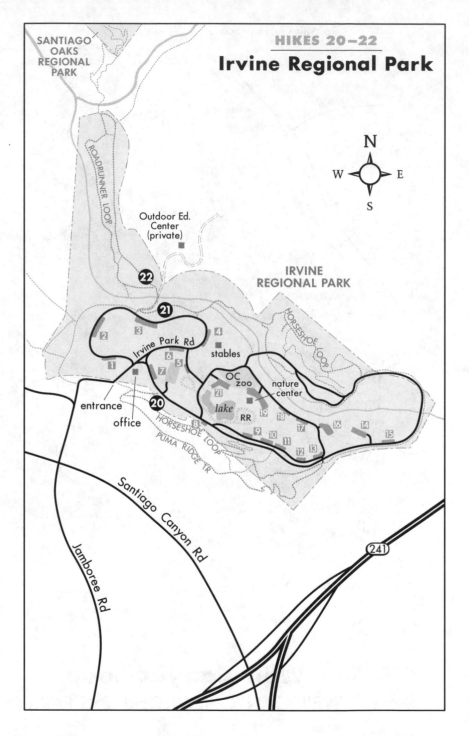

SANTIAGO
OAKS
REGIONAL
PARK

Irvine Regional Park

N
W ← → E
S

ROADRUNNER LOOP

Outdoor Ed.
Center
(private)

IRVINE
REGIONAL PARK

HORSESHOE LOOP

22

21

2   3
Irvine Park Rd   4

1   stables

6
7   5

entrance

office

20

OC
zoo
21   lake   nature
center

HORSESHOE LOOP
PUMA RIDGE TR

8   RR   19   18
9   10   11   17   16   14
12   13   15

Santiago Canyon Rd

Jamboree Rd

241

78

20. Puma Ridge—Horseshoe Loop

IRVINE REGIONAL PARK

Hiking distance: 2-mile loop
Hiking time: 1 hour
Configuration: loop
Elevation gain: 100 feet
Difficulty: easy
Exposure: exposed canyon slope with pockets of trees on lower trail
Dogs: allowed
Maps: U.S.G.S. Orange and Black Star Canyon
Irvine Regional Park map

Irvine Regional Park, located in the city of Orange, is nestled in Santiago Canyon at the base of the Santa Ana Mountains. The 475-acre park is tucked in a gorgeous valley with groves of majestic sycamores and 700-year-old live oaks. Transient Santiago Creek runs the length of the parkland. Dating back to 1897, it is the oldest regional park in California. It was used as a picnic grounds by early settlers for several decades before officially becoming a park.

Irvine Park offers many family-friendly amenities, including a two-acre fishing lake, the Orange County Zoo, the Irvine Park Railroad, a nature center, horse riding stables, and sheltered picnic areas. A multi-use trail network loops around the valley hills, connecting with the creek bottom and grassy parklands. This hike forms a loop on the south canyon wall, overlooking the park, the Santa Ana Mountains, and the San Gabriel Mountains.

To the trailhead

1 IRVINE PARK ROAD · ORANGE   33.796937, -117.755968

From the 55 (Costa Mesa) Freeway in Orange, take the Chapman Avenue exit. Drive 4.2 miles east to Jamboree Road (2.3 miles east of Cannon Street) and turn left. Continue 0.4 miles to the signed park entrance on the left. From the entrance station, curve right and drive 0.1 mile to the first parking lot (P-7) on the left. A parking fee is required.

The hike

Walk 70 yards east down the park road to the posted trailhead on the right. Take the dirt path up the hill to a trail split. Begin the loop to the right on the Puma Ridge Trail—the upper trail—and head up the spine of the hill to the 800-foot summit. Follow the ridge east along the south edge of the canyon, overlooking Irvine Park, the lake, the Santa Ana Mountains, and the San Gabriel Mountains. At the east end of the hill, descend along the ridge to a junction by a large boulder. Take the left fork and zigzag down to a junction at the park road.

For the return, bear left on the Horseshoe Loop Trail, an old dirt road. Meander west to a covered bench. From the cabana are views of the entire park, the trail system, and the Villa Park Dam in the west. Descend through ancient oaks and scattered palms, completing the loop at the far west end. ■

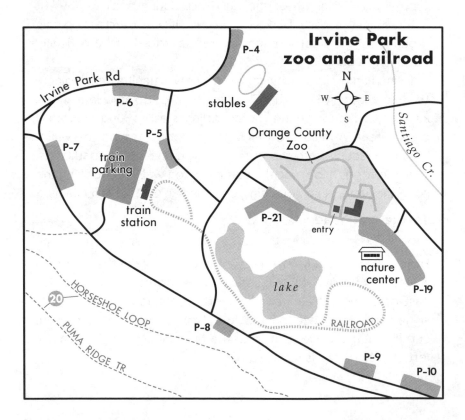

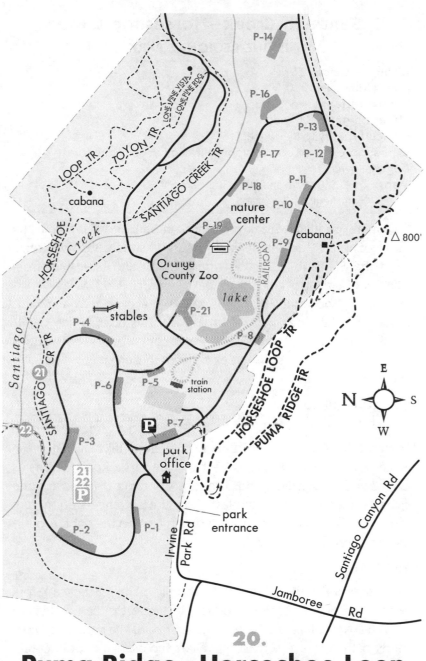

20.
Puma Ridge–Horseshoe Loop
IRVINE REGIONAL PARK

21. Santiago Creek—Horseshoe Loop

IRVINE REGIONAL PARK

Hiking distance: 2.5 miles round trip
Hiking time: 1 hour
Configuration: lollipop loop
Elevation gain: 100 feet
Difficulty: easy to moderate
Exposure: exposed canyon slope with section of mature forest
Dogs: allowed
Maps: U.S.G.S. Orange and Black Star Canyon
Irvine Regional Park map

Ephemeral Santiago Creek runs through Santiago Canyon in the heart of Irvine Regional Park. The park is situated downstream from the Santiago Reservoir (Irvine Lake) and upstream from Villa Park Dam (above Santiago Oaks Regional Park). Miles of hiking, biking, and equestrian trails follow the creekbed and loop around the hilly perimeter of the park. This hike, which parallels Santiago Creek, traverses the north canyon slope and returns along the broad, seasonal creek bottom through mature oak and sycamore groves.

To the trailhead

1 IRVINE PARK ROAD · ORANGE   33.799094, –117.756204

From the 55 (Costa Mesa) Freeway in Orange, take the Chapman Avenue exit. Drive 4.2 miles east to Jamboree Road (2.3 miles east of Cannon Street) and turn left. Continue 0.4 miles to the signed park entrance on the left. From the entrance station, turn left and drive 0.4 miles to the P-3 parking lot on the right. A parking fee is required.

The hike

Cross the park road and take the wide dirt path, reaching a Y-fork before crossing the rocky creekbed. To the left is the Roadrunner Loop (Hike 22). Take the Santiago Creek Trail to the right on a wide, sandy path. At the park road, curve left and cross the rocky creekbed. After crossing, curve right (east). Parallel the hills on the left and the creekbed on the right to a trail on the right, the return loop.

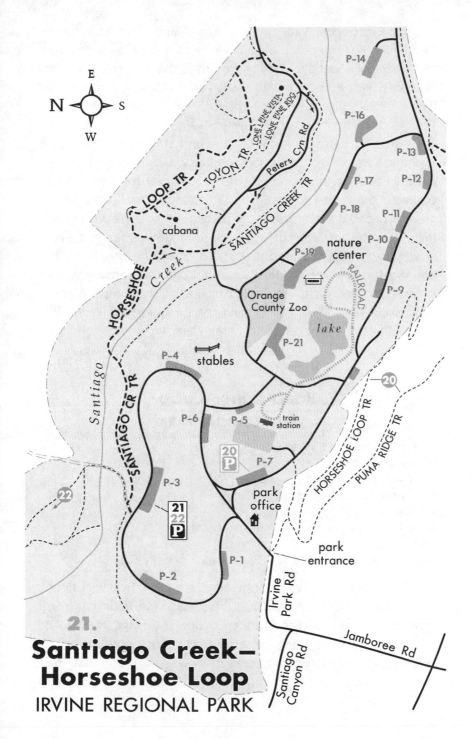

21.
Santiago Creek–
Horseshoe Loop
IRVINE REGIONAL PARK

Begin the loop, staying on the main trail, and ascend the south-facing hills. Loop around the side draw to a cabana on the right that overlooks Santiago Canyon. Return to the main trail and continue east. Pass a junction with the Toyon Trail to another junction. (For a shorter hike, take the right fork, returning to the canyon floor on the Toyon and Lone Pine Trails.)

Go left 30 yards to another fork, and stay to the right to a T-junction at the fenced park boundary. Descend to the park road, and follow the road 30 yards east (left) for a few yards. Curve to the right and pick up the Santiago Creek Trail, an old graveled road. Pass sculpted sandstone formations with caves, then take the left fork of the park road under oak and sycamore groves. Just before both park roads merge, take the well-defined footpath on the left. Stroll through the dense grove of ancient oaks and cross the road. Continue on the footpath to the Horseshoe Loop Trail, completing the loop. Return to the left along the edge of the Santiago Creek wash. ▪

22. Roadrunner Loop

IRVINE REGIONAL PARK

Hiking distance: 1.5-mile loop
Hiking time: 45 minutes
Configuration: loop
Elevation gain: 50 feet
Difficulty: easy
Exposure: mostly open hills with pockets of trees
Dogs: allowed
Maps: U.S.G.S. Orange and Black Star Canyon · Irvine Regional Park map

Irvine Regional Park was at one time a productive agricultural ranch dating back to the mid 1800s. James Irvine Jr. donated 160 acres of his oak woodland to the County of Orange in 1897. The shaded oak groves along the creekbed were already a popular picnicking area for early settlers. It was Irvine's intent that the trees should always be maintained. The area was renamed

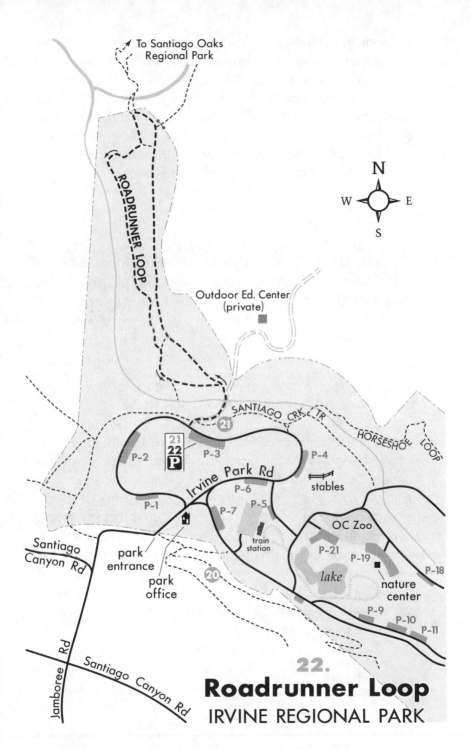

To Santiago Oaks
Regional Park

ROADRUNNER LOOP

N
W ← → E
S

Outdoor Ed. Center
(private)

SANTIAGO CRK. TR.

HORSESHOE LOOP

21

P-2

21
22
P

P-3

P-4

Irvine Park Rd

P-6

stables

P-1

P-7

P-5

P-21

OC Zoo

train
station

P-19

P-18

Santiago
Canyon Rd

park
entrance

park
office

20

lake

nature
center

P-9

P-10

P-11

Jamboree Rd

Santiago Canyon Rd

22.
Roadrunner Loop
IRVINE REGIONAL PARK

in his honor from Orange County Park to Irvine Park in 1926. The park was the filming site for many movies, including *Lassie Come Home* with Elizabeth Taylor in 1943.

Over the years, Irvine Park has grown to 475 acres, with a web of trails traversing the rolling foothills and creek bottom throughout the park. This hike explores the northwest corner of the park through a mix of ecosystems, meandering through the arid open hills, riparian creek bottom, and shady tree groves.

To the trailhead

1 IRVINE PARK ROAD · ORANGE   33.799094, -117.756204

From the 55 (Costa Mesa) Freeway in Orange, take the Chapman Avenue exit. Drive 4.2 miles east to Jamboree Road (2.3 miles east of Cannon Street) and turn left. Continue 0.4 miles to the signed park entrance on the left. From the entrance station, turn left and drive 0.4 miles to the P-3 parking lot on the right. A parking fee is required.

The hike

Cross the park road and take the wide dirt path to a Y-fork. To the right is the Santiago Creek Trail (Hike 21). Stay to the left and cross the rocky creekbed to a posted junction. Begin the Roadrunner Loop to the right, hiking counter-clockwise. Cross the open terrain through sage scrub, then drop down into an oak grove and a junction. Bear right and head north, crossing an open plateau through the rolling hills. Head up the rise to a private property gate by oaks and patches of prickly pear. Curve to the left and descend to an information kiosk. Go left again on the wide path to a fork. Take the footpath on the right, and climb the small hill to the willow trees. Weave through scattered eucalyptus, sycamore, and palm trees in a riparian corridor to a T-junction. Follow the right fork, then veer left at a road split, completing the loop. Return to the trailhead on the right. ▪

23. Peters Canyon Reservoir

PETERS CANYON REGIONAL PARK

Hiking distance: 2.5-mile loop
Hiking time: 1.5 hours
Configuration: loop
Elevation gain: 250 feet
Difficulty: easy
Exposure: mostly open with pockets of trees
Dogs: allowed
Maps: U.S.G.S. Orange · Peters Canyon Regional Park map

Peters Canyon Reservoir, built in 1931 by James Peters, is a 55-acre lake on the northern part of the 340-acre regional park. It is used for irrigation and is a vital habitat for fish and migrating waterfowl. The lake sits at an elevation of 550 feet and is fed by Handy Creek at the northeast corner. Peters Canyon Creek is the outlet stream. It drains through the parkland canyon before flowing into San Diego Creek and eventually into Upper Newport Bay.

The park has more than six miles of hiking, biking, and equestrian trails across gravel roads and paths. The routes weave through rolling hillsides, riparian woodlands, and freshwater marsh and grassland habitats. This hike circles the lake on rolling hillsides covered with coastal sage scrub, dotted with willows, sycamores, and cottonwoods.

To the trailhead

1019 CANYON VIEW AVE · ORANGE   33.784288, -117.762443

There are numerous routes to access Peters Canyon Regional Park. The park is located in Orange just south of Chapman Avenue between Newport Boulevard and Jamboree Road.

From the 55 (Costa Mesa) Freeway in Orange, take the Chapman Avenue exit. Drive 4.2 miles east to Jamboree Road (2.3 miles east of Cannon Street) and turn right (south). Continue 0.5 miles to Canyon View Avenue and turn right. Drive 0.1 mile to the park entrance on the left. Turn left into the parking lot. A parking fee is required.

The hike

From the kiosk west of the ranger office, take the signed trail to the right, heading towards Canyon View Avenue. Cross the concrete drain and curve left towards the main body of the reservoir. Pass two junctions with the Skylark Trail, staying left along the lake. Pass the Cactus Point Trail, an optional loop path that follows the curvature of the lake and rejoins the main trail at the top of the hill. Climb the hill on the main trail, and cross over the ridge with sweeping vistas. Descend along the park's west boundary, and ascend the hill to a junction and an overlook of the entire lake and dam. The left fork leads 30 yards to an overlook with a bench. Return to the junction and continue down the hillside to a T-junction on the floor of Peters Canyon. To extend the hike through Peters Canyon, continue with Hike 24 to the right (south).

For this hike, bear left on the Peters Canyon Trail on a gentle uphill grade. At the north end of the trail, descend into a lush wetland, returning to the Lake View Trail. The Willow Trail, a gorgeous riparian cut-across through a dense willow grove, intersects with the main route on the left for an optional route. The main trail skirts Jamboree Road and Canyon View Avenue through a forested canopy. Both trails merge and return to the east end of the parking lot behind the ranger office. ■

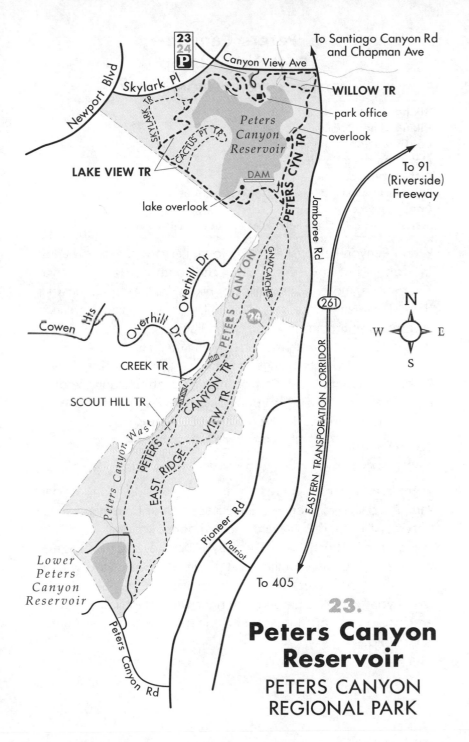

To Santiago Canyon Rd and Chapman Ave

WILLOW TR

park office

overlook

LAKE VIEW TR

Peters Canyon Reservoir

DAM

lake overlook

To 91 (Riverside) Freeway

Newport Blvd

Skylark Pl

SKYLARK TR

CACTUS PT TR

PETERS CYN TR

Canyon View Ave

23
24
P

Jamboree Rd

Overhill Dr

Overhill Dr

Cowen Hts

CREEK TR

SCOUT HILL TR

Peters Canyon Wash

PETERS CANYON TR

EAST RIDGE TR

VIEW TR

GNATCATCHER

261

N
W · E
S

EASTERN TRANSPORTATION CORRIDOR

Pioneer Rd

Patriot

To 405

Lower Peters Canyon Reservoir

Peters Canyon Rd

23.

Peters Canyon Reservoir

PETERS CANYON REGIONAL PARK

89

24. Peters Canyon—
East Ridge Loop

PETERS CANYON REGIONAL PARK

Hiking distance: 4 miles round trip
Hiking time: 2 hours
Configuration: lollipop loop
Elevation gain: 250 feet
Difficulty: moderate
Exposure: mostly open with pockets of trees
Dogs: allowed
Maps: U.S.G.S. Orange · Peters Canyon Regional Park map

Peters Canyon Regional Park is a long, narrow 354-acre park in the foothills of north Tustin along the south border of Orange. The park has more than six miles of hiking, biking, and equestrian trails that weave through rolling hillsides, riparian woodlands, and freshwater marsh and grassland habitats. The reservoir was built in 1931 to support the surrounding ranches.

This hike strolls the length of the park, from Peters Canyon Reservoir through Peters Canyon, making a return along the open East Ridge View Trail. The route passes through lush groves of willow, sycamore, cottonwood, and eucalyptus trees.

To the trailhead

1019 CANYON VIEW AVE · ORANGE   33.784288, –117.762443

There are numerous routes to access Peters Canyon Regional Park. The park is located in Orange just south of Chapman Avenue between Newport Boulevard and Jamboree Road.

From the 55 (Costa Mesa) Freeway in Orange, take the Chapman Avenue exit. Drive 4.2 miles east to Jamboree Road (2.3 miles east of Cannon Street) and turn right (south). Continue 0.5 miles to Canyon View Avenue and turn right. Drive 0.1 mile to the park entrance on the left. Turn left into the parking lot. A parking fee is required.

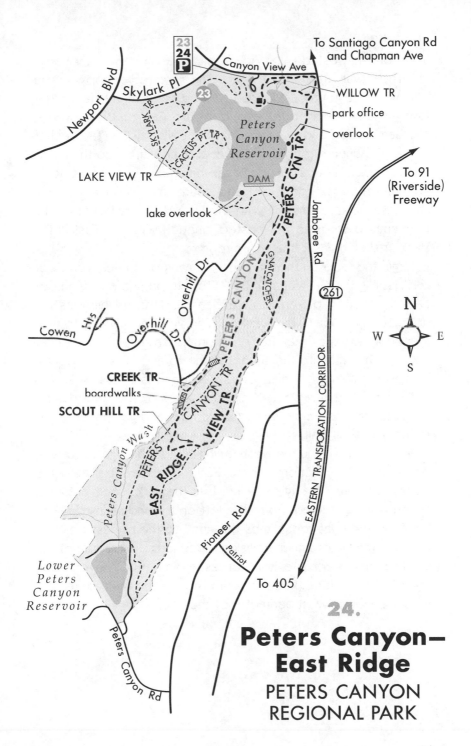

To Santiago Canyon Rd and Chapman Ave

Canyon View Ave

Newport Blvd

Skylark Pl

SKYLARK TR

CACTUS PT TR

WILLOW TR

park office

overlook

Peters Canyon Reservoir

LAKE VIEW TR

DAM

lake overlook

PETERS CYN TR

Jamboree Rd

To 91 (Riverside) Freeway

Overhill Dr

Overhill Dr

Cowen Hts

GNATCATCHER

PETERS CANYON

261

N W E S

CREEK TR

boardwalks

SCOUT HILL TR

CANYON TR

VIEW TR

PETERS CANYON

EAST RIDGE

Peters Canyon Wash

PETERS

EASTERN TRANSPORATION CORRIDOR

Pioneer Rd

Patriot

To 405

Lower Peters Canyon Reservoir

Peters Canyon Rd

24.

Peters Canyon– East Ridge
PETERS CANYON REGIONAL PARK

The hike

Begin on the posted Lake View Trail, located behind the ranger office. Walk northeast through the forested canopy to the Willow Trail, a gorgeous riparian cut-across through a dense willow grove on the right. The main trail skirts Canyon View Avenue and Jamboree Road, where the two trails rejoin. (Take either route.) Continue through a lush wetland, and climb up the hill to an overlook of Peters Canyon Reservoir and a bench at the north end of Peters Canyon Trail. Head south, overlooking the lake, and descend to a junction with the Lake View Trail at one mile. Continue 50 yards to the posted junction with the East Ridge View Trail on the left, the return route.

Begin the loop on the right fork, staying on the canyon floor and passing the Gnatcatcher Trail. Stroll through the canyon between the rolling, barren hills to the east and the lush hillsides and riparian vegetation to the west. At a grove of eucalyptus trees is a junction with the Creek Trail on the right, a hiking-only trail. Bear right on this trail into the shade of the forest. Cross a wooden footbridge over perennial Peters Canyon Wash. Pass an access trail from Overhill Drive, and cross a series of four boardwalks over the wetland. Rejoin Peters Canyon Trail and go right 20 yards to the Scout Hill Trail.

Veer left and climb the west-facing hillside through a eucalyptus grove to a T-junction with the East Ridge View Trail atop the ridge at 2.2 miles. The right fork leads to the park's south entrance at Peters Canyon Road. Go to the left on the undulating ridge to a Y-fork. The right fork climbs the knoll to the highest point of the trail. The Gnatcatcher Trail skirts around the west side of the knoll for an easier route. Both routes rejoin on the canyon floor, completing the loop. Retrace your steps to the right, or make a loop around the west perimeter of the lake. ▪

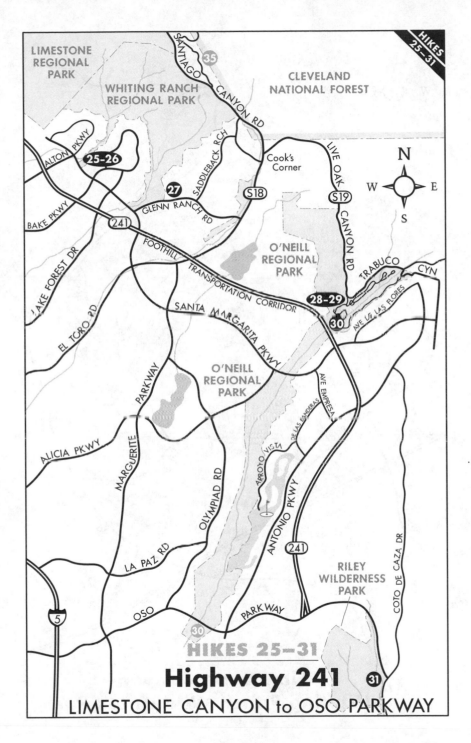

LIMESTONE
REGIONAL
PARK

WHITING RANCH
REGIONAL PARK

CLEVELAND
NATIONAL FOREST

SANTIAGO

35

CANYON RD

ALTON PKWY

25-26

27

SADDLEBACK RCH

Cook's
Corner

LIVE OAK

S18

S19

CANYON RD

N
W   E
S

BAKE PKWY

GLENN RANCH RD

241

FOOTHILL

TRABUCO

CYN

LAKE FOREST DR

TRANSPORTATION CORRIDOR

O'NEILL
REGIONAL
PARK

28-29

AVE LA LAS FLORES

30

EL TORO RD

SANTA MARGARITA PKWY

PARKWAY

O'NEILL
REGIONAL
PARK

AVE EMPRESA

MARGUERITE

ALICIA PKWY

ARROYO VISTA

AVE DE LAS BANDERAS

OLYMPIAD RD

ANTONIO PKWY

241

COTO DE CAZA DR

RILEY
WILDERNESS
PARK

LA PAZ RD

5

OSO

PARKWAY

30

31

HIKES 25–31

Highway 241

LIMESTONE CANYON to OSO PARKWAY

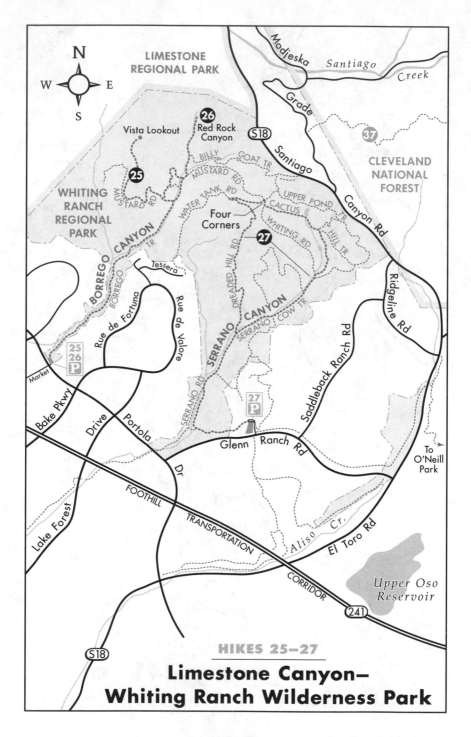

Limestone Canyon–
Whiting Ranch Wilderness Park

HIKES 25–27

25. Borrego Canyon to Vista Lookout
LIMESTONE CANYON—
WHITING RANCH WILDERNESS PARK

Hiking distance: 5.5 miles round trip
Hiking time: 2.5 hours
Configuration: out-and-back
Elevation gain: 800 feet
Difficulty: moderate to strenuous
Exposure: shady canyon and open hillside
Dogs: not allowed
Maps: U.S.G.S. El Toro
      Limestone-Whiting Wilderness Park map

Limestone-Whiting Wilderness Park encompasses 4,000 acres on the north end of Lake Forest and Foothill Ranch in the foothills of the Santa Ana Mountains. The park, an old cattle ranch, contains riparian and oak woodlands, rolling grasslands, scrub-covered slopes, and dramatic rock formations. Four seasonal streams— Borrego, Serrano, Glass, and Aliso Creek—wind through the parkland canyons. Twenty-six miles of graded roads and foot trails traverse throughout the park for hikers, bikers, and equestrians.

Borrego Canyon and Serrano Canyon are the two largest drainages in the parkland. This hike leads up Borrego Canyon to Vista Lookout, a 1,500-foot knoll on the northwest corner of the park. From the overlook are views of Red Rock Canyon, Limestone Canyon, and the Santa Ana and San Gabriel mountains. Viewing scopes atop the knoll highlight Old Saddleback, Luke Mesa, Caspers Wilderness Park, and Catalina Island.

The Santiago Fire burned 90% of the area in 2007, but the landscape has been steadily recovering.

To the trailhead

26701 PORTOLA PARKWAY · FOOTHILL RANCH   33.680983, -117.664442

From the I-5 (San Diego) Freeway in Lake Forest, take the El Toro Road exit. Drive 4.6 miles northeast to Portola Parkway and turn left. Continue 1.8 miles to Market Place, at the north end of Foothill Ranch Marketplace. Turn right and immediately left into the posted trailhead parking lot. A parking fee is required.

The hike

Walk to the far end of the parking lot to the posted trailhead by the rusted metal sculpture. Take the wide dirt path into the mouth of Borrego Canyon. Curve right through a trail gate and into a forest of oaks, sycamores, and lush riparian vegetation. Pass through a dense oak grove and continue past a cave in the cliffs on the right. Follow the east side of the drainage to just under one mile. Cross a footbridge over the stream, and continue up the canyon to a T-junction with Mustard Road/Trail at 1.5 miles. The right fork leads to Red Rock Canyon (Hike 26) and Four Corners (Hike 27).

For this hike, bear left, passing the Cattle Pond Loop Trail on the right. Wind up the open hillside on the west wall of the canyon. Top the ridge, leaving Borrego Canyon, and traverse the hillside to a trail split. The views range across Orange County, from Huntington Beach to San Clemente. Mustard Road veers left and descends into the next canyon. Take the right fork on the Vista Lookout Trail and climb to the ridge. Follow the level ridge to the lookout on the 1,500-foot knoll.

After studying the views and looking through the scoping tubes, return to the posted Cattle Pond Loop Trail below. Bear left and follow the contours of the hillside. Loop through a side ravine, returning to Borrego Canyon and Mustard Road. The right fork completes the loop down canyon, returning 1.5 miles to the trailhead.

To extend the hike into Red Rock Canyon, bear left on Mustard Road and continue with the next hike. ▨

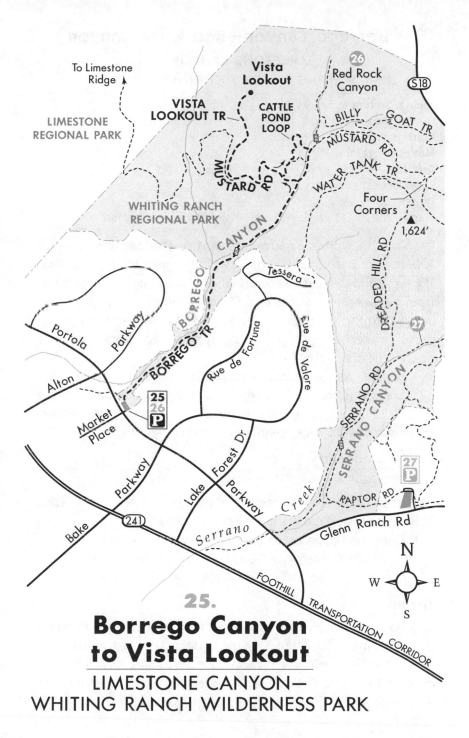

To Limestone
Ridge

LIMESTONE
REGIONAL PARK

Vista
Lookout

VISTA
LOOKOUT TR

CATTLE
POND
LOOP

Red Rock
Canyon

BILLY

GOAT TR

MUSTARD RD

WATER TANK TR

Four
Corners

1,624'

MUSTARD RD

WHITING RANCH
REGIONAL PARK

BORREGO CANYON

Tessera

DREADED HILL RD

Portola Parkway

BORREGO TR

Rue de Fortuna

Rue de Valore

SERRANO RD

SERRANO CANYON

Alton

25
26
P

Market
Place

Parkway

Lake Forest Dr.

Parkway

Creek

RAPTOR RD

27
P

Glenn Ranch Rd

Bake

241

Serrano

FOOTHILL TRANSPORTATION CORRIDOR

N
W E
S

25.
Borrego Canyon
to Vista Lookout

LIMESTONE CANYON—
WHITING RANCH WILDERNESS PARK

26. Borrego Canyon—Red Rock Canyon

LIMESTONE CANYON—
WHITING RANCH WILDERNESS PARK

Hiking distance: 5 miles round trip
Hiking time: 2.5 hours
Configuration: out-and-back
Elevation gain: 600 feet
Difficulty: moderate
Exposure: shaded canyon
Dogs: not allowed
Maps: U.S.G.S. El Toro · Limestone-Whiting Wilderness Park map

Red Rock Canyon is a narrow canyon surrounded by dramatic 100-foot red sandstone cliffs in Whiting Ranch Wilderness Park. The wind and water-carved formations cast a red terra cotta tint from oxidized iron in the rock. Shellfish and marine fossils can be seen in the fluted and chiseled sedimentary cliffs. To help preserve the fragile serrated outcroppings, Red Rock Canyon is open to hikers only.

This hike follows stream-fed Borrego Canyon to its upper reaches in Red Rock Canyon. The trail winds under a dense canopy of twisted live oaks, towering sycamores, and willows to the weathered rock sculptures in Red Rock Canyon.

To the trailhead

26701 PORTOLA PARKWAY · FOOTHILL RANCH   33.680983, -117.664442

From the I-5 (San Diego) Freeway in Lake Forest, take the El Toro Road exit. Drive 4.6 miles northeast to Portola Parkway and turn left. Continue 1.8 miles to Market Place, at the north end of Foothill Ranch Marketplace. Turn right and immediately left into the posted trailhead parking lot. A parking fee is required.

The hike

Walk to the far end of the parking lot to the posted trailhead by the rusted metal sculpture. Take the wide dirt path into the mouth of Borrego Canyon. Curve right through a trail gate and into a forest of oaks, sycamores, and lush riparian vegetation. Pass through a dense oak grove and continue past a cave in the cliffs on the

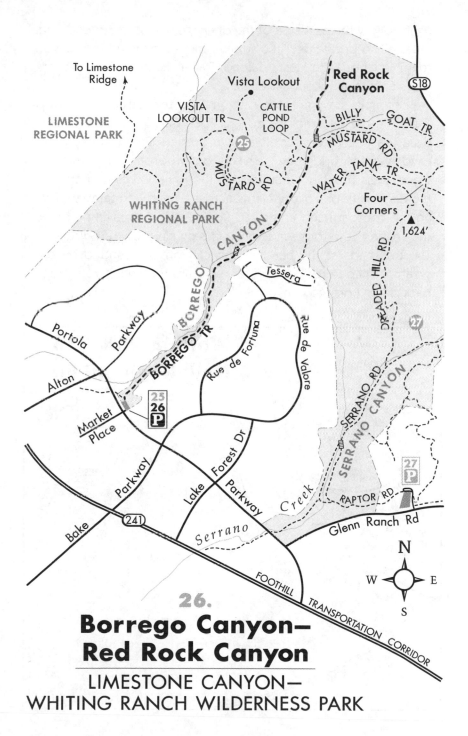

To Limestone
Ridge

LIMESTONE
REGIONAL PARK

Vista Lookout

Red Rock
Canyon

S18

VISTA
LOOKOUT TR

CATTLE
POND
LOOP

BILLY

GOAT TR

MUSTARD RD

25

MUSTARD RD

WATER TANK TR

WHITING RANCH
REGIONAL PARK

CANYON

Four
Corners

1,624'

BORREGO

Tessera

DREADED HILL RD

27

BORREGO TR

Rue de Fortuna

Rue de Valore

SERRANO RD

SERRANO CANYON

Portola

Parkway

Alton

Market
Place

25 26 P

27 P

Parkway

Lake Forest Dr

Parkway

Creek

RAPTOR RD

Bake

241

Serrano

Glenn Ranch Rd

N

W   E

S

FOOTHILL

TRANSPORTATION CORRIDOR

26.

Borrego Canyon–
Red Rock Canyon
LIMESTONE CANYON–
WHITING RANCH WILDERNESS PARK

right. Follow the east side of the drainage to just under one mile. Cross a footbridge over the stream, and continue up the canyon to a T-junction with Mustard Road/Trail at 1.5 miles. The left fork leads to Vista Lookout (Hike 25).

Bear right, staying in the canyon. Pass the Cattle Pond Loop Trail on the left to the posted Red Rock Trail. The main trail continues east up to the saddle at Four Corners. Bear left and cross a wooden footbridge on the hikers-only footpath. In a short distance, pass the Billy Goat Trail on the right. Continue north on the canyon floor. Follow cairns across a sandy streambed. Pick up the footpath and enter Red Rock Canyon, weaving through the eroded 100-foot sandstone cliffs on a narrow red dirt path. The trail ends at the head of the canyon, surrounded by the weather-shaped rock sculptures. Return by retracing your steps back down Borrego Canyon. ■

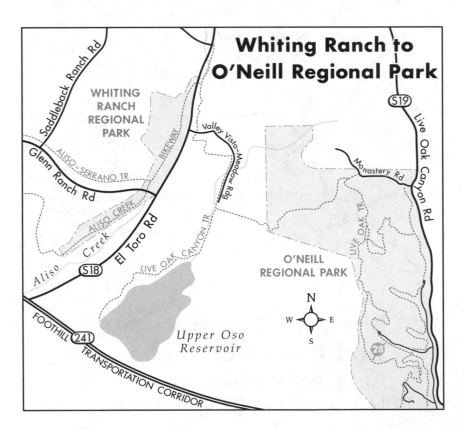

27. Serrano Canyon Loop to Four Corners

LIMESTONE CANYON—
WHITING RANCH WILDERNESS PARK

Hiking distance: 4.8 miles round trip
Hiking time: 2.5 hours
Configuration: lollipop loop
Elevation gain: 850 feet
Difficulty: moderate
Exposure: shaded canyon and open hillside
Dogs: not allowed
Maps: U.S.G.S. El Toro · Limestone-Whiting Wilderness Park map

Limestone-Whiting Wilderness Park is a popular hiking and biking corridor that provides easy access into the wilderness of the Santa Ana Mountains. Borrego Canyon and Serrano Canyon are the two largest canyons that drain through the parklands. This hike climbs up Serrano Canyon through dense oak woodland and riparian habitat to Four Corners, located on a saddle where four roads merge. It is the watershed divide of the two canyons. En route to Four Corners, a path leads through a lush, atmospheric draw with gnarled oaks (back cover photo). The hike returns down the Dreaded Hill Road, a steep fire road that connects Four Corners with Serrano Canyon.

To the trailhead

27901 GLEN RANCH RD · TRABUCO CANYON   33.675004, -117.641918

From the I-5 (San Diego) Freeway in Lake Forest, take the El Toro Road exit. Drive 4.6 miles northeast to Portola Parkway and turn left. Continue 0.8 miles to Glenn Ranch Road and turn right. Drive 0.6 miles to the trailhead parking lot on the left. A parking fee is required.

The hike

Take the well-posted trail and head west 100 yards on Raptor Road to the power lines. Curve right and descend into Serrano Canyon. Follow the canyon bottom through tall, dense chaparral and live oaks to a Y-fork at 0.2 miles. Curve right on the Live Oak Trail, and weave through the shade in a tunnel of large live oaks. At 0.4 miles, cross a bridge over the intermittent stream. Continue straight on Serrano Road to a Y-fork with the Dreaded Hill Road, the beginning of the loop.

Begin the loop to the right on the Serrano Cow Trail. Steadily climb to a junction. Take the left fork on the Whiting Road a short distance to the Sleepy Hollow Trail, a hiking-only path on the right. Bear right on the Sleepy Hollow Trail into the natural area, descending into the lush draw with towering gnarled oaks and grassland meadows. Climb a half mile north to the head of the atmospheric, stream-fed drainage. Exit the draw on the Cactus Hill Trail. Bear left for 50 yards, then veer left again, staying on the Cactus Hill Trail. Pass a pond on the right, and climb the narrow serpentine path to a T-junction with Whiting Road. Go to the right 70 yards to the bench at Four Corners. From the overlook are views into Red Rock Canyon, Serrano Canyon, Borrego Canyon, and across the Santa Ana Mountains.

Head west on the posted Water Tank Road to a ridge and a trail split. Bear left on Dreaded Hill Road. Cross a saddle overlooking Four Corners, and climb to the 1,624-foot summit. Top the summit and cross the saddle along a narrow ridge. Top the second summit and descend from the chaparral back down to the shady oak groves, completing the loop in Serrano Canyon. Return along the same trail one mile to the right. ▦

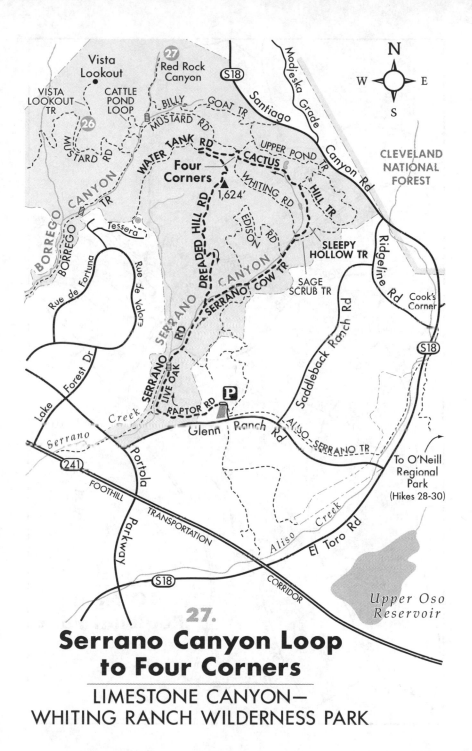

27.
Serrano Canyon Loop
to Four Corners

LIMESTONE CANYON—
WHITING RANCH WILDERNESS PARK

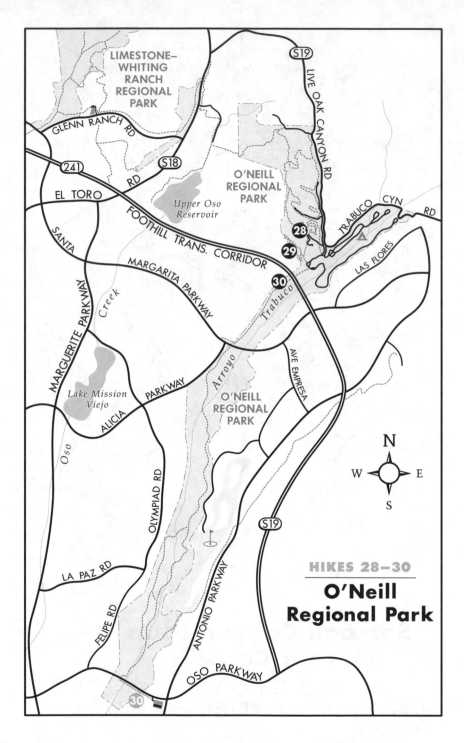

LIMESTONE–
WHITING
RANCH
REGIONAL
PARK

GLENN RANCH RD

S19

LIVE OAK CANYON RD

241

S18

RD

EL TORO

O'NEILL
REGIONAL
PARK

Upper Oso
Reservoir

FOOTHILL TRANS. CORRIDOR

TRABUCO CYN RD

28

29

LAS FLORES

30

Trabuco

SANTA

MARGARITA PARKWAY

Creek

MARGUERITE PARKWAY

AVE EMPRESA

Arroyo

Lake Mission
Viejo

PARKWAY

ALICIA

O'NEILL
REGIONAL
PARK

Oso

OLYMPIAD RD

S19

N
W E
S

HIKES 28–30

O'Neill
Regional Park

LA PAZ RD

FELIPE RD

ANTONIO PARKWAY

30

OSO PARKWAY

28. Live Oak Trail to Vista Point
O'NEILL REGIONAL PARK

Hiking distance: 3-mile loop
Hiking time: 1.5 hours
Configuration: loop
Elevation gain: 600 feet
Difficulty: moderate
Exposure: mostly open with pockets of trees
Dogs: allowed in campground and paved trails
Maps: U.S.G.S. Santiago Peak
O'Neill Regional Park and Wilderness Areas map

O'Neill Regional Park and Wilderness Area encompasses 3,358 acres between Mission Viejo and Rancho Santa Margarita in the foothills of the Santa Ana Mountains. The park, once part of the Rancho Trabuco lands, has several diverse ecosystems, including grassy meadows, oak and sycamore woodlands, rolling chaparral-covered hills, riparian habitats, and two heavily wooded canyons. Seasonal Arroyo Trabuco runs through the long and narrow park. An extensive hiking, biking, and equestrian trail system ranges over 23 miles.

This hike at the north end of the park follows the Live Oak Trail from the forested canyon, then heads up along the west canyon ridge to Vista Point. The 1,492-foot open summit has expansive views that range from the upper reaches of the Santa Ana Mountains to the ocean and from Old Saddleback to the San Joaquin Hills. A map atop the summit highlights the mountain ridgeline and peaks.

To the trailhead

30892 TRABUCO CANYON RD · TRABUCO CYN   33.650219, -117.603411

From the I-5 (San Diego) Freeway in Lake Forest, take the El Toro Road exit. Drive 7.4 miles northeast to the Y-fork of Santiago Canyon Road (S18) and Live Oak Canyon Road (S19), known as Cook's Corner. Bear right and take Live Oak Canyon Road 3.3 miles to the posted park entrance on the right. From the park entrance station, bear right and drive 0.2 miles to the posted Edna

Spaulding Trail and Live Oak Trail on the right. Park 50 yards ahead in the parking spaces on the right. A parking fee is required.

The hike

Begin at the posted Live Oak–Spaulding trailhead. Pass through the trail gate, and head up the canyon on a narrow asphalt road. At 100 yards is a junction in an oak grove with the Edna Spaulding Nature Trail on the left (Hike 29). Continue straight on the Live Oak Trail for 0.3 miles to a dirt path on the left. The paved path ends a short distance ahead at the back of the canyon. Take the footpath on the left, and climb the canyon's west wall to the head of the canyon. Veer left, dropping into the adjoining canyon to the oak-shaded floor by an old park road. Cross the road and pick up the Live Oak Trail, passing the Pawfoot Trail on the right. Climb up the north canyon wall, and curve around the hillside to sweeping views of the Santa Ana Mountains. Pass the Homestead Trail on the right, and crest the hill to 360-degree vistas of the mountains and surrounding geography. Drop down and pass the Coyote Canyon Trail on the right (the return route) to the base of the prominent 1,492-foot knoll with the communication tower.

Ascend the summit on the steep, narrow footpath along the park's west boundary. Atop the flat knoll is a bench, viewing scopes, and an interpretive map. Continuing north, the trail connects to Whiting Ranch Wilderness Park. From the east end of the knoll, the steep Valley Vista Trail drops into Live Oak Canyon. This more strenuous trail may be taken as an alternative return route, heading back down the canyon on the Hoffman Homestead Trail.

For an easier route, return south to the Coyote Canyon Trail. Take the Coyote Canyon Trail, now on the left, and weave 0.4 miles to the canyon floor. Near the park road, bear right, continuing on the Coyote Trail. Parallel the road on the hillside and through oak groves to the park entrance. Follow the park road a quarter mile back to the trailhead. Or, as another option, take the Pawfoot Trail to the right, and climb up to the junction with the Live Oak Trail, completing the loop. ▪

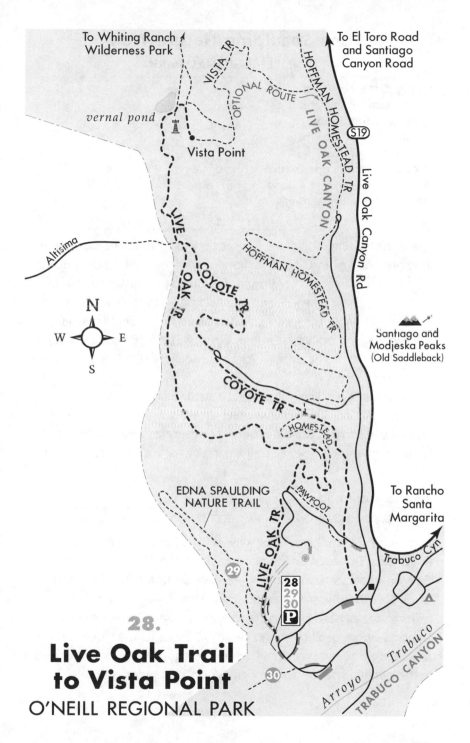

To Whiting Ranch
Wilderness Park

VISTA TR

OPTIONAL ROUTE

To El Toro Road
and Santiago
Canyon Road

HOFFMAN HOMESTEAD TR

LIVE OAK CANYON

S19

Live Oak Canyon Rd

vernal pond

Vista Point

LIVE OAK TR

COYOTE TR

Altisima

HOFFMAN HOMESTEAD TR

N
W   E
S

Santiago and
Modjeska Peaks
(Old Saddleback)

COYOTE TR

HOMESTEAD

EDNA SPAULDING
NATURE TRAIL

PAWFOOT

To Rancho
Santa
Margarita

LIVE OAK TR

Trabuco Cyn

29

28
29
30
P

30

28.

Live Oak Trail
to Vista Point

O'NEILL REGIONAL PARK

Arroyo

Trabuco

TRABUCO CANYON

29. Edna Spaulding Nature Trail

O'NEILL REGIONAL PARK

Hiking distance: 0.8-mile loop
Hiking time: 30 minutes
Configuration: loop
Elevation gain: 200 feet
Difficulty: very easy
Exposure: mostly open with pockets of trees
Dogs: allowed in campground and paved trails
Maps: U.S.G.S. Santiago Peak
O'Neill Regional Park and Wilderness Areas map

The Edna Spaulding Nature Trail is an easy, short walk along an interpretive trail in O'Neill Regional Park. The trail makes a loop along the east-facing canyon slope through coastal sage scrub and pockets of trees. From the hillside slopes is a view Old Saddleback Mountain, a crescent-shaped mountain formed from the two highest points in Orange County. The 5,687-foot Santiago Peak sits on the right, and 5,496-foot Modjeska Peak lies one mile away to its left.

The Edna Spaulding Nature Trail is named in honor of an Orange County science and botany teacher who created this trail for school use. Fifty acres have been set aside as a wilderness area to protect the hillside. A trail brochure is available at the park office.

To the trailhead

30892 TRABUCO CANYON RD · TRABUCO CYN   33.650219, -117.603411

From the I-5 (San Diego) Freeway in Lake Forest, take the El Toro Road exit. Drive 7.4 miles northeast to the Y-fork of Santiago Canyon Road (S18) and Live Oak Canyon Road (S19), known as Cook's Corner. Bear right and take Live Oak Canyon Road 3.3 miles to the posted park entrance on the right. From the park entrance station, bear right and drive 0.2 miles to the posted Edna Spaulding Trail and Live Oak Trail on the right. Park 50 yards ahead in the parking spaces on the right. A parking fee is required.

The hike

Begin at the posted Live Oak–Spaulding trailhead. Pass through the trail gate and head up the canyon on a narrow asphalt road. At 100 yards is a junction in an oak grove. The Live Oak Trail continues straight (Hike 28). Bear left on the Edna Spaulding Nature Trail. The loop begins at the base of the west canyon wall. Take the left fork, hiking clockwise, and climb the hillside to vistas of Trabuco Canyon and the Santa Ana Mountains. Head north along the park boundary just below the ridge. Traverse the hillside on a gentle uphill grade. Near the upper ridge are vistas of Santiago and Modjeska Peaks. Descend southeast into a pocket of live oaks near the canyon bottom. Complete the loop and bear left to the Live Oak Trail. Return to the trailhead on the right. ■

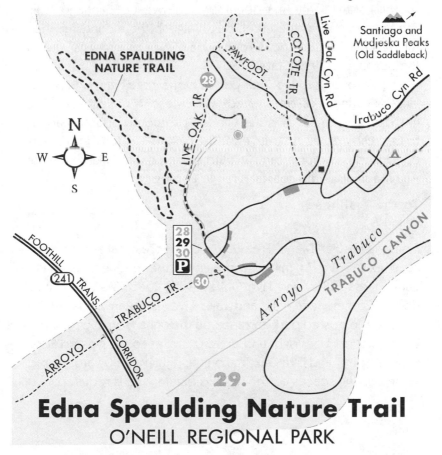

Edna Spaulding Nature Trail
O'NEILL REGIONAL PARK

30. Arroyo Trabuco Trail
O'NEILL REGIONAL PARK

Hiking distance: 12 miles round trip
(6 miles for a one-way shuttle hike)
Hiking time: 6 hours
Configuration: out-and-back or one-way shuttle
Elevation gain: 300 feet
Difficulty: moderate to strenuous
Exposure: a mix of open slopes and riparian woodlands
Dogs: allowed in campground and paved trails
Maps: U.S.G.S. Santiago Peak, Canada Gobernadora, San Juan Capistrano
O'Neill Regional Park and Wilderness Areas map

Arroyo Trabuco runs the length of O'Neill Regional Park in the foothills of the Santa Ana Mountains southwest of Santiago Peak. The headwaters of the creek begin high in the mountains, then run through Trabuco Canyon and O'Neill Regional Park en route to the ocean at Doheny State Beach.

The Arroyo Trabuco Trail parallels the creek through a six-mile-long finger of designated wilderness in O'Neill Park. The near-level trail meanders through the protected riparian habitat to Oso Parkway at its south end. The narrow stretch of undeveloped land is an important wildlife corridor that links the Santa Ana Mountains with coastal Orange County.

To the trailhead

30892 TRABUCO CANYON RD · TRABUCO CYN   33.650219, -117.603411

From the I-5 (San Diego) Freeway in Lake Forest, take the El Toro Road exit. Drive 7.4 miles northeast to the Y-fork of Santiago Canyon Road (S18) and Live Oak Canyon Road (S19), known as Cook's Corner. Bear right and take Live Oak Canyon Road 3.3 miles to the posted park entrance on the right. From the park entrance station, bear right and drive 0.2 miles to the posted Edna Spaulding Trail and Live Oak Trail on the right. Park 50 yards ahead in the parking spaces on the right. A parking fee is required.

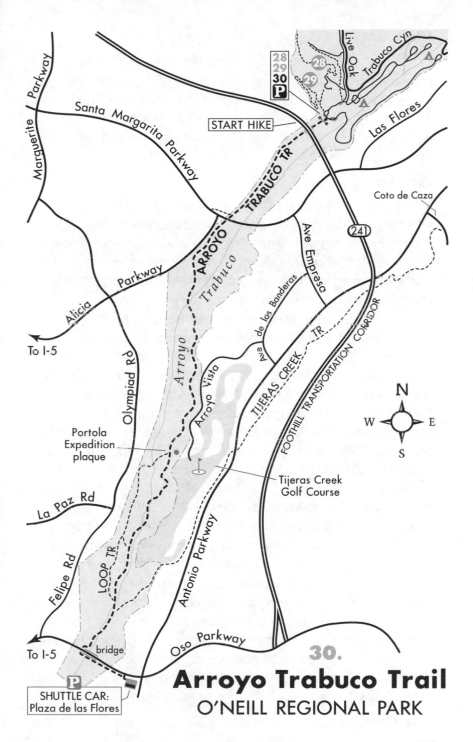

30.
Arroyo Trabuco Trail
O'NEILL REGIONAL PARK

Shuttle car

28562 Oso Pkwy · Rancho Santa Margarita   33.583512, -117.633282

From the I-5 (San Diego) Freeway in Mission Viejo, take the Oso Parkway exit. Drive 2.5 miles east to the Plaza turnoff, just after crossing the long bridge over Arroyo Trabuco and before Antonio Parkway. Turn right on Plaza and park in the Plaza De Las Flores Center on the left.

The hike

Walk south to the trailhead kiosk. Pass through the trail gate, and take the right fork through an oak and sycamore woodland. Cross under the towering Foothill Transportation Corridor Tollway (Highway 241), and stroll along the west side of the wide canyon. At 1.3 miles, a connector trail on the right leads up to Santa Margarita Parkway. Walk beneath the highway bridge and curve south, crossing over seasonal Arroyo Trabuco to the sloping hills on the east side of the canyon. Meander through groves of twisted live oaks and large-leafed sycamores along the canyon floor. Climb the gentle grade on the east slope to the mesa, parallel to Arroyo Vista on the left. Arroyo Vista ends at the Tijeras Creek Golf Club. Curve right to a Y-fork at a historic plaque that commemorates the Portola Expedition, which camped on this site in July 1769 while in search of mission locations. The Loop Trail descends into the lush canyon.

Stay atop the mesa on the Arroyo Trabuco Trail to the left, and slowly wind down to the canyon floor. Walk through the open meadows dotted with sycamores and oaks, then drop into the shady canyon bottom with palm trees, towering sycamores, and bamboo groves. Wind through the forest, crossing the creek three times where the two trails merge. Follow the wash 50 yards and pick up the trail, passing a second connector with the Loop Trail. Cross the creek two more times to the Oso Parkway bridge. A wide path heads up to the northwest corner of the bridge at the Oso Parkway trailhead. Return by retracing the route.

For the shuttle hike, cross the bridge and walk east 0.3 miles to the Plaza De Las Flores Center at Antonio Parkway. ▪

31. Riley Wilderness Park

Hiking distance: 3-mile loop
Hiking time: 1.5 hours
Configuration: loop
Elevation gain: 300 feet
Difficulty: easy to slightly moderate
Exposure: mostly open with pockets of trees
Dogs: not allowed
Maps: U.S.G.S. Canada Gobernadora
General Thomas F. Riley Wilderness Park map

Riley Wilderness Park in Wagon Wheel Canyon is a wildlife sanctuary south of Rancho Santa Margarita. The 475-acre park was part of a cattle ranch until 1983, when Orange County acquired the land. The park has two stream-fed canyons, rolling hills, and two overlooks. The seasonal creeks are lined with western sycamores and ancient coastal live oaks, while coastal sage scrub and grasslands carpet the hills. Five miles of hiking, biking, and equestrian trails weave through the park, connecting the canyons, hills, and overlooks.

This hike makes a loop through the heart of the park and includes two overlooks. Skink Vista Overlook and Horned Toad Vista Point offer views of the surrounding landscape, from the open canyons and dense tree groves to the mile-high peaks in the Santa Ana Mountains.

To the trailhead

30952 OSO PARKWAY · COTO DE CAZA   33.572667, –117.592818

From the I-5 (San Diego) Freeway in Mission Viejo, take the Oso Parkway exit. Drive 5.9 miles east to the park entrance on the right. (It is located just before Coto De Caza Drive, at the end of the road.) Turn right and drive 0.1 mile to the parking lot on the right. A parking fee is required.

The hike

From the northeast corner of the parking lot (by the metal gate), take the Wagon Wheel Trail. Head north into the canyon lined with oaks and sycamores. Cross the footbridge over the seasonal creek, and parallel Oso Parkway through mature live oaks to the posted Pheasant Run Trail at 0.4 miles. The Wagon Wheel Trail continues straight ahead along the road. Bear left and cross the rocky drainage. Loop back to the south and up the rolling grasslands. Cross a wooden bridge over a gully. Climb the exposed hillside and top the rolling hills to a T-junction. The Pheasant Run Trail returns to the parking lot on the left. Take the right fork on the Mule Deer Trail, meandering through the grasslands and coastal sage. Cross a footbridge over a wetland ravine, and weave up to the ridge and a junction with the Vista Ridge Trail. Detour right on the trail up to Skink Vista Point, a bald summit with an interpretive map. From the overlook is a view of the park's trail system and a sighting-tube that highlights Old Saddleback, the crescent-shaped formation composed of Santiago and Modjeska Peaks.

Return to the ridge and continue to the right on the Oak Canyon Trail. Curve left and descend into the oak-shaded riparian habitat, passing an old cattle pond on the left. Follow the west side of Oak Canyon to a posted junction, just beyond the oak canopy. Take the Horned Toad Trail to the right and climb up a side canyon on the looping trail. At the summit are views across southern Orange County. Descend to Oak Canyon and return to the trailhead and visitor center through open grasslands, passing junctions with the Sycamore Loop Trail and the Vista Ridge Trail. ▩

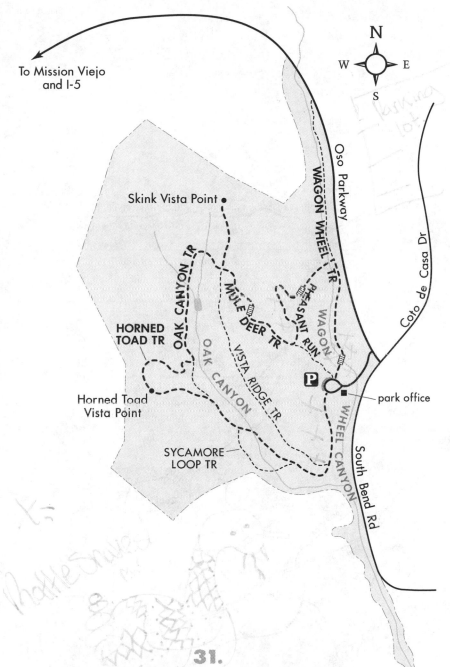

To Mission Viejo
and I-5

N
W · E
S

Oso Parkway

Coto de Casa Dr

WAGON WHEEL TR

Skink Vista Point ●

OAK CANYON TR

MULE DEER TR

PHEASANT RUN

WAGON

HORNED
TOAD TR

OAK CANYON

VISTA RIDGE TR

Horned Toad
Vista Point ●

park office

WHEEL CANYON

South Bend Rd

SYCAMORE
LOOP TR

31.
Riley Wilderness Park

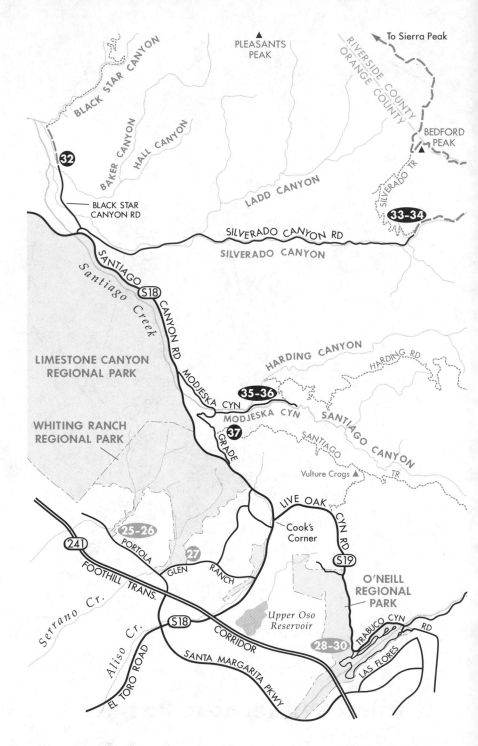

PLEASANTS PEAK

To Sierra Peak

RIVERSIDE COUNTY
ORANGE COUNTY

BLACK STAR CANYON

32

BAKER CANYON

HALL CANYON

BLACK STAR CANYON RD

LADD CANYON

BEDFORD PEAK

SILVERADO TR

33-34

SILVERADO CANYON RD

SILVERADO CANYON

Santiago Creek

SANTIAGO

S18

CANYON RD

LIMESTONE CANYON REGIONAL PARK

HARDING CANYON

HARDING RD

MODJESKA CYN

35-36

MODJESKA CYN

SANTIAGO CANYON

WHITING RANCH REGIONAL PARK

37

GRADE

SANTIAGO

TR

Vulture Crags ▲

LIVE OAK CYN RD

25-26

Cook's Corner

241

PORTOLA

27

GLEN

RANCH

S19

O'NEILL REGIONAL PARK

Serrano Cr.

FOOTHILL TRANS.

S18

CORRIDOR

Upper Oso Reservoir

28-30

TRABUCO CYN

RD

LAS FLORES

Aliso Cr.

EL TORO ROAD

SANTA MARGARITA PKWY

116

Santiago Canyon Road
SILVERADO CANYON ROAD to
TRABUCO CREEK ROAD

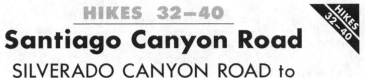

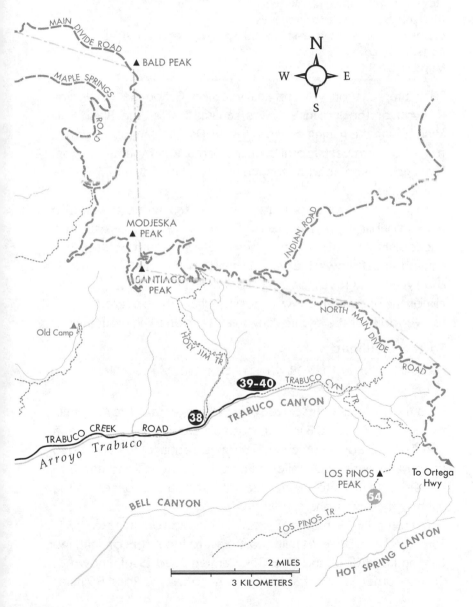

32. Black Star Canyon

Hiking distance: 6 miles round trip to switchbacks
15 miles round trip to Main Divide Road
Hiking time: 3—7 hours
Configuration: out-and-back
Elevation gain: 800—2,000 feet
Difficulty: moderate to strenuous
Exposure: mostly shady canyon with some open canyon sides
Dogs: allowed
Maps: U.S.G.S. Black Star Canyon

Black Star Canyon was originally called Cañon de los Indios (Canyon of the Indians). It was renamed after the Black Star Mine during the mining boom in the 1870s. The canyon stretches from the northwest foothills of the Santa Ana Mountains, from Santiago Canyon Road to the Main Divide Road at the Riverside County line.

This hike follows an old dirt road as it zigzags up the canyon through public and private land. (The road is a vehicle-restricted public right-of-way.) The hike begins at the mouth of Black Star Canyon and follows the canyon bottom through oak, willow, and sycamore groves, passing old ranch sites. En route, the trail climbs the north canyon wall, crossing chaparral-covered slopes to overlooks of the scenic canyon and surrounding mountains.

To the trailhead

SILVERADO CANYON ROAD—BLACK STAR CANYON ROAD · SILVERADO
33.764321, -117.678037

From the 55 (Costa Mesa) Freeway in Orange, take the Chapman Avenue exit. Drive 10.8 miles east to Silverado Canyon Road and turn left. (Chapman Avenue becomes Santiago Canyon Road en route.) Continue 0.1 mile to Black Star Canyon Road and turn left. Drive 1.1 miles to the vehicle gate. Park in the spaces on the right by the sandstone formation.

From the I-5 (San Diego) Freeway in Lake Forest, take the El Toro Road exit. Drive 7.4 miles northeast to the Y-fork of Santiago Canyon Road (S18) and Live Oak Canyon Road (S19), known as Cook's Corner. Bear left and take Santiago Canyon Road 5.9 miles

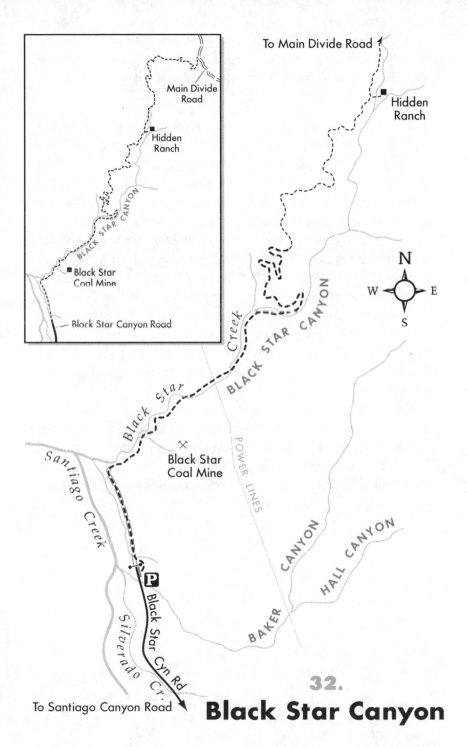

To Main Divide Road

Hidden Ranch

N
W — E
S

Main Divide Road

Hidden Ranch

BLACK STAR CANYON

Black Star Coal Mine

Black Star Canyon Road

Creek

Black Star

BLACK STAR CANYON

Black Star Coal Mine

POWER LINES

Santiago Creek

P

Black Star Cyn Rd

Silverado Cr.

BAKER CANYON

HALL CANYON

To Santiago Canyon Road

32.

Black Star Canyon

to Silverado Canyon Road and turn right. Continue 0.1 mile to Black Star Canyon Road and turn left. Drive 1.1 miles to the vehicle gate. Park in the spaces on the right by the sandstone formation.

The hike

Walk around the right side of the metal gate, and follow the partially paved road along the east side of the Santiago Creek drainage. At a half mile, the road bends 90 degrees to the right and enters the mouth of Black Star Canyon. Gently wind up the canyon through groves of oak, sycamore, and eucalyptus trees. Pass remnants of old homesites, and cross over to the north side of the canyon drainage between picturesque rock walls. Cross under towering power lines at two miles. A row of juniper and ponderosa pines line the road near a group of remote homes. Beyond the last home, make a horseshoe left bend, and climb up the canyon wall to overlooks. Follow the contours of the hillside up a dry side canyon filled with grass and chaparral. The road/ trail twists, turns, and doubles back to the cliffs high above Black Star Canyon and a series of overlooks. Choose your own turn-around point anywhere along the road.

The road continues climbing, then drops into Hidden Valley and the site of Hidden Ranch at 5 miles. Pass through the grassy upper valley on private land, staying on the road easement. Follow the ridge, overlooking Fremont Canyon to the west. The Main Divide Road is at 7.5 miles. The road lies just north of the buildings known as Beek's Place. ▧

33. Silverado Trail to Overlook
SILVERADO CANYON

Hiking distance: 4.6 miles round trip
Hiking time: 2.5 hours
Configuration: out-and-back
Elevation gain: 1,500 feet
Difficulty: moderate to strenuous
Exposure: exposed plateau
Dogs: allowed
Maps: U.S.G.S. Santiago Peak and Corona South
Cleveland National Forest map

Silverado Canyon is in the heart of the Santa Ana Mountains north of Santiago Peak. The canyon was originally called Cañada de la Madera (Timber Canyon) but was renamed during the boom and bust mining days in the late 1870s.

This hike up the Silverado Trail begins at the end of Silverado Canyon Road. The trail traverses the north wall of Silverado Canyon from the tree-shaded canyon bottom to the exposed sedimentary rock ridge, climbing the first 2.3 miles of an old

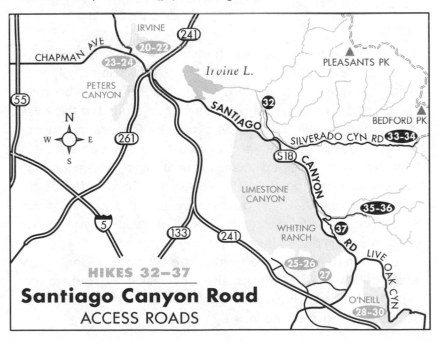

HIKES 32–37
Santiago Canyon Road
ACCESS ROADS

road to a 3,426-foot peak atop the ridge. From the overlook are sweeping views into Ladd Canyon, Silverado Canyon, Pleasants Peak, and 3,800-foot Bedford Peak. For even better views, the trail continues to Bedford Peak—Hike 34—where the panoramic views span to the ocean.

To the trailhead

31341 SILVERADO CANYON RD · SILVERADO   33.747386, -117.583448

From the 55 (Costa Mesa) Freeway in Orange, take the Chapman Avenue exit. Drive 10.8 miles east to Silverado Canyon Road and turn left. (Chapman Avenue becomes Santiago Canyon Road en route.) Continue 5.8 miles to the end of Silverado Canyon Road at the Forest Service gate. Park in the spaces on the left.

From the I-5 (San Diego) Freeway in Lake Forest, take the El Toro Road exit. Drive 7.4 miles northeast to the Y-fork of Santiago Canyon Road (S18) and Live Oak Canyon Road (S19), known as Cook's Corner. Bear left and take Santiago Canyon Road 5.9 miles to Silverado Canyon Road and turn right. Continue 5.8 miles to the end of Silverado Canyon Road at the Forest Service gate. Park in the spaces on the left.

The hike

Walk past the road gate, and follow one-lane Maple Springs Road 0.1 mile to a distinct footpath on the left. Bear sharply left, heading up the hillside and leaving the shaded canyon bottom. Curve to the right up a side canyon and loop around to the west canyon wall. Steadily climb to an overlook of Silverado Canyon. Curve right and continue winding up the mountain on the cliff-edge path. At 1.7 miles is a horseshoe right bend. Cross under the power lines to a wide, flat plateau on a ridge. To the left is a side path, which heads a short distance west to the summit of the 3,426-foot peak. There are great views into Ladd Canyon and of the surrounding peaks. This is the turn-around point.

To hike farther, continue northeast on the Silverado Trail to Bedford Peak (Hike 34). The 3,800-foot peak is adjacent to the Main Divide Road. It is located 1.2 miles ahead, with an additional 350 feet gained in elevation. ■

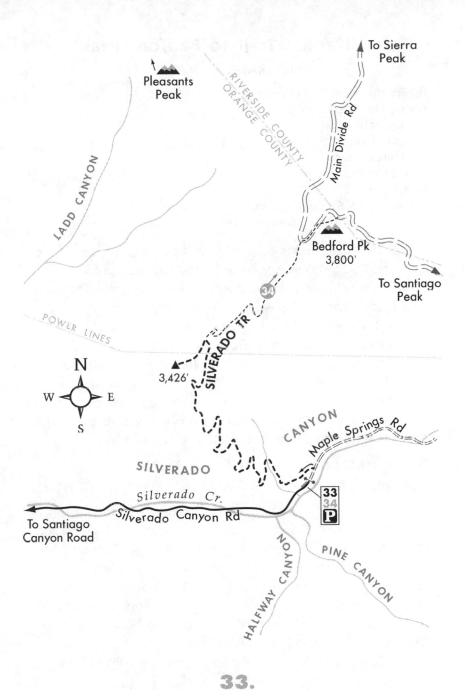

To Sierra Peak

Pleasants Peak

RIVERSIDE COUNTY
ORANGE COUNTY

Main Divide Rd

LADD CANYON

Bedford Pk
3,800'

To Santiago Peak

POWER LINES

N
W ⊕ E
S

3,426'

SILVERADO TR

34

CANYON

Maple Springs Rd

SILVERADO

Silverado Cr.

Silverado Canyon Rd

33
34
P

To Santiago Canyon Road

HALFWAY CANYON

PINE CANYON

33.
Silverado Trail to overlook

34. Silverado Trail to Bedford Peak

SILVERADO CANYON

Hiking distance: 7 miles round trip
Hiking time: 3.5 hours
Configuration: out-and-back
Elevation gain: 1,900 feet
Difficulty: strenuous
Exposure: exposed ridge
Dogs: allowed
Maps: U.S.G.S. Santiago Peak and Corona South
Cleveland National Forest map

Bedford Peak sits on the edge of Orange County just shy of the Riverside County boundary in the Santa Ana Mountains. From the 3,800-foot peak are vistas across the Santa Ana range, Temescal Valley, Lake Mathews, Silverado Canyon, Ladd Canyon, and the Orange County basin to the ocean.

This strenuous hike begins from the end of Silverado Canyon road. The route follows the Silverado Trail up a cliff-edge path to an overlook at 3,426 feet about midway to the peak (the end of the previous hike). The trail continues climbing another 1.2 miles to rounded Bedford Peak at the Main Divide Road, following the ridgeline between Silverado Canyon and Ladd Canyon.

To the trailhead

31341 SILVERADO CANYON RD · SILVERADO   33.747386, -117.583448

From the 55 (Costa Mesa) Freeway in Orange, take the Chapman Avenue exit. Drive 10.8 miles east to Silverado Canyon Road and turn left. (Chapman Avenue becomes Santiago Canyon Road en route.) Continue 5.8 miles to the end of Silverado Canyon Road at the Forest Service gate. Park in the spaces on the left.

From the I-5 (San Diego) Freeway in Lake Forest, take the El Toro Road exit. Drive 7.4 miles northeast to the Y-fork of Santiago Canyon Road (S18) and Live Oak Canyon Road (S19), known as Cook's Corner. Bear left and take Santiago Canyon Road 5.9 miles

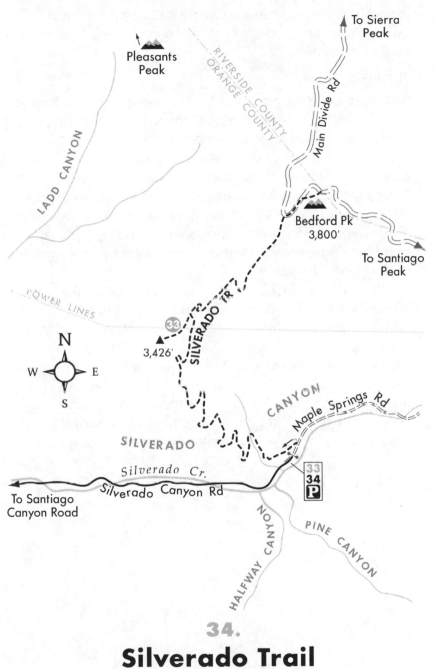

34.
Silverado Trail
to Bedford Peak

to Silverado Canyon Road and turn right. Continue 5.8 miles to the end of Silverado Canyon Road at the Forest Service gate. Park in the spaces on the left.

The hike

Walk past the road gate, and follow one-lane Maple Springs Road 0.1 mile to a distinct footpath on the left. Bear sharply left, heading up the hillside and leaving the shaded canyon bottom. Curve to the right up a side canyon and loop around to the west canyon wall. Steadily climb to an overlook of Silverado Canyon. Curve right and continue winding up the mountain on the cliff-edge path. At 1.7 miles is a horseshoe right bend. Cross under the power lines to a wide, flat plateau on a ridge. To the left is a side path, which heads a short distance west to the summit of the 3,426-foot peak.

After the overlook, continue on the main Silverado Trail, heading uphill on the cliff-side path along the canyon's northwest wall. Cross the head of the canyon, with a view down Silverado Canyon to the trailhead and across the Orange County basin. Loop to the left as the grade levels out, and follow the top-of-the-world path north. Descend a short distance to the Main Divide Road on a U-shaped bend. Take the dirt road to the right 0.2 miles to a Y-fork. Veer to the right on the side road up to Bedford Peak. After savoring the views, return along the same route. ■

35. Harding Road to Santiago Canyon Viewpoint

MODJESKA CANYON

Hiking distance: 3.2 miles round trip
Hiking time: 1.5 hours
Configuration: out-and-back
Elevation gain: 500 feet
Difficulty: easy to moderate
Exposure: exposed mountain slope
Dogs: allowed
Maps: U.S.G.S. Santiago Peak · Cleveland National Forest map

Harding Road (also called Harding Truck Trail) is a 9.5-mile vehicle-restricted road that begins in Modjeska Canyon and climbs to the Main Divide Road. Modjeska Canyon, an extension of Santiago Canyon, is located on the edge of the 400-square-mile Cleveland National Forest on the western slope of the Santa Ana Mountains. The canyon is named for Madame Modjeska, a Shakespearean actress who arrived in America from Poland in 1876. She made her home in the lush, wooded canyon from 1888 through 1906.

Harding Road begins by the Tucker Wildlife Sanctuary, a 12-acre research and interpretive center with weaving paths, ponds, and bridges alongside Santiago Creek. This hike follows the first 1.6 miles of the road, from Modjeska Canyon Road to an overlook of Santiago Canyon. For a more strenuous climb, the next hike continues from the overlook to the Harding Canyon Overlook (1.5 miles farther up the trail) and Laurel Spring (3.4 miles farther up the trail).

To the trailhead

29322 MODJESKA CANYON RD · SILVERADO   33.710468, -117.619083

From the 55 (Costa Mesa) Freeway in Orange, take the Chapman Avenue exit. Drive 13.6 miles east to Modjeska Canyon Road and turn left. The turnoff is located 2.8 miles past Silverado Canyon Road. (Chapman Avenue becomes Santiago Canyon Road en route.) Continue 0.9 miles to a junction with the Modjeska

Grade Road. Bear left and stay on Modjeska Canyon Road one mile to the Tucker Wildlife Sanctuary. Park in the spaces on the right.

From the I-5 (San Diego) Freeway in Lake Forest, take the El Toro Road exit. Drive 7.4 miles northeast to the Y-fork of Santiago Canyon Road (S18) and Live Oak Canyon Road (S19), known as Cook's Corner. Bear left, take Santiago Canyon Road 3 miles to Modjeska Canyon Road, and turn right. Continue 0.9 miles to a junction with the Modjeska Grade Road. Bear left and stay on Modjeska Canyon Road one mile to the Tucker Wildlife Sanctuary. Parking spaces are on the right.

The hike

Cross the paved road to the gated Harding Road. Head up the north wall of Santiago Canyon on the dirt road by a towering sedimentary rock formation on the left. Stay on the wide dirt road, passing a paved road on the right that leads to a water tank. Zigzag past the base of the outcropping to a side road on the left at 0.4 miles. Detour left 100 yards to an overlook of lower Harding Canyon. (The road descends to the canyon floor by the Modjeska Reservoir.)

Continue up Harding Road to a clearing on a point overlooking tree-filled Harding Canyon at 0.7 miles. From the clearing, the path twists and bends along the mountain contours, offering alternating views of Harding Canyon and Santiago Canyon. Descend around a deep rock gorge, and continue winding up the mountain to a horseshoe left bend at 1.6 miles. On the 1,908-foot bend is the Santiago Canyon Viewpoint by a grouping of five wooden poles that are known locally as the "goat shed." This is the turn-around point.

Hike 36 continues up Harding Road to the Harding Canyon Overlook and Laurel Spring. The overlook is 1.5 miles farther, gaining another 720 feet. The spring is 3.4 miles farther, gaining another 1,550 feet. ▪

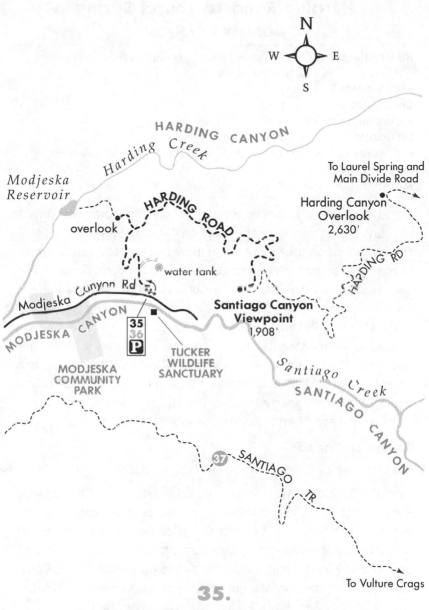

N
W · E
S

HARDING CANYON

Harding Creek

Modjeska Reservoir

To Laurel Spring and
Main Divide Road

Harding Canyon
Overlook
2,630'

overlook

HARDING ROAD

HARDING RD

water tank

Modjeska Canyon Rd

Santiago Canyon
Viewpoint
1,908'

MODJESKA CANYON

35
36
P

TUCKER
WILDLIFE
SANCTUARY

Santiago Creek

MODJESKA
COMMUNITY
PARK

SANTIAGO CANYON

37 SANTIAGO TR

To Vulture Crags

35.
Harding Road to
Santiago Canyon Viewpoint
MODJESKA CANYON

36. Harding Road to Laurel Spring
MODJESKA CANYON

Hiking distance: 6.2 miles round trip to Harding Canyon Overlook
10 miles round trip to Laurel Spring
Hiking time: 3—5 hours
Configuration: out-and-back
Elevation gain: 1,200 feet—2,300 feet
Difficulty: very strenuous
Exposure: exposed mountain slope with shady grove at Laurel Spring
Dogs: allowed
Maps: U.S.G.S. Santiago Peak · Cleveland National Forest map

This strenuous hike heads up Harding Road from Modjeska Canyon to Laurel Spring on the western slope of the Santa Ana Mountains. The trail winds up the mountain on the vehicle-restricted fire road to the ridge separating Harding Canyon and Santiago Canyon. The hike includes an optional turn-around point at Harding Canyon Overlook, which also offers great views of the rolling landscape.

At 3.1 miles, the trail reaches the 2,630-foot Harding Canyon Overlook, with vistas into both canyons. The views span to majestic Red Rock Canyon in the Whiting Ranch Wilderness, Irvine Lake, and Modjeska Peak. At five miles, the road reaches Laurel Spring, a thriving, shady oasis with giant bay laurel, toyon, and ferns amid a sea of arid chaparral and sage scrub.

To the trailhead

29322 MODJESKA CANYON RD · SILVERADO   33.710468, -117.619083

From the 55 (Costa Mesa) Freeway in Orange, take the Chapman Avenue exit. Drive 13.6 miles east to Modjeska Canyon Road and turn left. The turnoff is located 2.8 miles past Silverado Canyon Road. (Chapman Avenue becomes Santiago Canyon Road en route.) Continue 0.9 miles to a junction with the Modjeska Grade Road. Bear left and stay on Modjeska Canyon Road one mile to the Tucker Wildlife Sanctuary. Park in the spaces on the right.

From the I-5 (San Diego) Freeway in Lake Forest, take the El Toro Road exit. Drive 7.4 miles northeast to the Y-fork of Santiago Canyon Road (S18) and Live Oak Canyon Road (S19), known as

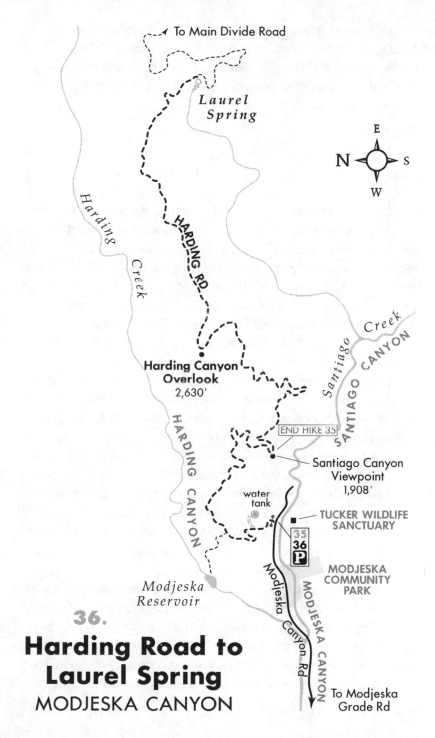

To Main Divide Road

Laurel Spring

E
N ✦ S
W

Harding Creek

HARDING RD.

Harding Canyon
Overlook
2,630'

Santiago Creek
SANTIAGO CANYON

HARDING CANYON

END HIKE 35

Santiago Canyon
Viewpoint
1,908'

water
tank

TUCKER WILDLIFE
SANCTUARY

35
36
P

MODJESKA
COMMUNITY
PARK

*Modjeska
Reservoir*

Modjeska Canyon Rd

MODJESKA CANYON

To Modjeska
Grade Rd

36.
Harding Road to
Laurel Spring
MODJESKA CANYON

Cook's Corner. Bear left, take Santiago Canyon Road 3 miles to Modjeska Canyon Road, and turn right. Continue 0.9 miles to a junction with the Modjeska Grade Road. Bear left and stay on Modjeska Canyon Road one mile to the Tucker Wildlife Sanctuary. Parking spaces are on the right.

The hike

Cross the paved road to the gated Harding Road. Head up the north wall of Santiago Canyon on the dirt road by a towering sedimentary rock formation on the left. Stay on the wide dirt road, passing a paved road on the right that leads to a water tank. Zigzag past the base of the outcropping to a side road on the left at 0.4 miles. Detour left 100 yards to an overlook of lower Harding Canyon. (The road descends to the canyon floor by the Modjeska Reservoir.) Continue up Harding Road to a clearing on a point overlooking tree-filled Harding Canyon at 0.7 miles. From the clearing, the path twists and bends along the mountain contours, offering alternating views of Harding Canyon and Santiago Canyon. Descend around a deep rock gorge, and continue winding up the mountain to a horseshoe left bend at 1.6 miles. On the 1,908-foot bend is the Santiago Canyon Viewpoint by a grouping of five wooden poles that are known locally as the "goat shed."

From the Santiago Canyon Viewpoint, steadily continue up Harding Road along the contours of the mountain. The southwest views span over the San Joaquin Hills and across the ocean to Palos Verdes while the north views reach to the San Gabriel Mountains. At just over 3 miles, curve right, looping around the 2,630-foot Harding Canyon Overlook, with far-reaching vistas from atop the south rim of Harding Canyon. This is the turnaround point for a 6.2-mile round-trip hike.

To continue up to Laurel Spring, follow the dramatic north-facing wall that lies 650 feet above the rugged canyon floor. At just under 5 miles, curve right around the head of a draw. A signed path veers off from the right side of the road, dropping down about 30 yards to the spring and a water trough at 3,456 feet. After enjoying the shady grove, return along the same route. ■

37. Santiago Trail to Vulture Crags
MODJESKA GRADE—SANTIAGO CANYON

Hiking distance: 6.6 miles round trip
Hiking time: 3 hours
Configuration: out-and-back
Elevation gain: 600 feet
Difficulty: moderate
Exposure: mostly exposed with pockets of trees
Dogs: allowed
Maps: U.S.G.S. El Toro and Santiago Peak
　　　Cleveland National Forest map

The Santiago Trail is an eight-mile fire road that parallels Santiago Canyon on the western slope of the Santa Ana Mountains. The ridgeline road connects the Modjeska Grade Road to the upper reaches of Santiago Canyon at Old Camp, a flat, grassy area in a maple and oak woodland with a seasonal creek. This hike follows the first three miles of the dirt road, straddling the south ridge of Santiago Canyon to picturesque Vulture Crags. The eroding conglomerate rock cliffs were once a nesting site for the endangered California condors.

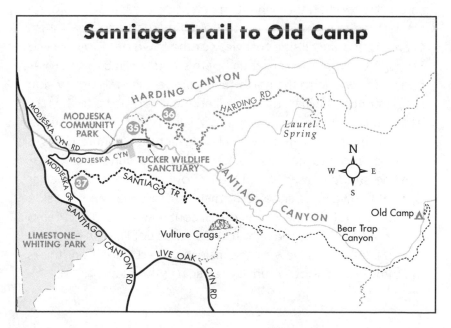

Santiago Trail to Old Camp

To the trailhead

From the 55 (Costa Mesa) Freeway in Orange, take the Chapman Avenue exit. Drive 15.3 miles east to Modjeska Grade Road and turn left. The turnoff is located 4.5 miles past Silverado Canyon Road. (Chapman Avenue becomes Santiago Canyon Road en route.) The trailhead is on the right at 0.5 miles on the crest of the grade. Parking is not allowed by the trailhead. Park on the shoulder of the Modjeska Grade Road 0.2—0.3 miles up the grade.

From the I-5 (San Diego) Freeway in Lake Forest, take the El Toro Road exit. Drive 7.4 miles northeast to the Y-fork of Santiago Canyon Road (S18) and Live Oak Canyon Road (S19), known as Cook's Corner. Bear left, take Santiago Canyon Road 1.2 miles to Modjeska Grade Road, and turn right. The trailhead is on the right at 0.5 miles on the crest of the grade. Parking is not allowed by the trailhead. Park on the shoulder of the Modjeska Grade Road 0.2—0.3 miles up the grade.

The hike

Follow the Modjeska Grade Road uphill a quarter mile to the gated dirt road on the right at the crest of the hill. Walk around the left side of the gate on the old fire road and head east. Curve around the hillside to a view of the town of Modjeska and Santiago Canyon. The serpentine path steadily climbs and crosses a narrow ridge to the north-facing slope. Several narrow side paths veer off the main trail and climb the steep slope to the left. At 2.5 miles, the trail is completely surrounded by mountains. Traverse the south canyon wall and descend to Vulture Crags, a multi-colored sedimentary rock wall. Loop around the formation and straddle a saddle on the narrow ridge to a spectacular view of the weather-chiseled formation. Cross the head of a side canyon to a Y-fork. The Santiago Trail continues east to Old Camp on the left fork. Take the right fork 50 yards uphill to an overlook atop a knoll with a view of the majestic tilted formation. This is the turn-around spot. Return by retracing your steps. ■

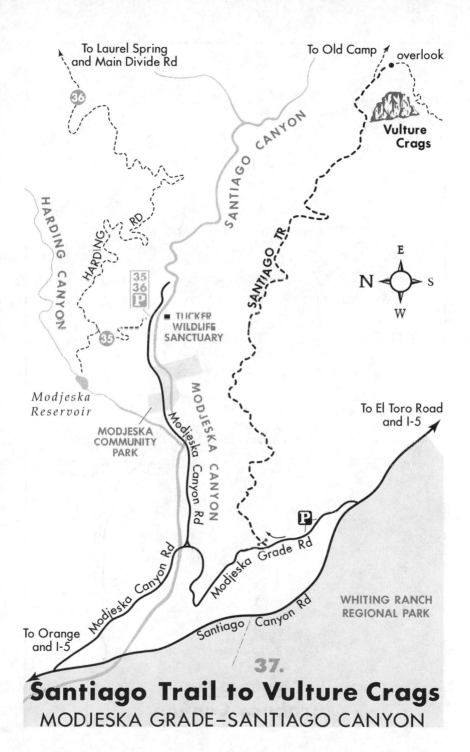

To Laurel Spring and Main Divide Rd

36

To Old Camp / overlook

Vulture Crags

SANTIAGO CANYON

HARDING CANYON

HARDING RD.

35 36 P

TUCKER WILDLIFE SANCTUARY

35

SANTIAGO TR.

Modjeska Reservoir

MODJESKA COMMUNITY PARK

MODJESKA CANYON

Modjeska Canyon Rd

E
N ⊕ S
W

To El Toro Road and I-5

P

Modjeska Grade Rd

WHITING RANCH REGIONAL PARK

Modjeska Canyon Rd

To Orange and I-5

Santiago Canyon Rd

37.

Santiago Trail to Vulture Crags
MODJESKA GRADE–SANTIAGO CANYON

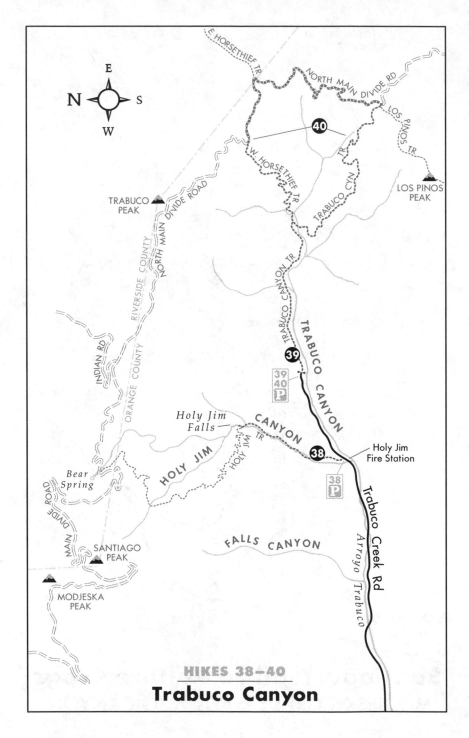

E
N · S
W

E. HORSETHIEF TR

NORTH MAIN DIVIDE RD

40

W. HORSETHIEF TR

LOS PINOS TR

TRABUCO PEAK

LOS PINOS PEAK

TRABUCO CYN. TR

RIVERSIDE COUNTY

NORTH MAIN DIVIDE ROAD

INDIAN RD

ORANGE COUNTY

TRABUCO CANYON TR

TRABUCO CANYON

39

39 40 P

Holy Jim Falls

CANYON TR

HOLY JIM

HOLY JIM

Holy Jim Fire Station

38

38 P

Bear Spring

DIVIDE ROAD

MAIN

SANTIAGO PEAK

FALLS CANYON

Trabuco Creek Rd

Arroyo Trabuco

MODJESKA PEAK

HIKES 38–40
Trabuco Canyon

38. Holy Jim Falls

HOLY JIM CANYON

Hiking distance: 2.6 miles round trip
Hiking time: 1.5 hours
Configuration: out-and-back
Elevation gain: 650 feet
Difficulty: easy to moderate
Exposure: shaded canyon
Dogs: allowed
Maps: U.S.G.S. Santiago Peak · Cleveland National Forest map

Holy Jim Canyon was named for a foul-mouthed beekeeper and shepherd named "Cussin'" Jim Smith who lived in the canyon during the 1890s. The canyon sits on the southeast flank of 5,687 foot Santiago Peak (Old Saddleback), the highest peak in the Santa Ana Mountains and Orange County. The eight-mile Holy Jim Trail climbs the canyon from Trabuco Canyon up to the peak. En route, the trail leads to Holy Jim Falls in a lush, narrow box canyon, then continues up to Bear Spring at the Main Divide Road. The popular trail parallels Holy Jim Creek in the lower portion of the picturesque, tree-filled drainage. The trail crosses the creek numerous times. This hike ends on a short spur by a pool at the

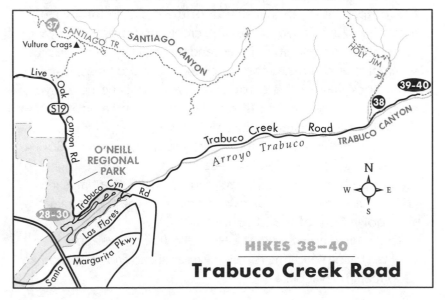

HIKES 38—40

Trabuco Creek Road

base of the 18-foot Holy Jim Falls, which cascades out of a notch in a fern-covered rock wall.

Trabuco Creek Road—the road to the trailhead—is rough but passable for most vehicles.

To the trailhead

TRABUCO CREEK ROAD · TRABUCO CANYON   33.676928, –117.517273

From the I-5 (San Diego) Freeway in Lake Forest, take the El Toro Road exit. Drive 7.4 miles northeast to the Y-fork of Santiago Canyon Road (S18) and Live Oak Canyon Road (S19), known as Cook's Corner. Bear right and take Live Oak Canyon Road 4.3 miles to the bridge over Trabuco Wash (located one mile past O' Neill Regional Park). Cross the bridge and immediately turn left onto an unsigned dirt road—Trabuco Creek Road. Continue 4.6 miles up the bumpy road to the trailhead parking area on the left, just after the Holy Jim Volunteer Fire Station.

The hike

Head north under a few oak trees on the dirt road. Follow the east edge of Holy Jim Creek, passing a series of cabins. Cross the creek two times to the Forest Service trailhead gate at a half mile by the last house. Rock-hop over the creek, and take the footpath along the west side of the drainage through lush, narrow Holy Jim Canyon. Cross the creek and traverse the west-facing canyon wall, steadily ascending through oaks, maples, sycamores, and ferns. Cross the creek two more times, just below a rock wall with a 6-foot waterfall. Continue up canyon, crossing the creek for the fifth and sixth times by a pool on the right. There is a posted junction 20 yards ahead. The Holy Jim Trail stays left and climbs the west canyon wall to Bear Spring and antenna-covered Santiago Peak. For this hike, bear right on the footpath and cross the creek three consecutive times into a lush, circular grotto in a narrow box canyon. The trail terminates at a pool in front of the 18-foot cataract.

To continue hiking, take the Holy Jim Trail to Bear Spring and the Main Divide Road. The road is 3.2 miles ahead and gains another 1,300 feet in elevation. ∎

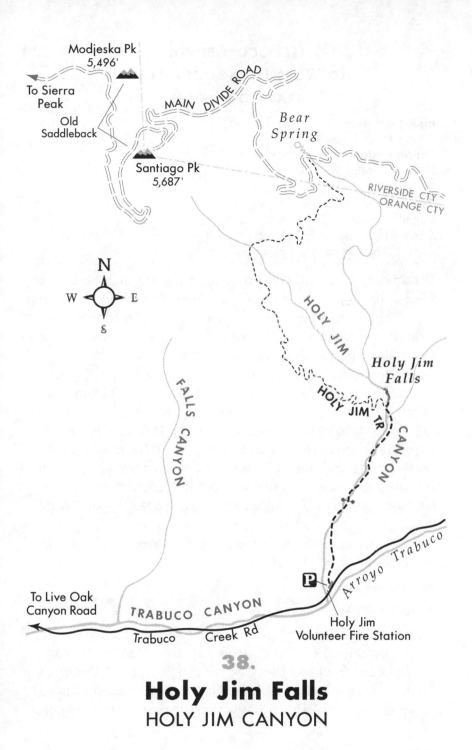

Modjeska Pk
5,496'

To Sierra
Peak

Old
Saddleback

MAIN DIVIDE ROAD

Bear
Spring

Santiago Pk
5,687'

RIVERSIDE CTY
ORANGE CTY

N
W ✦ E
S

HOLY JIM

Holy Jim
Falls

FALLS CANYON

HOLY JIM TR

CANYON

Arroyo Trabuco

P

To Live Oak
Canyon Road

TRABUCO CANYON

Trabuco   Creek Rd

Holy Jim
Volunteer Fire Station

38.

Holy Jim Falls
HOLY JIM CANYON

39. Trabuco Canyon to West Horsethief Trail

TRABUCO CANYON

Hiking distance: 3.6 miles round trip
Hiking time: 2 hours
Configuration: out-and-back
Elevation gain: 900 feet
Difficulty: moderate
Exposure: shady streamside canyon
Dogs: allowed
Maps: U.S.G.S. Santiago Peak and Alberhill
       Cleveland National Forest map

Stream-fed Trabuco Canyon runs from the North Main Divide Road in the upper mountains by Los Pinos Peak to the foothills near O'Neill Regional Park. The Trabuco Canyon Trail follows the main canyon for four miles between two peaks in the Santa Ana Mountains—Trabuco Peak and Los Pinos Peak. The creekside trail travels through a varied forest of spruce, Coulter pine, maple, coastal live oaks, sycamores, alders, madrone, and California bay laurel.

This hike follows the first 1.8 miles of the Trabuco Canyon Trail to the junction with the West Horsethief Trail. The primitive path parallels the north side of Trabuco Creek along the sunny, south canyon slope. Hike 40 continues from this junction for a longer (and more strenuous) 10-mile loop up to the North Main Divide Road.

Trabuco Creek Road—the road to the trailhead—is rough but passable for most vehicles.

To the trailhead

TRABUCO CREEK ROAD · TRABUCO CANYON   33.682408, -117.504388

From the I-5 (San Diego) Freeway in Lake Forest, take the El Toro Road exit. Drive 7.4 miles northeast to the Y-fork of Santiago Canyon Road (S18) and Live Oak Canyon Road (S19), known as Cook's Corner. Bear right and take Live Oak Canyon Road 4.3 miles to the bridge over Trabuco Wash (one mile past O' Neill Regional

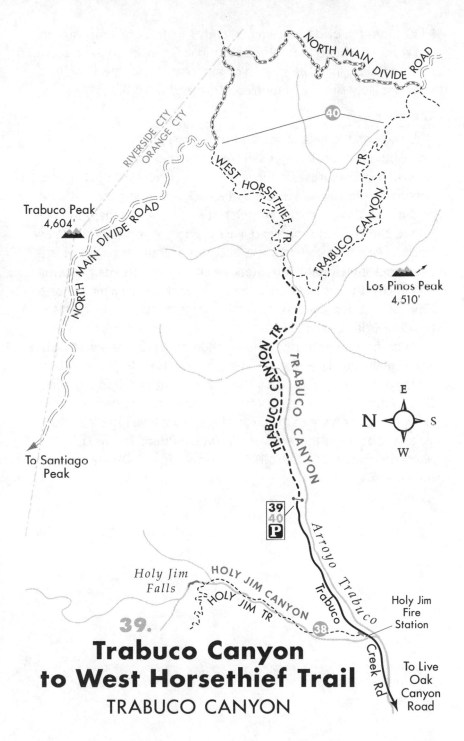

NORTH MAIN DIVIDE ROAD

40

RIVERSIDE CTY
ORANGE CTY

WEST HORSETHIEF TR

TRABUCO CANYON TR

NORTH MAIN DIVIDE ROAD

Trabuco Peak
4,604'

Los Pinos Peak
4,510'

TRABUCO CANYON TR

TRABUCO CANYON

To Santiago
Peak

E

N   S

W

39
40
P

Arroyo Trabuco

Holy Jim
Falls

HOLY JIM CANYON

HOLY JIM TR

Trabuco

38

Holy Jim
Fire
Station

39.

Creek Rd

To Live
Oak
Canyon
Road

Trabuco Canyon
to West Horsethief Trail
TRABUCO CANYON

Park). Cross the bridge and immediately turn left onto an unsigned dirt road—Trabuco Creek Road. Continue 5.6 miles up the bumpy road to the trailhead at the end of the road. It is located one mile after the Holy Jim Fire Station and trailhead (Hike 38).

The hike

Walk through the gate at the end of the road. Head up the north side of the canyon, and parallel Trabuco Creek amidst the mature oaks and sycamores. Continue east on a gentle uphill grade, passing an old rusted vehicle and a rock wall lining the left side of the trail. Cross a rocky stretch between two washes, and return to the shaded woodland. Pass a side canyon on the left as Trabuco Peak comes into view. Just beyond the talus slope is a deep rock cave on the left. Steadily climb the north canyon wall high above the creek to an unsigned T-junction at 1.8 miles. For a view of Trabuco Canyon, continue 30 yards to the right. This is the turn-around point.

To extend the hike from the junction, both routes lead to the North Main Divide Road. The West Horsethief Trail heads left, zigzagging up the canyon to the divide south of Trabuco Peak. The Trabuco Canyon Trail continues to the right, weaving up the canyon to the divide at the base of Los Pinos Peak. The two trails make a loop with the North Main Divide Road. The next hike— Hike 40—continues on this 6.4-mile loop for a 10-mile, round-trip hike. ▪

40. Trabuco Canyon—
West Horsethief Loop
to North Main Divide Road
TRABUCO CANYON

Hiking distance: 10 miles round trip
Hiking time: 5 hours
Configuration: lollipop loop
Elevation gain: 2,300 feet
Difficulty: very strenuous
Exposure: a mix of shaded canyon and exposed mountain slopes
Dogs: allowed
Maps: U.S.G.S. Santiago Peak and Alberhill
Cleveland National Forest map

The 40-mile-long Main Divide Road traverses the crest of the Santa Ana Mountains, from Sierra Peak in the north to the Ortega Highway in the south. From the dirt road are gorgeous vistas of the Santa Ana range, Lake Elsinore, Temecula Valley, and Orange County. This remote loop hike climbs up to the North Main Divide Road between Trabuco Peak and Los Pinos Peak. The hike steadily switchbacks out of the canyon up to the road via the West Horsethief Trail, an early trade route used by the Gabrieleno Indians that connects the inland valleys to the coast. The trail was also used by horse thieves during the Spanish period. After enjoying the far-reaching views from the divide road, the hike returns back into the canyon on the Trabuco Canyon Trail.

Trabuco Creek Road—the road to the trailhead—is rough but passable for most vehicles.

To the trailhead

TRABUCO CREEK ROAD · TRABUCO CANYON   33.682408, -117.504388

From the I-5 (San Diego) Freeway in Lake Forest, take the El Toro Road exit. Drive 7.4 miles northeast to the Y-fork of Santiago Canyon Road (S18) and Live Oak Canyon Road (S19), known as Cook's Corner. Bear right and take Live Oak Canyon Road 4.3 miles to the bridge over Trabuco Wash (one mile past O' Neill Regional Park). Cross the bridge and immediately turn left onto an unsigned dirt road—Trabuco Creek Road. Continue 5.6 miles up the bumpy road to the trailhead at the end of the road. It is located one mile after the Holy Jim Trailhead (Hike 38).

The hike

Walk through the gate at the end of the road. Head up the north side of the canyon, and parallel Trabuco Creek amidst the mature oaks and sycamores. Continue east on a gentle uphill grade, passing an old rusted vehicle and a rock wall lining the left side of the trail. Cross a rocky stretch between two washes, and return to the shaded woodland. Pass a side canyon on the left as Trabuco Peak comes into view. Just beyond the talus slope is a deep rock cave on the left. Climb the north canyon wall high above the creek to an unsigned T-junction at 1.8 miles.

Begin the loop to the left on the West Horsethief Trail. Switchback up the canyon, steadily climbing through sage scrub beneath Trabuco Peak to the north. The zigzagging path ascends the south-facing mountain slope, gaining 1,300 feet in 1.5 miles. En route, the landscape changes from a tall conifer and oak forest to exposed scrub brush and chaparral. Near the top, follow the ridge through Coulter pines, reaching the North Main Divide Road at 3.3 miles. To the left, the road leads 1.3 miles north to 4,604-foot Trabuco Peak.

Take the right fork and weave along the ridge past the East Horsethief Trail on the left. Continue on the undulating road while overlooking Trabuco Canyon. Arrive at Los Pinos (Munhall) Saddle at the base of Los Pinos Peak at just under six miles. The North Main Divide Road continues over the saddle to the left down to the Falcon Campground.

Leave the road and take the posted Trabuco Canyon Trail to the right, passing the Los Pinos Trail (Hike 54) on the left. Walk down canyon through a tunnel of live oak and Douglas fir, staying left at a junction one mile down. Continue downhill through bay laurel and arid sage scrub, completing the loop. Return 1.8 miles to the left. ∎

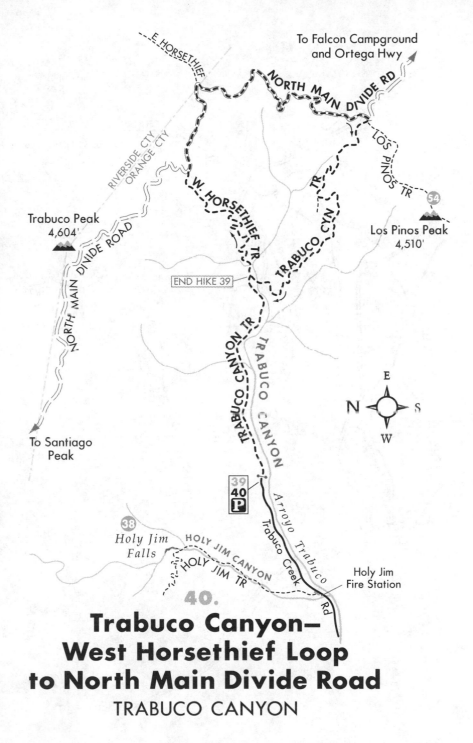

To Falcon Campground
and Ortega Hwy

E. HORSETHIEF

NORTH MAIN DIVIDE RD

LOS PINOS TR

RIVERSIDE CTY
ORANGE CTY

W. HORSETHIEF TR

TRABUCO CYN TR

54

Trabuco Peak
4,604'

Los Pinos Peak
4,510'

NORTH MAIN DIVIDE ROAD

END HIKE 39

TRABUCO CANYON TR

TRABUCO CANYON

E

N · S

W

To Santiago
Peak

39
40
P

Arroyo Trabuco

38

Holy Jim
Falls

HOLY JIM CANYON

Trabuco Creek

Holy Jim
Fire Station

HOLY JIM TR

Trabuco Rd

40.
Trabuco Canyon–
West Horsethief Loop
to North Main Divide Road
TRABUCO CANYON

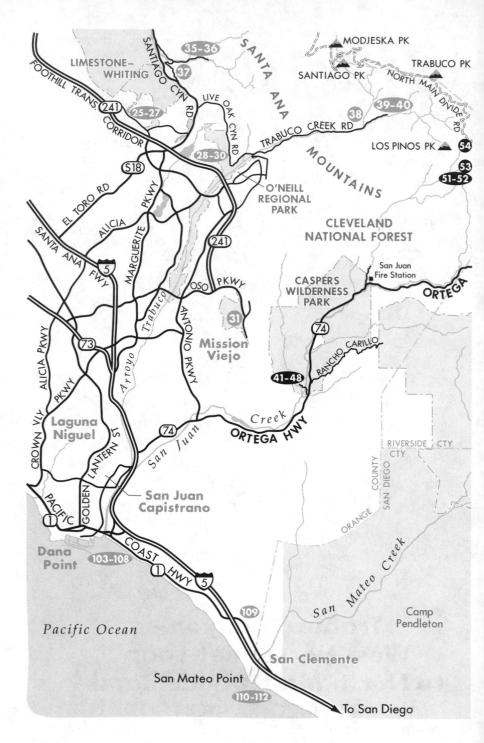

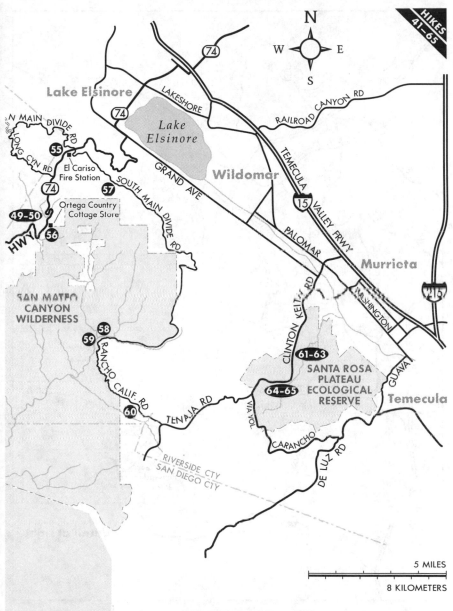

HIKES 41–65
Ortega Highway
Lower Santa Ana Mountains

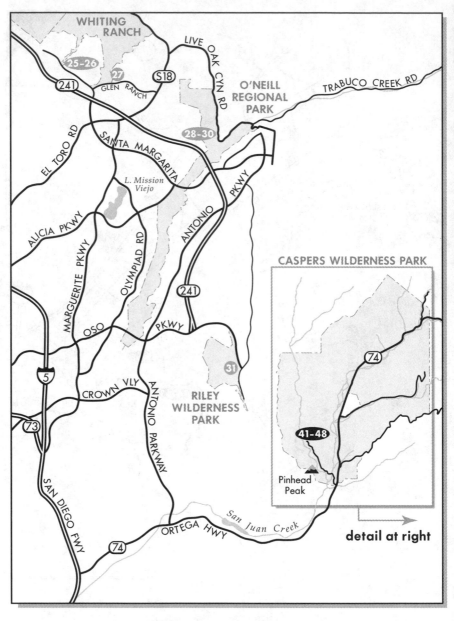

WHITING RANCH

25-26

27

241

GLEN RANCH

S18

LIVE OAK CYN RD

O'NEILL REGIONAL PARK

TRABUCO CREEK RD

28-30

EL TORO RD

SANTA MARGARITA

L. Mission Viejo

ANTONIO

PKWY

ALICIA PKWY

MARGUERITE PKWY

OLYMPIAD RD

OSO

PKWY

241

5

73

CROWN VLY

ANTONIO PARKWAY

RILEY WILDERNESS PARK

31

SAN DIEGO FWY

ORTEGA HWY

San Juan Creek

74

CASPERS WILDERNESS PARK

74

41-48

Pinhead Peak

detail at right

HIKES 41–48

Ronald W. Caspers Wilderness Park

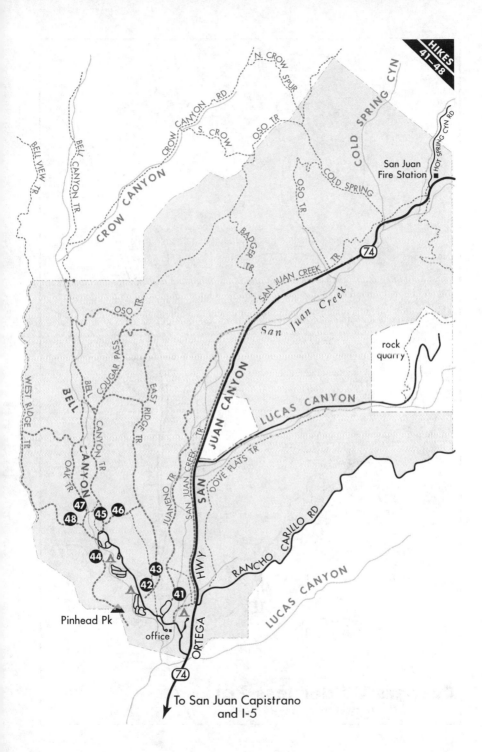

N. CROW SPUR

COLD SPRING CYN

HOT SPRING CYN RD

San Juan
Fire Station

CROW CANYON RD

S. CROW

OSO TR

CROW CANYON

BELL VIEW TR

BELL CANYON TR

OSO TR

COLD SPRING

OSO TR

BADGER TR

74

SAN JUAN CREEK TR

San Juan Creek

rock
quarry

LUCAS CANYON

OSO TR

COUGAR PASS

BELL CANYON TR

EAST RIDGE TR

WEST RIDGE TR

BELL CANYON

OAK TR

San Juan Creek

SAN JUAN CANYON

JUANENO TR

SAN JUAN CREEK TR

DOVE FLATS TR

RANCHO CARILLO RD

47
48
45 46

44

43

42

41

Pinhead Pk

office

HWY

ORTEGA

LUCAS CANYON

74

To San Juan Capistrano
and I-5

149

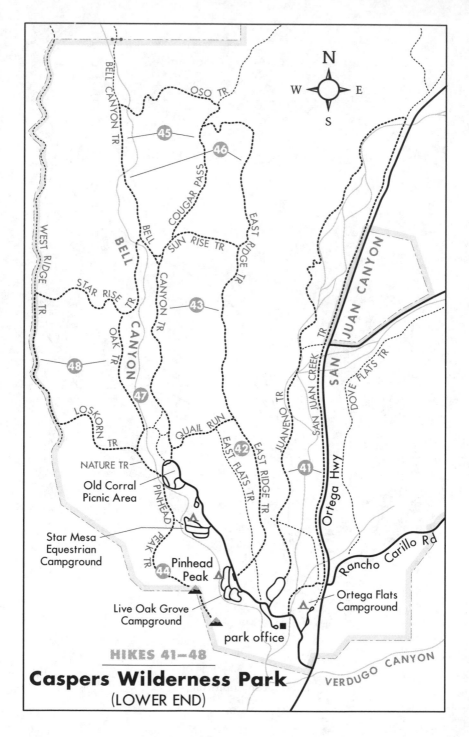

N
W E
S

BELL CANYON TR

OSO TR

45

46

COUGAR PASS

WEST RIDGE TR

BELL

CANYON

SUN RISE TR

EAST RIDGE TR

STAR RISE TR

BELL CANYON TR

43

OAK TR

48

47

LOSKORN TR

QUAIL RUN

EAST FLATS TR

42

EAST RIDGE TR

JUANENO TR

SAN JUAN CREEK TR

SAN JUAN CANYON

DOVE FLATS TR

41

Ortega Hwy

NATURE TR

Old Corral
Picnic Area

PINHEAD

Star Mesa
Equestrian
Campground

PEAK TR

44

Pinhead
Peak

Live Oak Grove
Campground

park office

Rancho Carillo Rd

Ortega Flats
Campground

HIKES 41–48

Caspers Wilderness Park
(LOWER END)

VERDUGO CANYON

41. Juaneno Trail—San Juan Creek Loop

RONALD W. CASPERS WILDERNESS PARK

Hiking distance: 6.5-mile loop (with optional cut-across path)
Hiking time: 3 hours
Configuration: loop
Elevation gain: 150 feet
Difficulty: moderate
Exposure: mostly exposed foothills with pockets of shade
Dogs: not allowed
Maps: U.S.G.S. Canada Gobernadora
Ronald W. Caspers Wilderness Park map

Caspers Wilderness Park is among Orange County's premier un-developed parklands. The land was once a working ranch. Old ranch roads, fire roads, footpaths, and cow paths now form an extensive trail system through 8,000 acres of primitive terrain. More than 30 miles of equestrian, biking, and hiking trails criss-cross the natural landscape, connecting open ridgetops with wildflower meadows and cool, moss-covered creek bottoms.

The Juaneno Trail is named for the Juaneno Indians, who flour-ished in the area until the 1770s (after which Spain took con-trol of the land). The footpath meanders along the west edge of San Juan Canyon and traverses the lower edge of 900-foot sedimentary cliffs. The return path on the San Juan Creek Trail parallels the Ortega Highway through the creek basin. The park has very diverse eco-systems, and this hike features the varied terrain. The habitats range from arid, sandy creek bottoms with cholla and prickly pear cactus to lush, grassy meadows and oak woodlands. A cut-across path, about midway through the loop, offers an optional shorter loop.

Access to the park is via the Ortega Highway, a scenic highway that runs from San Juan Capistrano to I-15. The highway parallels San Juan Creek past Caspers Wilderness Park and into the Santa Ana Mountains, passing through the Cleveland National Forest. The road emerges on the other side of the range at Lake Elsinore. Drive carefully, as the road has a reputation of being one of the most dangerous in the state.

To the trailhead

33401 Ortega Hwy · San Juan Capistrano   33.538053, -117.553775

From the I-5 (San Diego) Freeway in San Juan Capistrano, take the Ortega (74) Highway exit. Drive 7.7 miles east to the posted park entrance and turn left. From the park entrance station, continue 0.4 miles to the San Juan Meadows Day Use Area on the right. Turn right and continue 0.2 miles to the posted trailhead at the far end of the road. An entrance fee is required.

The hike

Take the posted trail north, and head up the slope overlooking San Juan Canyon. Traverse the hillside through oak and sycamore groves, descending to the grassy canyon floor and the unpaved Pump House Road. The right fork leads to the San Juan Creek Trail (the return trail). Continue north along the base of the eroding cliffs, gently rising along the lower slopes and dropping to the canyon floor. Stay on the west side of the drainage above the rocky wash. At a mile, cross the drainage, moving away from the sandstone cliffs, and wind through the sandy canyon bottom. Cross back over the creekbed, returning to the base of the cliffs and into the oak woodland. At 1.4 miles, pass the Mesa Trail cut-across (for the optional shorter loop), and continue under the oak canopy. Follow the contours of the hills, perched on the cliffs. Loop around a side canyon beneath the rock wall, and descend to the canyon floor. Steadily alternate between meadows and woodlands to a wooden footbridge at three miles. Climb and weave through side ravines, returning to the canyon bottom. Curve slowly to the right as the valley narrows and the mountains bend east towards the Ortega Highway. The trail ends at a T-junction on the north side of the highway bridge over San Juan Creek.

Bear right on the San Juan Creek Trail and cross the creek bottom. Head south, parallel to the highway. The trail stays close to the highway but is frequently buffered by oak groves and low rolling hills, dropping below the highway. It is an easy and direct return route to Ortega Flats, adjacent to the trailhead and park road at San Juan Meadow. ▦

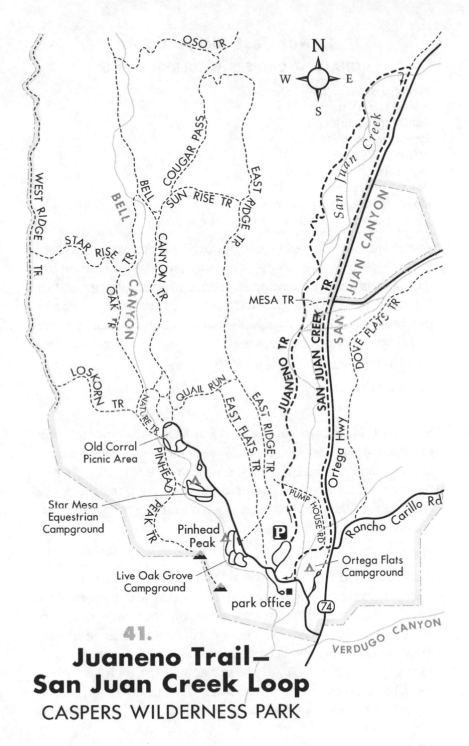

41.
Juaneno Trail—
San Juan Creek Loop
CASPERS WILDERNESS PARK

42. Lower East Ridge Loop

RONALD W. CASPERS WILDERNESS PARK

Hiking distance: 1.8-mile loop
Hiking time: 1 hour
Configuration: loop
Elevation gain: 300 feet
Difficulty: easy
Exposure: exposed hillside
Dogs: not allowed
Maps: U.S.G.S. Canada Gobernadora
 Ronald W. Caspers Wilderness Park map

East Ridge runs north and south through Caspers Wilderness Park between Bell Canyon on the west and San Juan Canyon on the east. This is a short, easy, open loop trail on the lower end of East Ridge. The hike follows the 700-foot ridge along a graded dirt road—the East Ridge Trail—through exposed sage scrub and chaparral. The loop returns along the west-facing slope on a footpath through grassland meadows.

To the trailhead

33401 ORTEGA HWY · SAN JUAN CAPISTRANO   33.540459, -117.556693

From the I-5 (San Diego) Freeway in San Juan Capistrano, take the Ortega (74) Highway exit. Drive 7.7 miles east to the posted park entrance and turn left. From the park entrance station, continue 0.6 miles to the parking spaces on the left by a restroom, directly across the road from the posted East Ridge Trailhead. An entrance fee is required.

The hike

Cross the road to the posted trailhead by the coast live oak trees. Climb the hillside 0.2 miles to a junction with the East Flats Trail on the left (the return trail). Begin the loop straight ahead and continue up the hillside. Curve north along the spine of East Ridge, overlooking San Juan Canyon, Bell Canyon, and the surrounding peaks, including Old Saddleback. The path levels out for 0.3 miles, then climbs the shoulder to the upper ridge. Follow the 700-foot ridgeline to a posted junction with the Quail Run

Trail on the left. Leave the ridge and steeply descend 200 yards down the Quail Run Trail to the East Flats Trail. Bear left on the footpath and cross the grassy plateau, an ancient river terrace. At the south end of the flat, gradually slope downward, completing the loop. Return to the left. ■

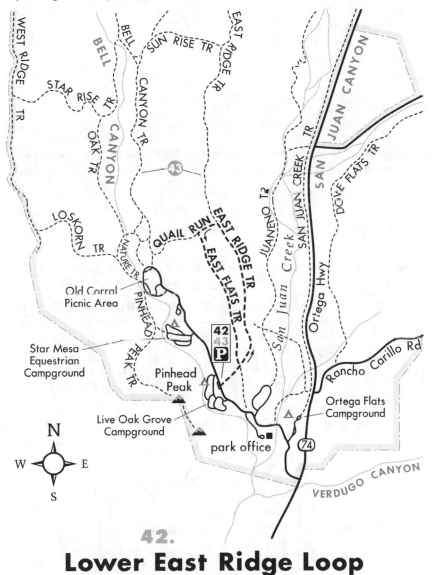

42.
Lower East Ridge Loop
CASPERS WILDERNESS PARK

43. Lower Bell Canyon— East Ridge Loop

RONALD W. CASPERS WILDERNESS PARK

Hiking distance: 4.3-mile loop
Hiking time: 2 hours
Configuration: loop
Elevation gain: 400 feet
Difficulty: moderate
Exposure: exposed hillside with pockets of shade on return
Dogs: not allowed
Maps: U.S.G.S. Canada Gobernadora
Ronald W. Caspers Wilderness Park map

Caspers Wilderness Park is Orange County's largest park. The park's 8,000 acres of protected wilderness lie in the lower foothills of the western side of the Santa Ana Mountains, adjacent to the Cleveland National Forest. The former ranchland became established as a regional park in 1974, expanding to its current size over the next decade.

East Ridge is a long, open ridge that straddles San Juan Canyon to the east and Bell Canyon to the west. East Ridge offers panoramic mountain vistas as well as views into the forested Bell Canyon below. This hike climbs East Ridge on a graded fire road, overlooking the two

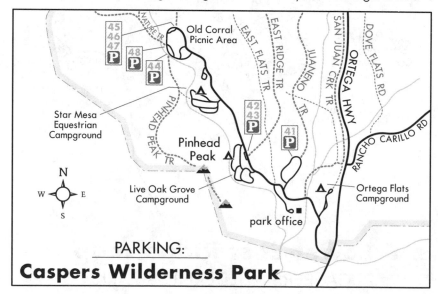

PARKING:

Caspers Wilderness Park

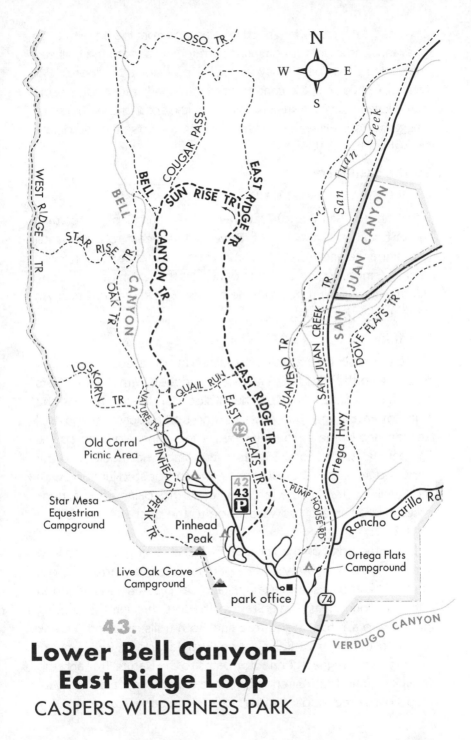

43.

Lower Bell Canyon– East Ridge Loop

CASPERS WILDERNESS PARK

canyons. At the loop's far end, the trail drops from the ridge through grasslands and chaparral communities, returning back to the trailhead under the riparian oak and sycamore canopy along the floor of Bell Canyon. Bell Canyon, the centerpiece of the park, received its name from a legend that its former Native American occupants would strike a large boulder within the canyon, causing the noise to reverberate throughout the canyon.

To the trailhead

33401 ORTEGA HWY · SAN JUAN CAPISTRANO   33.540459, -117.556693

From the I-5 (San Diego) Freeway in San Juan Capistrano, take the Ortega (74) Highway exit. Drive 7.7 miles east to the posted park entrance and turn left. From the park entrance station, continue 0.6 miles to the parking spaces on the left by a restroom, directly across the road from the posted East Ridge Trailhead. An entrance fee is required.

The hike

Cross the road to the posted trailhead by the coastal live oak trees. Climb the hillside 0.2 miles to a junction with the East Flats Trail on the left. Continue up the hillside, curving north along the spine of East Ridge. The views extend up San Juan Canyon, Bell Canyon, and to the surrounding peaks, including Old Saddleback. The path levels out for 0.3 miles, then climbs the shoulder to the upper ridge. Follow the 700-foot ridge to a posted junction with the Quail Run Trail on the left. Stay atop the rolling ridge for another mile on an easy upward slope to the posted Sun Rise Trail on the left.

Leave the ridge on the Sun Rise Trail, and steeply descend 200 yards to an open grassy plateau, an ancient river terrace. Cross the terrace and descend again to a lower plateau and a junction with the Cougar Pass Trail. Stay to the left through the sloping meadow to a Y-fork at the tree line. Both trails drop into an oak forest to the floor of Bell Canyon. Bear left down Bell Canyon, passing two unsigned connector paths to the Nature Trail and the Quail Run Trail. The trail ends one mile down canyon at the park road. Follow the road 0.8 miles back to the parking area. ■

44. Pinhead Peak

RONALD W. CASPERS WILDERNESS PARK

Hiking distance: 1.6 miles round trip
Hiking time: 1 hour
Configuration: out-and-back
Elevation gain: 250 feet
Difficulty: easy
Exposure: mostly exposed hillside
Dogs: not allowed
Maps: U.S.G.S. Canada Gobernadora
Ronald W. Caspers Wilderness Park map

Pinhead Peak is a 662-foot peak on the southwest corner of Caspers Wilderness Park. From the peak are panoramic vistas in every direction, including Bell Canyon, San Juan Canyon, Lucas Canyon, Verdugo Canyon, and the mile-high twin peaks of Modjeska Peak and Santiago Peak (Old Saddleback). This short, scenic hike (less than a mile one way) begins in Bell Canyon and climbs up a small side canyon to the scrub-covered ridge.

To the trailhead

33401 ORTEGA HWY · SAN JUAN CAPISTRANO   33.548390, -117.563002

From the I-5 (San Diego) Freeway in San Juan Capistrano, take the Ortega (74) Highway exit. Drive 7.7 miles east to the posted park entrance and turn left. From the park entrance station, continue 1.4 miles to the end of the park road by the Bell Canyon Trailhead. Turn left and continue 0.2 miles to the parking area on the left. An entrance fee is required.

The hike

Walk 20 yards south on the gravel road to the posted trailhead on the right. Cross the rocky wash and enter the sycamore and oak woodland. Stroll through the grassy meadow toward the prominent peak and a posted junction. The left fork recrosses the wash to the Star Mesa Equestrian Campground. Curve right, staying on the Pinhead Peak Trail. Curve around the base of the rounded mountain in a meadow surrounded by rolling hills. Head up the sloping draw to the back of the small valley. Climb up the draw to a ridge and an overlook of Bell Canyon, San Juan Canyon, and the Santa Ana Mountains. Follow the ridge southeast through sage scrub and prickly pear cactus. Pass a barbed wire fence at the park's southwest boundary, and cross a saddle to Pinhead Peak. The trail continues a few hundred yards southwest along the sloping ridge to another peak. After enjoying the vistas, return along the same route. ■

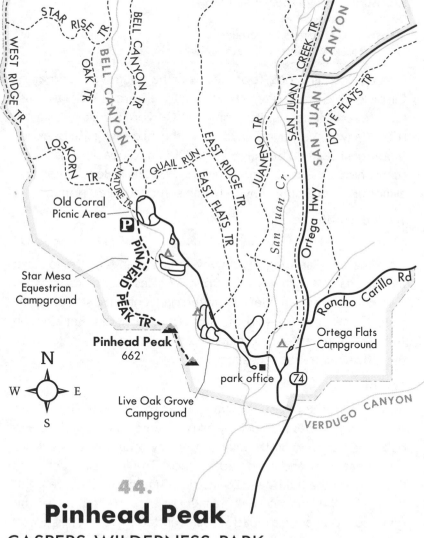

44.
Pinhead Peak
CASPERS WILDERNESS PARK

45. Upper Bell Canyon

RONALD W. CASPERS WILDERNESS PARK

Hiking distance: 4.8-mile loop
Hiking time: 2.5 hours
Configuration: lollipop
Elevation gain: 300 feet
Difficulty: moderate
Exposure: mostly wooded canyon with open plateau
Dogs: not allowed
Maps: U.S.G.S. Canada Gobernadora
Ronald W. Caspers Wilderness Park map

Caspers Wilderness Park is an 8,000-acre undeveloped parkland in the western foothills of the Santa Ana Mountains. The rugged sanctuary has rich and varied habitats, including rolling hills, grasslands, oak and sycamore woodlands, tranquil creeks, and lush riparian canyons and ravines. Over 30 miles of multi-use trails crisscross the terrain, making the area accessible to hikers, bikers, and equestrians.

This hike follows Bell Canyon, the centerpiece of the park. The route stays in the tree-filled canyon for most of hike's length, then makes a loop at the north end along the open East Ridge.

To the trailhead

33401 ORTEGA HWY · SAN JUAN CAPISTRANO   33.548390, -117.563002

From the I-5 (San Diego) Freeway in San Juan Capistrano, take the Ortega (74) Highway exit. Drive 7.7 miles east to the posted park entrance and turn left. From the park entrance station, continue 1.4 miles to the end of the park road by the Bell Canyon Trailhead. Park on the left. An entrance fee is required.

The hike

Take the signed trail north from the end of the park road. Pass the Quail Run trail at 80 yards and two unsigned Nature Trail connector paths on the left. Views extend from the sandstone cliffs on the west canyon wall to the prominent formation of Old Saddleback in the north. Follow the east edge of Bell Canyon to a posted trail split with the Sun Rise Trail on the right at one mile.

Begin the loop to the left, staying in the canyon. Drop down into the oak-filled canyon bottom, passing a junction with the Star Rise Trail. Walk past an old ranch gate, and stroll through an oak and sycamore woodland. Cross a rock wash to the west edge of the canyon to a bench and a junction at 1.9 miles.

Bear right on the Oso Trail, leaving the canyon floor. Ascend the west-facing hillside, cross a sloping plateau, and climb again to the upper plateau, an ancient river terrace. Cross the grassy plateau to a trail split at 2.6 miles at the base of East Ridge by an emergency phone. The Oso Trail continues left (northeast) to Cold Spring Canyon and the Forest Service station at Hot Springs Canyon Road.

Take the right fork on the Cougar Pass Trail, and descend along the west edge of an oak-filled drainage. Climb out of the canyon to a trail fork at 2.9 miles with the East Ridge Trail on the left. Stay on the Cougar Pass Trail to the right. Follow the sinuous path across the rolling plateau, 200 feet below East Ridge. Descend along a smaller ridge to the lower sloping plateau and a junction with the Sun Rise Trail. Bear right, strolling through the meadow to a Y-fork at the tree line. Both forks drop into the oak forest to the floor of Bell Canyon, completing the loop. Return to the left one mile, back down Bell Canyon. ■

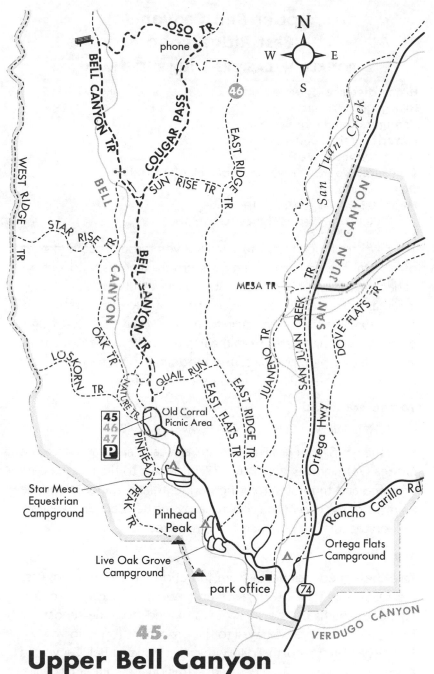

OSO TR
phone

BELL CANYON TR

COUGAR PASS

46

EAST RIDGE TR

N
W   E
S

BELL

SUN RISE TR

WEST RIDGE TR

STAR RISE TR

San Juan Creek

CANYON

OAK TR

BELL CANYON TR

MESA TR

SAN JUAN CANYON

SAN JUAN CREEK TR

DOVE FLATS TR

LOSKORN TR

QUAIL RUN

NATURE TR

EAST FLATS TR

EAST RIDGE TR

JUANENO TR

SAN JUAN CREEK

45
46
47
P

Old Corral
Picnic Area

PINHEAD PEAK TR

Ortega Hwy

Star Mesa
Equestrian
Campground

Pinhead
Peak

Roncho Carillo Rd

Live Oak Grove
Campground

Ortega Flats
Campground

park office

74

VERDUGO CANYON

45.

Upper Bell Canyon
CASPERS WILDERNESS PARK

46. Upper Bell Canyon—
East Ridge Loop

RONALD W. CASPERS WILDERNESS PARK

Hiking distance: 5.5-mile loop
Hiking time: 3 hours
Configuration: loop
Elevation gain: 500 feet
Difficulty: moderate
Exposure: wooded canyon and open plateau on return
Dogs: not allowed
Maps: U.S.G.S. Canada Gobernadora
Ronald W. Caspers Wilderness Park map

This hike strolls up stream-fed Bell Canyon through native groves of coastal live oak, towering western sycamores, and rich riparian woodlands. The area is abundant with wildlife, including mountain lions (rare), bobcats, deer, coyote, fox, rabbits, hawks, and vultures. The route then climbs the canyon wall to East Ridge, offering sweeping vistas from the Pacific Ocean to Santiago Peak in the Santa Ana Mountains. The moderate loop trail offers an excellent cross-section of the park's eco-systems.

To the trailhead

33401 ORTEGA HWY · SAN JUAN CAPISTRANO   33.548390, -117.563002

From the I-5 (San Diego) Freeway in San Juan Capistrano, take the Ortega (74) Highway exit. Drive 7.7 miles east to the posted park entrance and turn left. From the park entrance station, continue 1.4 miles to the end of the park road by the Bell Canyon Trailhead. Park on the left. An entrance fee is required.

The hike

Take the signed trail north from the end of the park road. Pass the Quail Run Trail at 80 yards and two unsigned Nature Trail connector paths on the left. Views extend from the sandstone cliffs on the west canyon wall to the prominent formation of Old Saddleback in the north. Follow the east edge of Bell Canyon to a posted trail split with the Sun Rise Trail on the right at one mile.

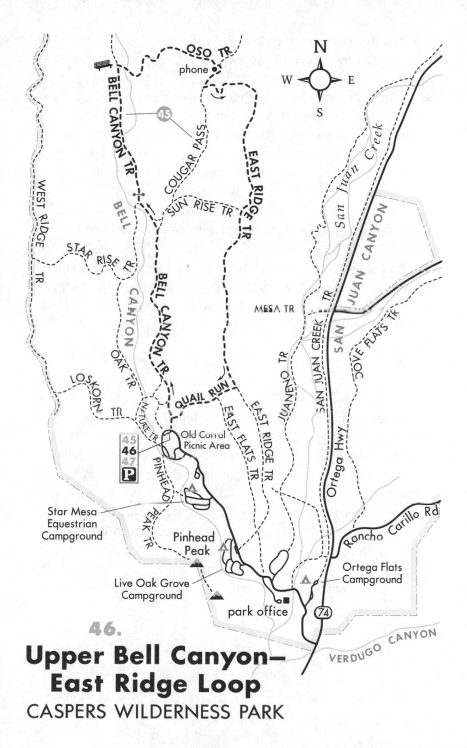

OSO TR

phone

N

W — E

S

BELL CANYON TR

45

COUGAR PASS

EAST RIDGE TR

SUN RISE TR

WEST RIDGE TR

STAR RISE TR

BELL CANYON

San Juan Creek

SAN JUAN CANYON

MESA TR

BELL CANYON TR

JUANENO TR

SAN JUAN CREEK TR

DOVE FLATS TR

OAK TR

LOSKORN TR

QUAIL RUN

EAST FLATS TR

EAST RIDGE TR

SAN

Ortega Hwy

NATURE TR

45
46
47

P

Old Corral
Picnic Area

Star Mesa
Equestrian
Campground

PINHEAD PEAK TR

Rancho Carillo Rd

Pinhead
Peak

Live Oak Grove
Campground

Ortega Flats
Campground

park office

74

VERDUGO CANYON

46.

Upper Bell Canyon—
East Ridge Loop

CASPERS WILDERNESS PARK

Head left, staying in the canyon. Drop down into the oak-filled canyon bottom, passing a junction with the Star Rise Trail. Walk past an old ranch gate, and stroll through an oak and sycamore woodland. Cross a rocky wash to the west edge of the canyon to a bench and a junction at 1.9 miles.

Bear right on the Oso Trail, leaving the canyon floor. Ascend the west-facing hillside, cross a sloping plateau, and climb again to the upper plateau, an ancient river terrace. Cross the grassy plateau to a trail split at 2.6 miles at the base of East Ridge by an emergency phone. The Oso Trail continues left (northeast) to Cold Spring Canyon and the Forest Service station at Hot Springs Canyon Road.

Take the right fork on the Cougar Pass Trail, and descend along the west edge of an oak-filled drainage. Climb out of the canyon to a trail fork at 2.9 miles with the East Ridge Trail on the left. The Cougar Pass Trail continues to the right (south), returning to Bell Canyon (Hike 45).

Take the left fork on the East Ridge Trail, and steeply climb up to the ridge, passing an old barbed wire fence. At the 900-foot ridge between Bell Canyon and San Juan Canyon, catch your breath and admire the sweeping views across the wilderness park, from the inland Santa Ana Mountains to the sea. Follow the rolling ridge south 1.5 miles on an easy downward slope. Pass the Sun Rise Trail on the right, and continue to the Quail Run Trail on the right.

Bear right and sharply descend from the ridge. The path levels out and passes the East Flats Trail, a footpath on the left. Continue straight ahead, winding downhill and reentering forested Bell Canyon to a T-junction on the canyon floor. Bear left 80 yards, returning to the trailhead. ▩

47. Bell Canyon—Oak Trail Loop

RONALD W. CASPERS WILDERNESS PARK

Hiking distance: 2.5-mile loop
Hiking time: 1.5 hours
Configuration: loop
Elevation gain: 100 feet
Difficulty: easy
Exposure: many shady pockets between open canyon slopes
Dogs: not allowed
Maps: U.S.G.S. Canada Gobernadora
    Ronald W. Caspers Wilderness Park map

Caspers Wilderness Park straddles San Juan Canyon east of San Juan Capistrano, stretching to the Riverside County line. The primitive park is adjacent to the Cleveland National Forest and is preserved to pre-ranching conditions. The parkland is a protected oasis with a varied terrain, including undisturbed forested canyons and chaparral-cloaked ridges.

This is an easy and scenic hike that meanders up fertile Bell Canyon, a quiet, natural canyon in the heart of the park. The hike forms a loop with the Oak Trail, a footpath on the west side of the canyon. The loop weaves through impressive sycamores and ancient oak woodlands.

To the trailhead

33401 ORTEGA HWY · SAN JUAN CAPISTRANO   33.548390, -117.563002

From the I-5 (San Diego) Freeway in San Juan Capistrano, take the Ortega (74) Highway exit. Drive 7.7 miles east to the posted park entrance and turn left. From the park entrance station, continue 1.4 miles to the end of the park road by the Bell Canyon Trailhead. Park on the left. An entrance fee is required.

The hike

Take the signed trail north from the end of the park road. Pass the Quail Run Trail at 80 yards and two unsigned Nature Trail connector paths on the left. Old Saddleback, the saddle-shaped formation of Modjeska Peak and Santiago Peak, can be seen in the distance. Follow the east edge of Bell Canyon to a posted trail split with the Sun Rise Trail on the right at one mile. Stay left in the oak-filled canyon for 0.1 mile to the Star Rise Trail on the left.

Bear left (the far end of the loop), and cross the rocky wash. Follow the gentle downhill slope through oaks and sycamores. Curve right to a posted junction with the Oak Trail. The Star Rise Trail continues up to the west ridge. Bear left and meander under the shade of mature twisted oaks. Recross the rocky wash to a junction. Both routes return to the trailhead. The right fork leads through the old oak forest to a junction with the Loskorn Trail on the right. Bear left, returning to the parking area. Complete the loop at the trailhead, 0.1 mile to the left. ■

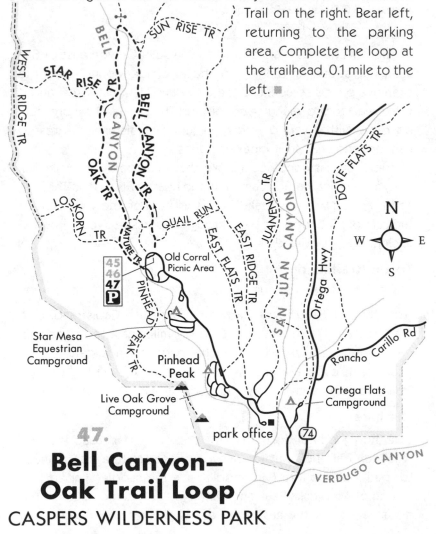

47.
Bell Canyon–
Oak Trail Loop
CASPERS WILDERNESS PARK

48. Bell Canyon—
West Ridge Loop

RONALD W. CASPERS WILDERNESS PARK

Hiking distance: 3.4-mile loop
Hiking time: 1.5 hours
Configuration: loop
Elevation gain: 400 feet
Difficulty: easy to slightly moderate
Exposure: a mix of shaded canyon and open ridge
Dogs: not allowed
Maps: U.S.G.S. Canada Gobernadora
     Ronald W. Caspers Wilderness Park map

Caspers Wilderness Park, in the foothills of the western Santa Anas, offers a wide cross-section of terrain, from riparian canyon bottoms to arid grassland and chaparral communities. This moderate-length loop at the lower end of Bell Canyon offers both.

The West Ridge Trail parallels the west edge of Caspers Wilderness Park 400 feet above Bell Canyon. The hike begins on the canyon floor under towering sycamores and ancient stands of contorted, picturesque oaks. The trail climbs the sandstone cliffs on the west wall of Bell Canyon to the open ridge. From West Ridge are vistas into Canada Gobernadora (the undeveloped canyon to the west), Bell Canyon (filled with oaks and sycamores), and Santiago and Modjeska Peaks.

To the trailhead

33401 ORTEGA HWY • SAN JUAN CAPISTRANO   33.548390, -117.563002

From the I-5 (San Diego) Freeway in San Juan Capistrano, take the Ortega (74) Highway exit. Drive 7.7 miles east to the posted park entrance and turn left. From the park entrance station, continue 1.4 miles to the end of the park road by the Bell Canyon Trailhead. Turn left and continue 0.1 mile to the Nature Trail on the right. Park 20 yards ahead in the parking spaces on either side of the road. An entrance fee is required.

The hike

Walk back to the posted Nature Trail on the left. Take the trail through groves of oaks, sycamores, and patches of prickly pear cactus to the west edge of Bell Canyon. Cross the rocky wash and stroll through grasslands under a forested canopy to a Y-fork. The Oak Trail, the return route, curves right. Take the Dick Loskorn Trail to the left. Climb the south slope of a side canyon, weaving through stately oaks. Across the narrow draw lie eroded sandstone cliffs with caves. Near the top are vistas across Bell Canyon and Caspers Park to the rugged Santa Ana Mountains. Pass the fragile sedimentary formations to a T-junction on the west ridge of Bell Canyon at 0.8 miles.

Bear right on the West Ridge Trail, a fire road that straddles Bell Canyon and Canada Gobernadora along the park boundary. From the trail are 360-degree vistas. Follow the gently rolling ridge north 0.7 miles, crossing a long, sloping saddle. At the north tip of the saddle is a posted junction.

Leave the ridge and bear right on the Star Rise Trail. Gradually descend through sage scrub and chaparral, returning to the shaded oak forest and a junction with the Oak Trail. Bear right on the footpath under the shade of mature twisted oaks. Cross a rocky wash to a junction. Both routes lead to the trailhead. The right fork completes the loop at the Loskorn Trail. ▪

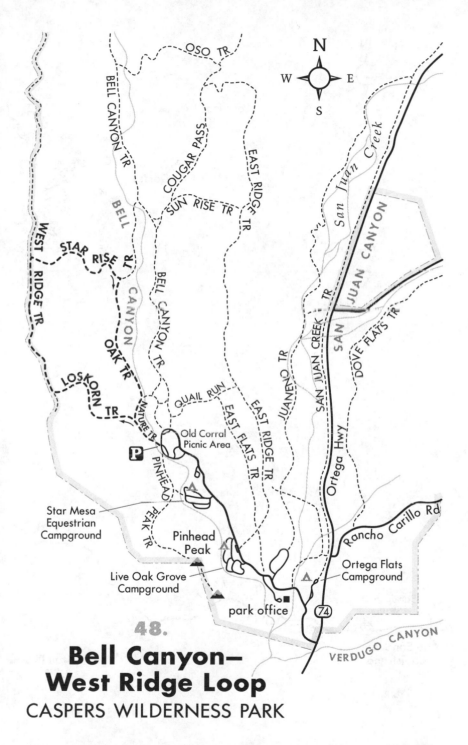

OSO TR

BELL CANYON TR

COUGAR PASS

SUN RISE TR

EAST RIDGE TR

BELL

WEST RIDGE TR

STAR RISE TR

CANYON

OAK TR

BELL CANYON TR

LOSKORN TR

NATURE TR

QUAIL RUN

EAST FLATS TR

EAST RIDGE TR

JUANENO TR

SAN JUAN CREEK TR

San Juan Creek

SAN JUAN CANYON

SAN

DOVE FLATS TR

Ortega Hwy

P

Old Corral
Picnic Area

PINHEAD PEAK TR

Star Mesa
Equestrian
Campground

Pinhead
Peak

Live Oak Grove
Campground

park office

Rancho Carillo Rd

Ortega Flats
Campground

74

VERDUGO CANYON

48.

Bell Canyon–
West Ridge Loop
CASPERS WILDERNESS PARK

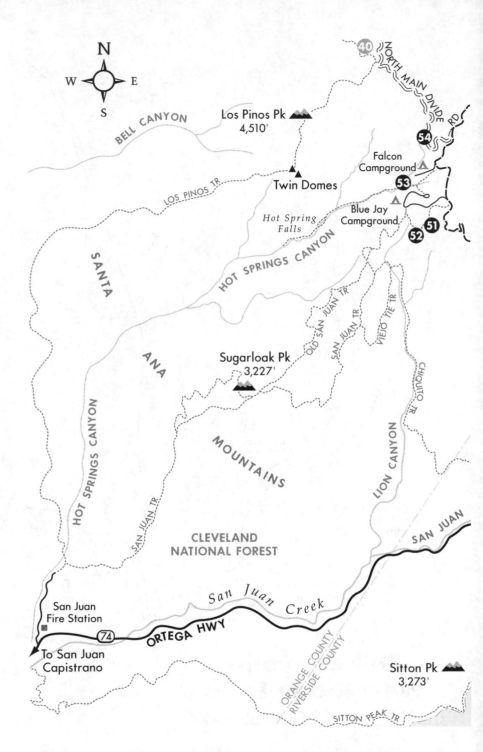

N
W   E
S

BELL CANYON

Los Pinos Pk
4,510'

LOS PINOS TR

Twin Domes

Hot Spring
Falls

SANTA

ANA

MOUNTAINS

HOT SPRINGS CANYON

HOT SPRINGS CANYON

Sugarloaf Pk
3,227'

OLD SAN JUAN TR

SAN JUAN TR

VIEJO TIE TR

LION CANYON

CHIQUITO TR

SAN JUAN TR

CLEVELAND
NATIONAL FOREST

SAN JUAN

NORTH MAIN DIVIDE RD

40

54

Falcon
Campground

53

Blue Jay
Campground

52 51

San Juan Creek

San Juan
Fire Station

74 ORTEGA HWY

To San Juan
Capistrano

ORANGE COUNTY
RIVERSIDE COUNTY

Sitton Pk
3,273'

SITTON PEAK TR

172

Upper Ortega Highway

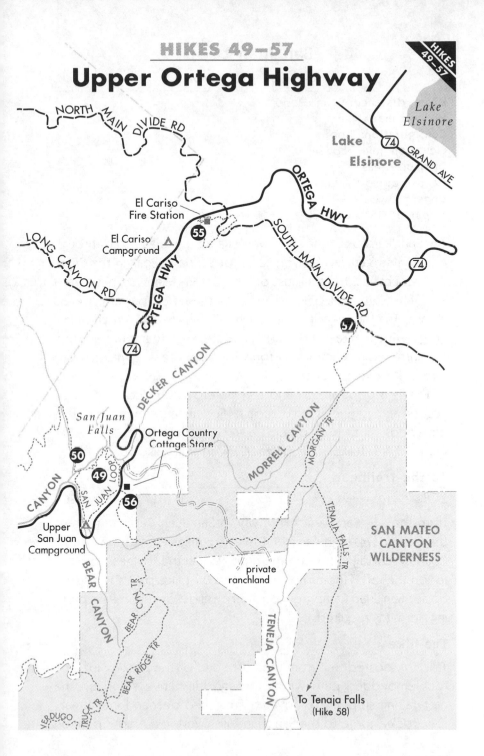

HIKES
49–57

Lake
Elsinore

NORTH MAIN DIVIDE RD

Lake
Elsinore

74

GRAND AVE

ORTEGA HWY

El Cariso
Fire Station

El Cariso
Campground

55

ORTEGA HWY

SOUTH MAIN DIVIDE RD

74

LONG CANYON RD

74

DECKER CANYON

57

San Juan
Falls

Ortega Country
Cottage Store

MORRELL CANYON

MORGAN TR

50

49

SAN JUAN LOOP

56

Upper
San Juan
Campground

BEAR CANYON

BEAR CYN TR

BEAR RIDGE TR

CANYON

TENAJA FALLS TR

SAN MATEO
CANYON
WILDERNESS

private
ranchland

TENEJA CANYON

VERDUGO

TRUCK TR

To Tenaja Falls
(Hike 58)

173

49. San Juan Loop
ORTEGA CORRIDOR

Hiking distance: 2.1-mile loop
Hiking time: 1 hour
Configuration: loop
Elevation gain: 350 feet
Difficulty: easy
Exposure: mostly forested
Dogs: allowed
Maps: U.S.G.S. Sitton Peak · Cleveland National Forest map

The San Juan Loop is an easy, well-signed trail that strolls through a scenic stream-fed canyon south of Santiago Peak in the Santa Ana Mountains. The trail, just off the Ortega Highway, has a variety of habitats, including oak woodlands and chaparral-covered slopes. The loop leads to San Juan Falls, a seasonal waterfall in a gorge with granite-lined pools. En route, six streams merge from the surrounding canyons to form San Juan Creek, a major tributary of Arroyo Trabuco.

This is a popular trail and can be crowded due to its easy access and gentle, scenic terrain. For an extended (and less crowded) hike, two other trails connect to the loop—the Chiquito Trail (Hike 50) and Bear Canyon Trail (Hike 56).

To the trailhead

34950 ORTEGA HWY · LAKE ELSINORE   33.612790, -117.426309

From the I-5 (San Diego) Freeway in San Juan Capistrano, take the Ortega (74) Highway exit. Drive 19.6 miles east to the Ortega Country Cottage Store on the right. Park in the trailhead parking lot on the left. (The turnoff is located 0.7 miles past the posted Upper San Juan Campground.) A pre-paid Adventure Pass parking permit is required.

The hike

Take the posted trail from the north end of the parking lot. The rock-embedded path winds through tall native scrub on the east-facing slope. Cross over the hill, and descend into a narrow, rocky gorge to the San Juan Falls overlook. A spur path on the right descends to the granite-walled canyon floor, upstream from the ephemeral 15-foot waterfall and pools. Continue on the main trail, traversing the cliffs and steadily dropping down to the rocky canyon floor. Stroll through San Juan Canyon under the oak canopy to a posted junction at 1.2 miles. The Chiquito Trail (Hike 50) heads up the unnamed drainage to the north.

For this hike, stay left on the San Juan Loop through stately live oaks toward the Ortega Highway. Curve south into Bear Canyon, parallel to the highway but separated by the creek and a forested draw. Pass rock formations under the shade of centuries-old oaks. Skirt the edge of Upper San Juan Campground, and make a horseshoe left bend, passing a few campground connector paths. Climb the exposed path and complete the loop at the south end of the parking lot. ■

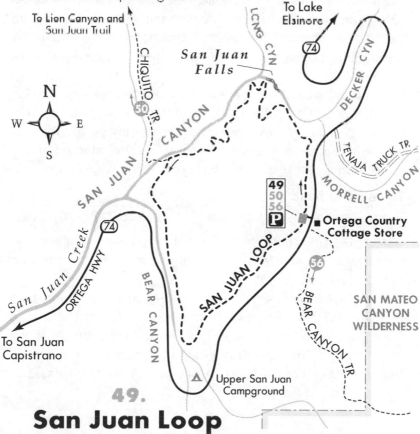

49.

San Juan Loop

50. Lower Chiquito Trail

San Juan Canyon to the Lion Canyon Overlook

ORTEGA CORRIDOR

Hiking distance: 8 miles round trip to overlook
11.2 miles one-way to Blue Jay Campground (shuttle)
Hiking time: 4—5.5 hours
Configuration: out-and-back (or shuttle from Hike 51)
Elevation gain: 900—1,900 feet
Difficulty: strenuous
Exposure: mostly forested canyon
Dogs: allowed
Maps: U.S.G.S. Sitton Peak and Alberhill
Cleveland National Forest map

The Chiquito Trail is an 8.2-mile trail that connects San Juan Canyon and the Ortega Highway with the San Juan Trail by the Blue Jay Campground. The heart of the trail follows the lush, forested canyon bottom of Lion Canyon between Los Pinos Peak and Sitton Peak.

This hike begins from the lower (south) trailhead on the San Juan Loop Trail and climbs to a spectacular overlook of Lion Canyon, San Juan Canyon, and the surrounding peaks. The trail can be hiked as an 11.2-mile one-way shuttle, starting at the upper trailhead at Hike 51 and hiking down into Lion Canyon.

To the trailhead

34950 ORTEGA HWY · LAKE ELSINORE   33.612790, -117.426309

LOWER TRAILHEAD PARKING. Park at the lower trailhead on the Ortega Highway to hike the out-and-back trail to the Lion Canyon overlook.

From the I-5 (San Diego) Freeway in San Juan Capistrano, take the Ortega (74) Highway exit. Drive 19.6 miles east to the Ortega Country Cottage Store on the right. Park in the trailhead parking lot on the left. (The turnoff is located 0.7 miles past the posted Upper San Juan Campground.) A pre-paid Adventure Pass parking permit is required.

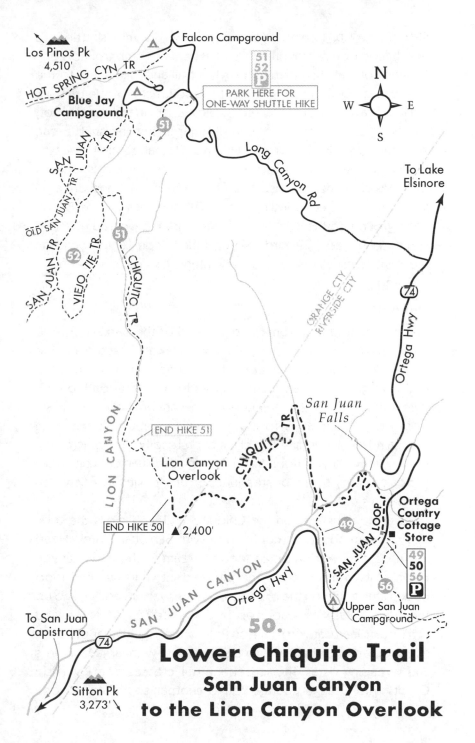

Los Pinos Pk
4,510'

Falcon Campground

HOT SPRING CYN TR

Blue Jay
Campground

51
52
P
PARK HERE FOR
ONE-WAY SHUTTLE HIKE

N
W · E
S

51

SAN JUAN TR

Long Canyon Rd

To Lake
Elsinore

OLD SAN JUAN TR

SAN JUAN TR

51

52

VIEJO TIE TR

CHIQUITO TR

ORANGE CTY
RIVERSIDE CTY

74

Ortega Hwy

LION CANYON

END HIKE 51

Lion Canyon
Overlook

END HIKE 50   ▲ 2,400'

CHIQUITO TR

San Juan
Falls

49

SAN JUAN LOOP

Ortega
Country
Cottage
Store

49
50
56
P

56

SAN JUAN CANYON

Ortega Hwy

To San Juan
Capistrano

74

Upper San Juan
Campground

Sitton Pk
3,273'

50.
Lower Chiquito Trail
San Juan Canyon
to the Lion Canyon Overlook

SHUTTLE CAR DIRECTIONS. For a one-way, 11.2-mile shuttle hike that heads down canyon, start at Blue Jay Campground/Long Canyon Road at the north end of the trail and hike south to the San Juan Loop/Ortega Highway at the south end of the trail.

First, leave a shuttle car at the lower trailhead parking lot, following the directions above. After parking the shuttle car, continue east on the Ortega Highway for another 4 miles to the North Main Divide Road on the left. (The turnoff is located 0.3 miles past the El Cariso Fire Station.) Turn left and drive 5.1 miles on the paved, winding mountain road, passing the Falcon Campground, to the Blue Jay Campground. The posted trailhead and parking area is 70 yards beyond the Falcon Campground on the right (west). A pre-paid Adventure Pass parking permit is required.

The hike

Take the posted trail from the north end of the parking lot. The rock-embedded path winds through tall native scrub on the east-facing slope. Cross over the hill, and descend into a narrow, rocky gorge to the San Juan Falls overlook. A spur path on the right descends to the granite-walled canyon floor, upstream from the ephemeral 15-foot waterfall and pools. Continue on the main trail, traversing the cliffs and steadily dropping down to the rocky canyon floor. Stroll through San Juan Canyon under the oak canopy to the posted junction at 1.2 miles. The San Juan Loop stays to the left.

Take the right fork on the Chiquito Trail, and cross the tributary stream above its confluence with San Juan Creek. Head north, parallel to an unnamed feeder stream on the rocky canyon floor. At two miles, cross the intermittent drainage, and loop back to the south on the dry west canyon wall. Steadily climb up the mountain as views open up of the entire canyon below and across San Juan Canyon to Sitton Peak in the south. Near the summit, loop around the point to a sitting area with large boulders and sweeping vistas. The serpentine trail crosses from Riverside County into Orange County. Round another south-facing ridge just north of a 2,400-foot knob that is topped with a jumble of huge, sculpted boulders. Curve to the east wall of vast Lion Canyon at four miles. This is the turn-around spot.

From here, the trail descends to the densely forested canyon bottom, then continues up canyon to the San Juan Trail and Blue Jay Campground at the upper end of the canyon. To hike the entire trail as a shuttle, however, it is easier to start at the upper end and hike south. ▪

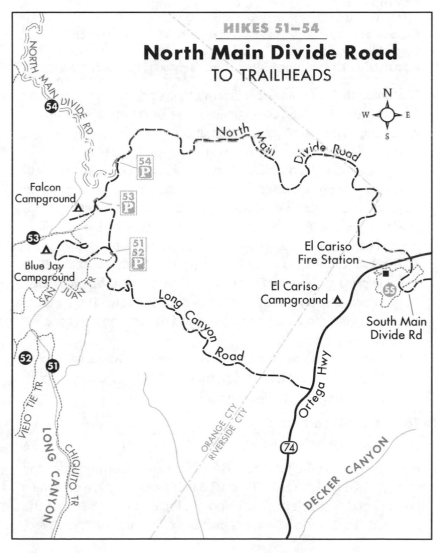

51. Upper Chiquito Trail

San Juan Trail to Lion Canyon

ORTEGA CORRIDOR

Hiking distance: 8.8 miles round trip through Lion Canyon
11.2 mile one-way shuttle
Hiking time: 4.5—5.5 hours
Configuration: out-and-back (or shuttle with Hike 50)
Elevation gain: 1,000—1,900 feet
Difficulty: strenuous to very strenuous
Exposure: a mix of open mountain slopes and forested canyon
Dogs: allowed
Maps: U.S.G.S. Alberhill and Sitton Peak · Cleveland National Forest map

The Chiquito Trail is an 8.2-mile trail that connects the San Juan Trail and the Blue Jay Campground (the upper trailhead at the north end) with San Juan Canyon and the Ortega Highway (the lower trailhead at the south end). The trail passes through a variety of habitats and plant communities, descending from arid chaparral-covered slopes with awesome vistas to streamside riparian woodlands with oaks and sycamores. The heart of the trail follows the lush, forested canyon bottom of Lion Canyon, which lies between Los Pinos Peak and Sitton Peak.

This hike begins from the upper (north) trailhead at the Blue Jay Campground on the San Juan Trail. The trail drops into Lion Canyon and closely follows the riparian drainage. The hike returns along the same trail, turning around before the trail ascends back out of the canyon.

The trail can also be hiked as an 11.2-mile one-way shuttle with Hike 50, ending at the Ortega Country Cottage Store at the south trailhead on the Ortega Highway.

To the trailhead

LONG CANYON ROAD · LAKE ELSINORE   33.652358, -117.448432

From the I-5 (San Diego) Freeway in San Juan Capistrano, take the Ortega (74) Highway exit. Drive 23.6 miles east to the North Main Divide Road on the left. (The turnoff is located 0.3 miles past the El Cariso Fire Station.) Turn left and drive 5.1 miles on the paved,

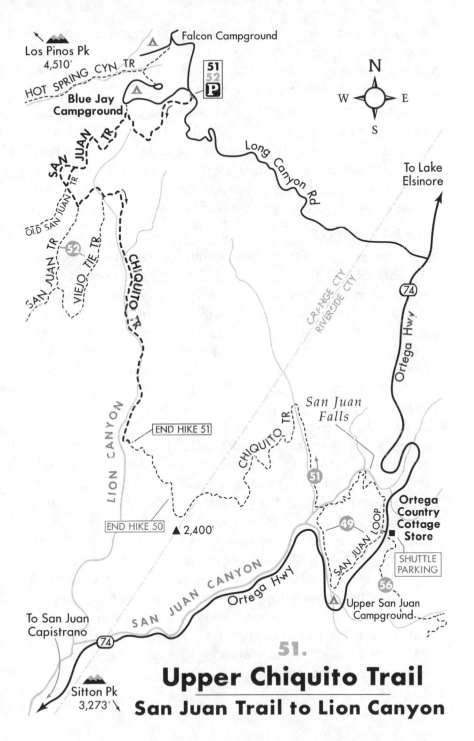

Los Pinos Pk
4,510'

Falcon Campground

HOT SPRING CYN TR

Blue Jay
Campground

51
52
P

N
W E
S

SAN JUAN TR

Long Canyon Rd

To Lake
Elsinore

OLD SAN JUAN TR

52

SAN JUAN TR

VIEJO TIE TR.

CHIQUITO TR

ORANGE CTY
RIVERSIDE CTY

74

Ortega Hwy

LION CANYON

END HIKE 51

CHIQUITO TR

San Juan
Falls

51

49

SAN JUAN LOOP

Ortega
Country
Cottage
Store

SHUTTLE
PARKING

END HIKE 50

▲ 2,400'

56

SAN JUAN CANYON

Ortega Hwy

Upper San Juan
Campground

To San Juan
Capistrano

74

Sitton Pk
3,273'

51.
Upper Chiquito Trail
San Juan Trail to Lion Canyon

winding mountain road, passing the Falcon Campground, to the Blue Jay Campground. The posted trailhead and parking area is 70 yards beyond the Falcon Campground on the right (west). A pre-paid Adventure Pass parking permit is required.

SHUTTLE CAR DIRECTIONS. From the I-5 (San Diego) Freeway in San Juan Capistrano, take the Ortega (74) Highway exit. Drive 19.6 miles east to the Ortega Country Cottage Store on the right. Park in the trailhead parking lot on the left. (The turnoff is located 0.7 miles past the posted Upper San Juan Campground.) A pre-paid Adventure Pass parking permit is required.

The hike

From the posted trailhead, walk south and curve west below the edge of Blue Jay Campground. Cross the head of two forested canyons, traversing the cliffside path. Weave in and out of shady oak groves, exposed sage scrub, and chaparral-clad slopes, overlooking Lion Canyon to Sitton Peak in the south. At 1.3 miles is a trail split. The shorter and steeper Old San Juan Trail bears left, and the longer but easier San Juan Trail stays to the right. Both paths crisscross at 1.7 miles. From the crossing, continue straight on the San Juan Trail 0.1 mile to a junction with the Chiquito Trail on the left.

Bear left and descend into forested Lion Canyon to a posted junction with the Viejo Tie Trail on the right at 2.4 miles (Hike 52). Stay on the Chiquito Trail, and continue down the stream-fed canyon through stands of large oaks. Follow the east side of the rocky drainage, crossing the seasonal stream four times. A few miles down the canyon the trail veers left, leaving the canyon floor and climbing up the east canyon wall. This is the turn-around point for an 8.8-mile round-trip hike. Return along the same trail.

For the shuttle hike, zigzag up the east wall of Lion Canyon to the ridge, with a spectacular view of Lion Canyon, San Juan Canyon, and the surrounding peaks. Continue on the Chiquito Trail to the San Juan Loop, referencing Hike 50 to the south trailhead on the Ortega Highway. ■

52. Upper Lion Canyon— Chiquito Basin Loop

ORTEGA CORRIDOR

Hiking distance: 6 miles round trip
Hiking time: 3 hours
Configuration: lollipop
Elevation gain: 700 feet
Difficulty: moderate
Exposure: mostly forested with some exposed slopes
Dogs: allowed
Maps: U.S.G.S. Alberhill · Cleveland National Forest map

This hike circles a 3,000-foot knoll between Lion Canyon and Chiquito Basin by Sugarloaf Peak. The peak lies in the Santa Ana Mountains between Santiago Peak and the Ortega Highway. It is accessed from the North Main Divide Road, which travels along the length of the Santa Anas. The route begins at the head of Lion Canyon by the Blue Jay Campground, following the San Juan Trail. The hike makes a loop around the knoll on the Chiquito Trail and the 1.2-mile Viejo Tie Trail. Throughout the hike are sweeping vistas of the forested canyons, folded ridges, and surrounding peaks.

To the trailhead

Long Canyon Road · Lake Elsinore   33.652358, -117.448432

From the I-5 (San Diego) Freeway in San Juan Capistrano, take the Ortega (74) Highway exit. Drive 23.6 miles east to the North Main Divide Road on the left. (The turnoff is located 0.3 miles past the El Cariso Fire Station.) Turn left and drive 5.1 miles on the paved, winding mountain road, passing the Falcon Campground, to the Blue Jay Campground. The posted trailhead and parking area is 70 yards beyond the Falcon Campground on the right (west). A pre-paid Adventure Pass parking permit is required.

The hike

From the posted trailhead, walk south and curve west below the south edge of Blue Jay Campground. Cross the head of two forested canyons, traversing the cliffside path. Weave in and out of shady oak groves, exposed sage scrub, and chaparral-clad slopes, overlooking Lion Canyon to Sitton Peak. At 1.3 miles is a trail split. The shorter and steeper Old San Juan Trail bears left, and the longer but easier San Juan Trail stays to the right. Both paths crisscross at 1.7 miles. From the crossing, continue straight on the San Juan Trail 0.1 mile to the San Juan–Chiquito Trail junction at 1.8 miles.

Begin the loop on the Chiquito Trail to the left, hiking clockwise. Descend 0.6 miles into forested Lion Canyon to the posted junction with the Viejo Tie Trail. The main trail continues down the canyon (Hike 51). Bear right on the Viejo Tie Trail, and head up and over a small rise. Climb the east wall of Lion Canyon under the shade of oaks on the narrow, undulating path. Loop around the south face of the mountain, and leave Lion Canyon to the west wall of Chiquito Basin, overlooking 3,227-foot Sugarloaf Peak. Weave north through scattered boulders just below the ridge to a posted junction with the San Juan Trail. Veer to the right on the cliffside path, and continue 0.6 miles through the forest, completing the loop at the San Juan–Chiquito Trail junction. Retrace your steps 1.8 miles back to Blue Jay Campground. ∎

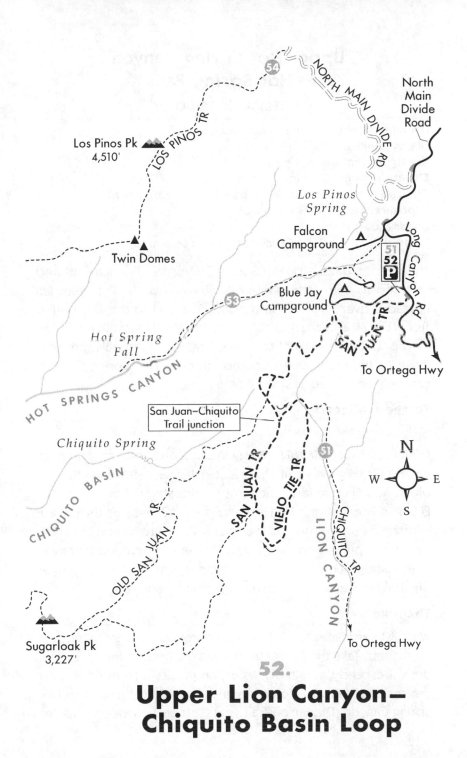

54

NORTH MAIN DIVIDE RD

North
Main
Divide
Road

Los Pinos Pk
4,510'

LOS PINOS TR

*Los Pinos
Spring*

Falcon
Campground

Long Canyon Rd

51
52
P

Twin Domes

53

Blue Jay
Campground

SAN JUAN TR

To Ortega Hwy

*Hot Spring
Fall*

HOT SPRINGS CANYON

San Juan–Chiquito
Trail junction

Chiquito Spring

CHIQUITO BASIN

SAN JUAN TR

VIEJO TIE TR

51

N
W E
S

OLD SAN JUAN TR

LION CANYON

CHIQUITO TR

Sugarloak Pk
3,227'

To Ortega Hwy

52.

Upper Lion Canyon–
Chiquito Basin Loop

53. Upper Hot Spring Canyon to Hot Spring Falls

ORTEGA CORRIDOR

Hiking distance: 3 miles round trip
Hiking time: 1.5 hours
Configuration: out-and-back
Elevation gain: 500 feet
Difficulty: easy to moderate with some technical sections
Exposure: mostly forested canyon
Dogs: allowed
Maps: U.S.G.S. Alberhill · Cleveland National Forest map

The 25-foot waterfall in Hot Spring Canyon sits in a multi-colored rock grotto with ferns and moss-covered walls. The waterfall cascades over two tiers into pools. The trail to the falls begins from the Falcon Campground along the North Main Divide Road on the southeast flank of Los Pinos Peak. The informal path stays close to the creek as it descends through Hot Spring Canyon, crossing the creekbed several times.

To the trailhead

LONG CANYON ROAD · LAKE ELSINORE   33.657747, -117.450835

From the I-5 (San Diego) Freeway in San Juan Capistrano, take the Ortega (74) Highway exit. Drive 23.6 miles east to the North Main Divide Road on the left. (The turnoff is located 0.3 miles past the El Cariso Fire Station.) Turn left and drive 4.7 miles on the paved, winding mountain road to the Falcon Campground on the right. Park in the pullout on the right, near the campground entrance. (The campground is closed to camping during the winter.) A pre-paid Adventure Pass parking permit is required.

The hike

Walk 30 yards into the Falcon Campground to the posted trail on the left. Take the footpath, skirting the north edge of a minor draw. Descend through oak trees, and cross a footbridge over the seasonal drainage to an unsigned Y-fork at the head of Hot Spring Canyon. The Falcon Trail veers left and connects with the

Blue Jay Campground. Stay to the right, crisscrossing the Hot Spring Canyon drainage under towering oaks. Pass through fields of rock outcroppings as the canyon deepens. Follow the north wall of the canyon, and drop down to the canyon bottom on the rocky path. The trail alternates between the rocky streambed and the north canyon wall. Pass an intersecting stream-fed canyon from the north and a series of seasonal pools. As the canyon widens, cross the sycamore-lined drainage two times beneath the 3,000-foot, two-domed mountain on the right, with a ridge dropping into the canyon. The trail soon emerges at the brink of the falls, dropping through a notch in the rock to the water-carved pools. Descend to the base of the falls and the pools. After enjoying the area, return along the same path. ■

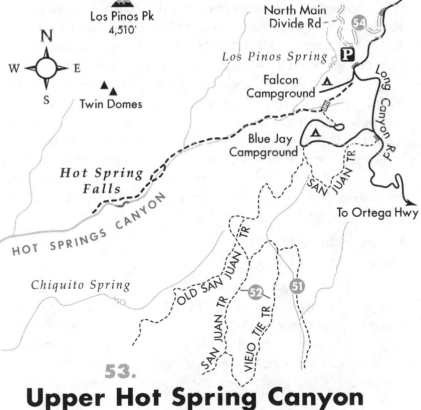

53.
Upper Hot Spring Canyon to Hot Spring Falls

54. Los Pinos Peak from North Main Divide Road

ORTEGA CORRIDOR

Hiking distance: 4.8 miles round trip
Hiking time: 2.5 hours
Configuration: out-and-back
Elevation gain: 1,100 feet
Difficulty: strenuous
Exposure: exposed ridgeline fire road
Dogs: allowed
Maps: U.S.G.S. Alberhill · Cleveland National Forest map

At an elevation of 4,510 feet, Los Pinos Peak is the fourth highest peak in the Santa Ana Mountains, topped only by Santiago Peak, Modjeska Peak, and Trabuco Peak. Los Pinos Peak can be accessed from three different routes—from the lower Los Pinos Trail in Hot Spring Canyon (by the San Juan Fire Station), from Trabuco Canyon (Hike 40), and from the North Main Divide Road.

This hike follows the shortest access route from the North Main Divide Road. The road up to the peak can be driven, but it is not recommended, as it is a steep, narrow, and winding road. The trail includes a strenuous ascent, but from atop the peak are sweeping 360-degree vistas from the mountains to the Pacific Ocean. The panoramic views span to the San Jacinto, San Bernardino, and San Gabriel Mountains; Catalina Island; and San Clemente Island.

To the trailhead

NORTH MAIN DIVIDE ROAD · LAKE ELSINORE   33.662373, -117.447897

From the I-5 (San Diego) Freeway in San Juan Capistrano, take the Ortega (74) Highway exit. Drive 23.6 miles east to the North Main Divide Road on the left. (The turnoff is located 0.3 miles past the El Cariso Fire Station.) Turn left and drive 4.2 miles on the paved, winding mountain road to the wide pullout on the right. Park in the turnout. A pre-paid Adventure Pass permit is required.

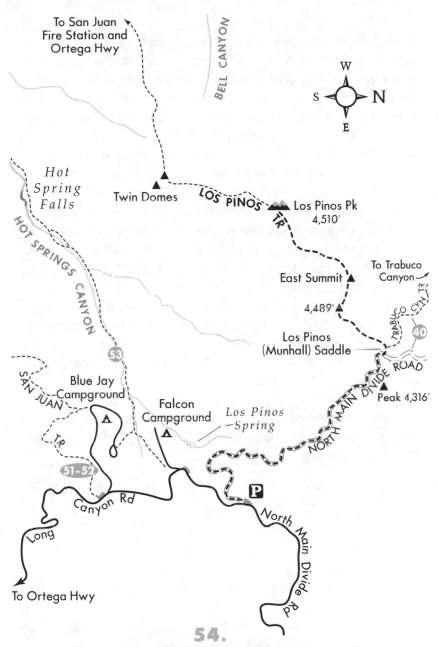

To San Juan
Fire Station and
Ortega Hwy

BELL CANYON

W N S E

Hot
Spring
Falls

Twin Domes

LOS PINOS TR

Los Pinos Pk
4,510'

HOT SPRINGS CANYON

East Summit

4,489'

To Trabuco
Canyon

TRABUCO CYN TR

40

Los Pinos
(Munhall) Saddle

53

SAN JUAN TR

Blue Jay
Campground

Falcon
Campground

Los Pinos
Spring

NORTH MAIN DIVIDE ROAD

Peak 4,316'

51-52

Canyon Rd

P

North Main Divide Rd

Long

To Ortega Hwy

54.

Los Pinos Peak
from North Main Divide Road

The hike

The North Main Divide Road continues from the south end of the pullout, a dirt road with an open gate. Head up the road, overlooking Hot Spring Canyon to the southwest (Hike 53), forested Falcon Campground, layers of mountains across the San Mateo Canyon Wilderness, and east across Temecula Valley. Skirt around the west side of the mountain and the west side of Peak 4,316 to Los Pinos (Munhall) Saddle, located on a large flat with a metal railing and a trail split. The North Main Divide Road continues to the right to Trabuco Peak and the Main Divide Road. Leave the road and take the posted Trabuco Canyon Trail a few yards left to the posted Los Pinos Trail on the left. Bear left up the rocky footpath through oaks, ponderosa pine, and tall scrub. Cross over a 4,489-foot knoll, with views of Trabuco Peak, Trabuco Canyon, and the Saddleback Valley. Follow the saddle on the exposed ridge to a second peak, then cross a third saddle to the lower, east summit. Make the short but steep final ascent to Los Pinos Peak. Leave the trail 20 yards left to the boulders atop the 4,510-foot summit, with two U.S. Geologic Survey pins embedded in the rock. This is the turn-around point.

To hike farther, the Los Pinos Trail continues 8 miles southwest to the San Juan Fire Station. The trail follows a roller-coaster route across ridges, peaks, and saddles, overlooking Lion Canyon, Bell Canyon, and Hot Spring Canyon. ▄

55. El Cariso Nature Trail

ORTEGA CORRIDOR

EL CARISO FIRE STATION and VISITOR CENTER

Hiking distance: 1.5-mile loop
Hiking time: 45 minutes
Configuration: loop
Elevation gain: 100 feet
Difficulty: easy
Exposure: a mix of woodland and chaparral-covered slopes
Dogs: allowed
Maps: U.S.G.S. Alberhill · Cleveland National Forest map

The El Cariso Nature Trail is a self-guiding loop that begins at the El Cariso Fire Station and visitor center on the Ortega Highway. The easy trail circles a knoll with north, west, and south vistas, meandering through Coulter pines, incense cedar, cypress, oaks, manzanita, coastal sage, and scrub oak. An interpretive pamphlet describes the surrounding geology, plants, and animals. Before setting out, ask for the self-guiding pamphlet at the visitor center.

To the trailhead

32353 ORTEGA HWY · LAKE ELSINORE   33.651169, -117.412950

From the I-5 (San Diego) Freeway in San Juan Capistrano, take the Ortega (74) Highway exit. Drive 23.3 miles east to the El Cariso Fire/Ranger Station and visitor center on the right. Park in the spaces in front of the center.

The hike

From the west (right) side of the El Cariso Visitor Center, walk up the stone steps to the signed trail. Follow the dirt path up the west-facing hillside on an easy grade through a grove of oaks and pines. Views extend across the rolling hills and surrounding mountain peaks. Cross over the summit to the south-facing slope, overlooking the San Mateo Canyon Wilderness and Santa Margarita Mountains. Descend along the backside of the hill, passing an old mine shaft with a three-foot-high tunnel. Continue east to the South Main Divide Road (also called Killen Trail). Cross the paved road and pick up the signed trail. Stroll through a grove of Coulter pines to the trail's east end. Descend and loop back to the left. Head west, parallel to the Ortega Highway, and re-cross the South Main Divide Road. Wind back through sage scrub and chaparral, skirting the edge of a picnic area to a service road. Bear right on the road for 100 yards, and complete the loop at the visitor center. ■

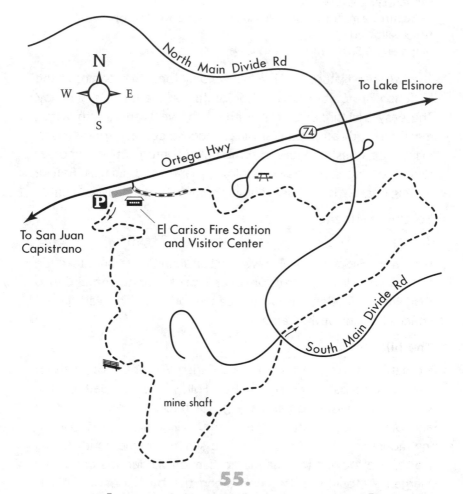

55.
El Cariso Nature Trail
EL CARISO FIRE STATION and VISITOR CENTER

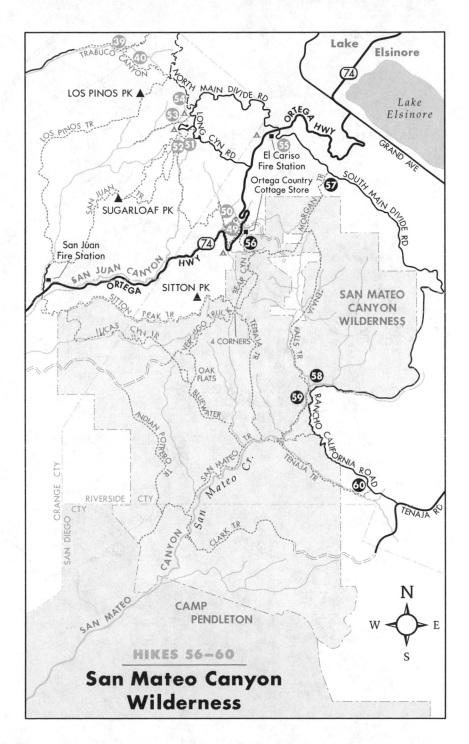

LOS PINOS PK ▲

TRABUCO CANYON
39
40

NORTH MAIN DIVIDE RD

54
53

Lake
Elsinore
74

Lake
Elsinore

LOS PINOS TR

LONG CYN RD

52 51

ORTEGA HWY

GRAND AVE

El Cariso
Fire Station
55

Ortega Country
Cottage Store

57

SOUTH MAIN DIVIDE RD

SAN JUAN TR

SUGARLOAF PK ▲

50
49

74

56

MORGAN TR

San Juan
Fire Station

SAN JUAN CANYON HWY

ORTEGA

SITTON PK ▲

BEAR CYN

SITTON PEAK TR

LUCAS CYN TR

VERDUGO TRUCK

4 CORNERS

TENAJA TR

TENAJA

FALLS TR

SAN MATEO
CANYON
WILDERNESS

58

OAK
FLATS

BLUEWATER

59

RANCHO CALIFORNIA ROAD

INDIAN POTRERO TR

SAN MATEO TR

San Mateo Cr.

TENAJA TR

60

TENAJA RD

ORANGE CTY

RIVERSIDE CTY

CLARK TR

SAN DIEGO CTY

SAN MATEO CANYON

CAMP
PENDLETON

SAN MATEO

N
W   E
S

HIKES 56–60

San Mateo Canyon
Wilderness

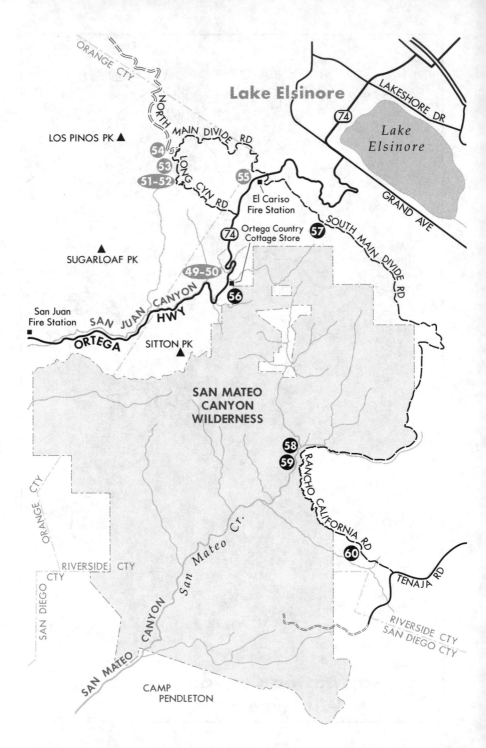

Lake Elsinore

LAKESHORE DR

74

Lake
Elsinore

GRAND AVE

LOS PINOS PK ▲

ORANGE CTY

NORTH MAIN DIVIDE RD

54

53

51–52

LONG CYN RD

55

El Cariso
Fire Station

74

Ortega Country
Cottage Store

57

SOUTH MAIN DIVIDE RD

SUGARLOAF PK ▲

49–50

SAN JUAN CANYON HWY

San Juan
Fire Station

SAN JUAN

ORTEGA

56

SITTON PK ▲

SAN MATEO
CANYON
WILDERNESS

58

59

RANCHO CALIFORNIA RD

ORANGE CTY

San Mateo Cr.

60

TENAJA RD

RIVERSIDE CTY

SAN DIEGO CTY

SAN MATEO CANYON

San Mateo Canyon

RIVERSIDE CTY
SAN DIEGO CTY

CAMP
PENDLETON

San Mateo Canyon Wilderness

Santa Rosa Plateau Ecological Reserve

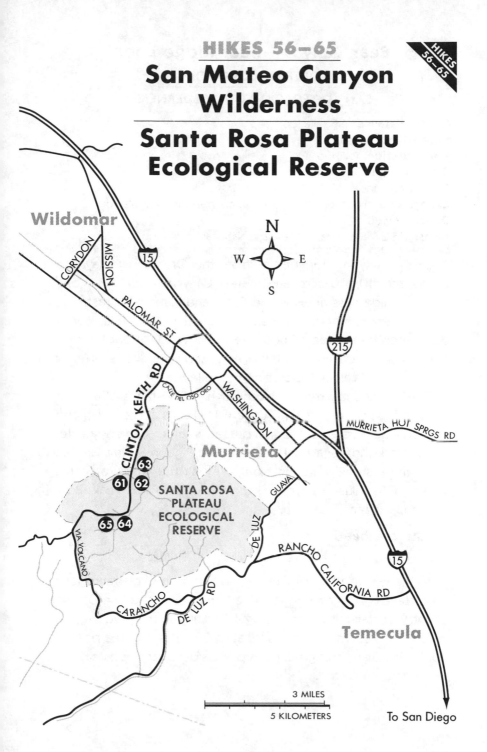

56. Bear Canyon—Bear Ridge Loop
ORTEGA CORRIDOR
SAN MATEO CANYON WILDERNESS

Hiking distance: 6.6-mile loop
Hiking time: 3 hours
Configuration: lollipop
Elevation gain: 800 feet
Difficulty: moderate
Exposure: a mix of forest and open chaparral-covered hillside
Dogs: allowed
Maps: U.S.G.S. Sitton Peak · Cleveland National Forest map

The Bear Canyon Loop begins from the Ortega Highway and enters the 40,000-acre San Mateo Canyon Wilderness, one of four wilderness areas in the Cleveland National Forest. The forest is the southernmost national forest in California. It was designated by President Theodore Roosevelt in 1908. The wilderness area is covered with chaparral and sage, with scattered oak woodlands along the slopes and valleys.

This backcountry trail winds through shady stands of ancient oaks and exposed chaparral-covered hillsides at the north end of the wilderness area. The trail passes weather-carved granite, grassy parklands, seasonal streams, and Pigeon Spring, an oak glen with a stone watering trough. Along the way are scenic views of San Juan Canyon, Sitton Peak, Los Pinos Peak, Bear Canyon, and Tenaja Canyon.

To the trailhead

34950 ORTEGA HWY · LAKE ELSINORE   33.612790, -117.426309

From the I-5 (San Diego) Freeway in San Juan Capistrano, take the Ortega (74) Highway exit. Drive 19.6 miles east to the Ortega Country Cottage Store on the right. Park in the trailhead parking lot on the left. (The turnoff is located 0.7 miles past the posted Upper San Juan Campground.) A pre-paid Adventure Pass parking permit is required.

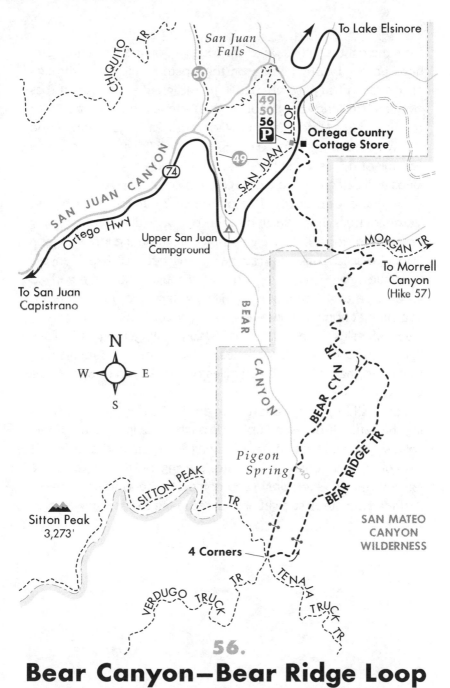

56.
Bear Canyon—Bear Ridge Loop
SAN MATEO CANYON WILDERNESS

The hike

From the right (south) side of the Ortega Country Cottage Store, head up the brushy hillside on the posted trail. Climb through chaparral and sage scrub, passing large granite boulders. Cross over the small ridge high above the Ortega Highway, and enter the signed San Mateo Canyon Wilderness. Pass a junction on the left with the Morgan Trail (Hike 57) at one mile, and cross over a few minor ridges. Crest the upper ridge and walk through grasslands and oak groves to a posted junction at 2.1 miles.

Begin the loop to the right on the Bear Canyon Trail (the old Verdugo Truck Trail). Stroll through oak woodlands on an easy downward slope. Pass the watering trough on the left at Pigeon Spring, a shady oak-covered flat at the head of Bear Canyon. Continue a half mile south, and pass through a gate in a barbed wire fence to 4 Corners at 3.1 miles, where five trails intersect. The intersection is at the far end of the loop. The sharp right fork leads 1.5 miles to the summit of Sitton Peak, gaining 1,100 feet. The Verdugo Truck Trail continues straight ahead. The Tenaja Trail, slightly to the left, heads five miles down canyon to San Mateo Creek.

For this hike, take the left fork on the Bear Ridge Trail, starting the return loop. Head uphill through manzanita to the ridge. Follow the ridge north, overlooking Bear Canyon and Tenaja Canyon. Pass through a trail gate, staying on the ridge. Curve left into the forested draw, and complete the loop at 4.5 miles. Retrace your steps straight ahead, returning to the highway. ▩

57. Morgan Trail—Morrell Canyon
South Main Divide Road to Ortega Highway
SAN MATEO CANYON WILDERNESS

Hiking distance: 10.2 miles round trip
5.1 miles one-way shuttle
(to the Ortega Country Cottage Store)
Hiking time: 2.5 to 5 hours
Configuration: out-and-back
Elevation gain: 900 feet (900 foot loss if doing shuttle)
Difficulty: strenuous (moderate for shuttle hike)
Exposure: a mix of forested canyon bottom and open canyon slopes
Dogs: allowed
Maps: U.S.G.S. Alberhill and Sitton Peak
Cleveland National Forest map

The Morgan Trail, originally a Juaneno Indian route, crosses the north end of the San Mateo Canyon Wilderness, one of four wilderness areas in the Cleveland National Forest. The trail connects the South Main Divide Road with the Bear Canyon Trail by the Ortega Country Cottage Store. The path descends through stream-fed Morrell Canyon in a lush oak, sycamore, and willow woodland with large granite boulders and grassy meadows. Beyond the canyon, the trail follows a low rolling ridge, providing vistas across the wilderness to the surrounding peaks. On the road to the trailhead are hang-gliding launches and bird's-eye views of Lake Elsinore to the north.

This trail can be hiked as a 5.1-mile one-way shuttle. The shuttle hike loses 900 feet in elevation (rather than gaining it on the return), ending at the Ortega Country Cottage Store on Ortega Highway.

To the trailhead

SOUTH MAIN DIVIDE RD · LAKE ELSINORE   33.633830, -117.382917

From the I-5 (San Diego) Freeway in San Juan Capistrano, take the Ortega (74) Highway exit. Drive 23.6 miles east to the posted South Main Divide Road (also called Killen Trail) on the right. (The turnoff is located 0.3 miles past the El Cariso Fire/Ranger Station.) Turn right and continue 2.5 miles on the paved road to the posted trailhead parking area on the right. A pre-paid Adventure Pass parking permit is required.

SHUTTLE CAR DIRECTIONS: From the I-5 (San Diego) Freeway in San Juan Capistrano, take the Ortega (74) Highway exit. Drive 19.6 miles east to the Ortega Country Cottage Store on the right. Park in the trailhead parking lot on the left. (The turnoff is located 0.7 miles past the posted Upper San Juan Campground.) A pre-paid Adventure Pass parking permit is required.

The hike

From the posted trailhead, drop down the slope to the Morrell Canyon drainage. Walk down canyon through the oak woodland with moss-covered rocks, sycamores, and poison oak. Pass a couple of side drainages to seasonal Morrell Canyon Creek at 1.2 miles. Cross the creek and enter the north end of the San Mateo Canyon Wilderness. Climb out of the lush canyon bottom to the dryer and exposed east slope of the canyon. Wind through tall brush and over small dips and rises amid a natural rock garden. Follow the open, rolling terrain and pastureland, enjoying the great vistas across the Santa Anas. Continue to a posted Y-fork at 2.3 miles. The left fork is the northern access into San Mateo Canyon and heads five miles south to Tenaja Falls (Hike 58).

Stay to the right and parallel an old barbed wire fence. Skirt the north edge of Potrero De La Cienega and Round Potrero, large private ranchlands surrounded by the wilderness. Cross two ranch access roads, and continue west through oak groves to a T-junction with the Bear Canyon Trail at 4.1 miles. The left fork leads to the Bear Canyon Loop (Hike 52) and Sitton Peak.

Bear right and descend on the rocky footpath through tall scrub and oak trees. Leave the wilderness and cross over a few minor hills to the cliffs above the Ortega Highway. Descend to the highway on the south side of the Ortega Country Cottage Store at 5.1 miles. ■

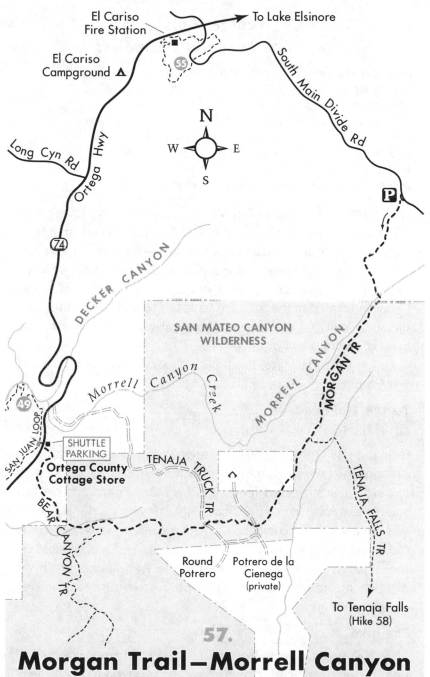

El Cariso
Fire Station

To Lake Elsinore

El Cariso
Campground △

South Main Divide Rd

Long Cyn Rd

Ortega Hwy

N
W   E
S

74

DECKER CANYON

SAN MATEO CANYON
WILDERNESS

Morrell   Canyon   Creek

MORRELL CANYON

MORGAN TR

P

49

SAN JUAN LOOP

SHUTTLE
PARKING

Ortega County
Cottage Store

TENAJA TRUCK TR

BEAR CANYON TR

Round
Potrero

Potrero de la
Cienega
(private)

TENAJA FALLS TR

To Tenaja Falls
(Hike 58)

57.

Morgan Trail–Morrell Canyon
SAN MATEO CANYON WILDERNESS

58. Tenaja Falls

SAN MATEO CANYON WILDERNESS

Hiking distance: 1.5 miles round trip
Hiking time: 1 hour
Configuration: out-and-back
Elevation gain: 240 feet
Difficulty: easy (with some technical sections across slippery rocks)
Exposure: mostly chaparral-covered slope
Dogs: allowed
Maps: U.S.G.S. Sitton Peak · Cleveland National Forest map

Tenaja Falls is located in San Mateo Canyon at an elevation of 1,570 feet. *Tenajas* are pools in basalt-lined creekbeds that hold water throughout the summer. When the water is flowing, Tenaja Falls is quite picturesque. The creek drops 160 feet over five tiers, cascading over polished granite into a series of pools (tenajas) formed in the smooth, sculpted rock. This path follows the west canyon wall on the chaparral-covered slope to the brink of the falls and pools.

For an extended hike, the trail continues down canyon along San Mateo Creek—Hike 59.

To the trailhead

CLEVELAND FOREST ROAD · FALLBROOK   33.548979, –117.394458

From the I-15 (Temecula Valley) Freeway in Wildomar, just north of Murrieta, take the Clinton Keith Road exit. Drive 7 miles south to a stop sign at posted Tenaja Road. (Clinton Keith Road merges into Tenaja Road en route.) Turn right, staying on Tenaja Road, and drive 4.3 miles to Rancho California Road, which is posted as Cleveland Forest Road. Turn right and carefully drive 5.3 miles on the winding, one-lane paved road to the well-marked trailhead and parking area on the left. A pre-paid Adventure Pass parking permit is required.

The hike

Walk 100 yards downhill on the posted trail to a signed junction. The left fork leads down San Mateo Canyon to Fisherman's Camp and Tenaja Canyon (Hikes 59 and 60). Take the right fork past a metal gate on the Tenaja Falls Trail, and head up canyon through an oak woodland. Cross San Mateo Creek on a concrete spillway, and meander up the west side of the creek. Climb the east-facing canyon wall on the wide, rocky path. Curve around a bend to a view of Tenaja Falls, cascading off a water-carved notch in the rock. Traverse the sloping hillside and loop back to the lip of the falls. At the top of the waterfall is a concrete spillway and a series of pools in the polished rock. The rocks are slippery, so use caution. The main trail crosses the creek above the falls and continues north up the canyon along the east side of the creek for 3.6 miles to the Morgan Trail at the north end of the San Mateo Canyon Wilderness. ■

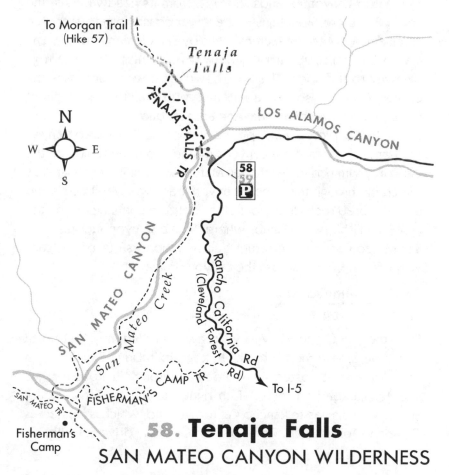

58. Tenaja Falls
SAN MATEO CANYON WILDERNESS

59. Upper San Mateo Canyon

San Mateo Creek—Fisherman's Camp Loop

SAN MATEO CANYON WILDERNESS

Hiking distance: 5.2-mile loop
Hiking time: 2.5 hours
Configuration: loop
Elevation gain: 500 feet
Difficulty: moderate
Exposure: riparian woodlands with exposed road on return
Dogs: allowed
Maps: U.S.G.S. Sitton Peak · Cleveland National Forest map

San Mateo Canyon extends 15 miles, from its headwaters in the upper Santa Ana Mountains to the lower coastal plain, where the creek empties into the Pacific Ocean by San Clemente. Upper San Mateo Canyon can be accessed via several trails off the Ortega Highway to the north. This hike, however, directly accesses the canyon from the south via I-15 and Murrieta. The more direct route utilizes a winding, one-lane access road.

The trail explores the upper canyon in the San Mateo Canyon Wilderness, where three canyons merge. From the trailhead, the path drops immediately into San Mateo Canyon. The trail parallels the creek through the remote canyon, passing several pools and multi-colored rock formations. The footpath continues along the creek to Fisherman's Camp, where Tenaja Canyon merges with San Mateo Canyon. The return trail switchbacks out of the canyon, offering views across the canyon drainages.

To the trailhead

CLEVELAND FOREST ROAD · FALLBROOK   33.548979, –117.394458

From the I-15 (Temecula Valley) Freeway in Wildomar, just north of Murrieta, take the Clinton Keith Road exit. Drive 7 miles south to a stop sign at posted Tenaja Road. (Clinton Keith Road merges into Tenaja Road en route.) Turn right, staying on Tenaja Road, and drive 4.3 miles to Rancho California Road, which is posted as Cleveland Forest Road. Turn right and carefully drive 5.3 miles on

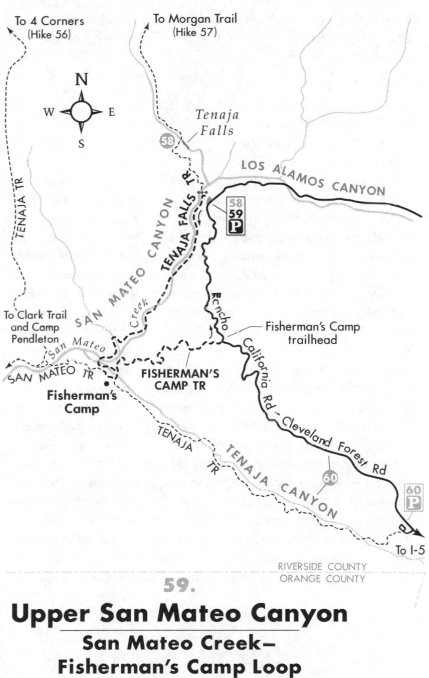

To 4 Corners
(Hike 56)

To Morgan Trail
(Hike 57)

N
W E
S

*Tenaja
Falls*

58

LOS ALAMOS CANYON

58
59 P

SAN MATEO CANYON

Creek

TENAJA FALLS TR

Rancho

Fisherman's Camp
trailhead

To Clark Trail
and Camp
Pendleton

SAN

San Mateo

SAN MATEO TR

Fisherman's
Camp

FISHERMAN'S
CAMP TR

California Rd - Cleveland Forest Rd

TENAJA TR

TENAJA CANYON

60

60 P

To I-5

RIVERSIDE COUNTY
ORANGE COUNTY

59.

Upper San Mateo Canyon

San Mateo Creek–
Fisherman's Camp Loop
SAN MATEO CANYON WILDERNESS

the winding, one-lane paved road to the well-marked trailhead and parking area on the left. A pre-paid Adventure Pass parking permit is required.

The hike

Walk 100 yards downhill on the posted trail to a signed junction. The right fork heads up canyon to Tenaja Falls (Hike 58). Bear left and head down San Mateo Canyon, passing moss-covered rocks under the shade of oaks. Follow the east side of the drainage on an easy downhill grade. At 0.8 miles, cross the creek and traverse the west canyon wall, leaving the oak groves to the exposed chaparral and sage-covered hill. Pass a series of pools on the left surrounded by metamorphic rock. Rock-hop over the creek to the east bank, and follow the edge of the rock-walled canyon past more pools. Cross the creek a third time, and curve around a wooded side canyon. Descend to the canyon floor, and follow rock cairns to where Tenaja Canyon merges with San Mateo Canyon. Cross both creeks above their confluence. Curve left into Tenaja Canyon for a short distance to a junction at 2 miles. Detour on the right fork, crossing the creek into Fisherman's Camp and a junction. The abandoned, streamside camp sits on the grassy canyon floor in an oak-filled flat. At the camp, the San Mateo Trail bears right and heads west, staying in San Mateo Canyon. The Tenaja Trail bears left in Tenaja Canyon (Hike 60).

Backtrack to the junction across the creek to start the return loop. Take the Fisherman's Camp Trail to the right (east), climbing the canyon wall to an overlook of the two canyons. Curve right and continue eastbound on the old camp road. Steadily climb to the rim of the canyon. Drop over to the east-facing slope, reaching the undeveloped Fisherman's Camp trailhead on Rancho California Road at 3.6 miles. Bear left and weave 1.6 miles downhill on the road, completing the loop. ▦

60. Tenaja Canyon

Tenaja Trail—Fisherman's Camp Loop

SAN MATEO CANYON WILDERNESS

Hiking distance: 7.9-mile loop
Hiking time: 4 hours
Configuration: loop
Elevation gain: 900 feet
Difficulty: moderate to strenuous
Exposure: riparian woodlands with exposed road on return
Dogs: allowed
Maps: U.S.G.S. Wildomar and Sitton Peak
Cleveland National Forest map

The Tenaja Trail stretches 8.5 miles across the central San Mateo Canyon Wilderness, connecting Bear Canyon in the north (off of the Ortega Highway) with Tenaja Canyon in the south. This hike makes a loop along the lush southern section of the trail through V-shaped Tenaja Canyon. The trail heads down Tenaja Canyon to Fisherman's Camp, where the mouth of the canyon merges with San Mateo Canyon. The abandoned Fisherman's Camp, once accessible by vehicle, sits in a broad grassy meadow among sycamores and 900-year-old oaks. Three trails merge at the camp. Tenaja Falls Trail heads up canyon along San Mateo Canyon to Tenaja Falls (Hike 58). The San Mateo Trail continues down canyon to the Clark Trail in San Diego County. The Fisherman's Camp Trail—the return trail for this loop—switchbacks out of the canyon on the old vehicle access road to views across the canyons.

To the trailhead

CLEVELAND FOREST ROAD · FALLBROOK   33.510016, -117.366193

From the I-15 (Temecula Valley) Freeway in Wildomar, just north of Murrieta, take the Clinton Keith Road exit. Drive 7 miles south to a stop sign at posted Tenaja Road. (Clinton Keith Road merges into Tenaja Road en route.) Turn right, staying on Tenaja Road, and drive 4.3 miles to Rancho California Road, which is posted as Cleveland Forest Road. Turn right and drive 0.9 miles to the large trailhead parking lot on the left. An Adventure Pass parking permit is required.

The hike

From the kiosk, head west on the well-defined footpath. Descend on the sandy trail through chaparral and sage brush to the oak woodland in Tenaja Canyon. Cross the seasonal creek, passing moss-covered granite boulders, and traverse the lush south wall of the canyon. The undulating path loops around a small rock-walled box canyon lined with ferns and towering sycamores. Loop around a second side canyon and continue northwest, perched on the rock wall. Return to the canyon floor and cross the drainage. Follow the northeast canyon wall a quarter mile and recross Tenaja Creek, returning to the north-facing slope.

Drop into Fisherman's Camp and a junction at 3.5 miles. The San Mateo Trail bears left, heading west down canyon along San Mateo Canyon. Take the right fork. Cross the grassy meadow and seasonal Tenaja Creek to a Y-fork just across the creek. The left fork continues up San Mateo Canyon to Tenaja Falls (Hike 58). Take the right fork on the Fisherman's Camp Trail, climbing the canyon wall to an over-look of the two canyons. Curve right and continue eastbound on the old vehicle road to the camp. Steadily climb to the rim of the canyon. Drop over to the east-facing slope, reaching the undeveloped Fisherman's Camp Trailhead on Rancho California Road at 5.1 miles.

Bear right and weave one mile up the narrow, serpentine road to a short dirt road on the right with sweeping vistas across Tenaja Canyon. Continue uphill on the main road for 100 yards, topping the hill as the road levels out. Follow the gentle downward slope 1.8 miles farther, completing the loop at the trailhead. ▩

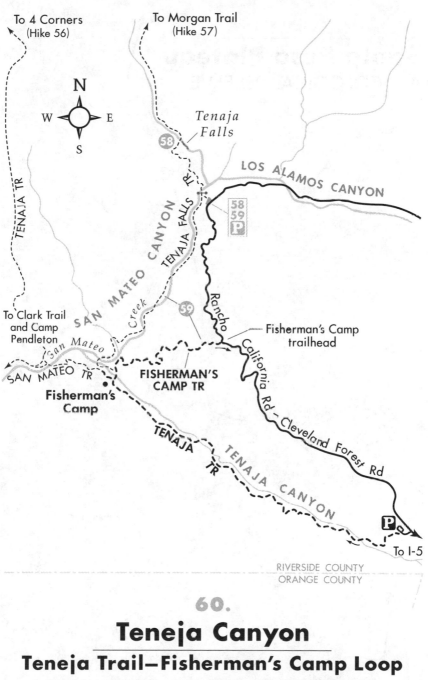

To 4 Corners
(Hike 56)

To Morgan Trail
(Hike 57)

N
W ⟷ E
S

Tenaja Falls

58

LOS ALAMOS CANYON

58 59 P

SAN MATEO CANYON

TENAJA TR

TENAJA FALLS TR

Creek

59

Rancho

To Clark Trail
and Camp
Pendleton

San Mateo

Fisherman's Camp
trailhead

SAN MATEO TR

California Rd

FISHERMAN'S
CAMP TR

Fisherman's
Camp

TENAJA TR

Cleveland Forest Rd

TENAJA CANYON

P

To I-5

RIVERSIDE COUNTY
ORANGE COUNTY

60.
Teneja Canyon
Teneja Trail—Fisherman's Camp Loop
SAN MATEO CANYON WILDERNESS

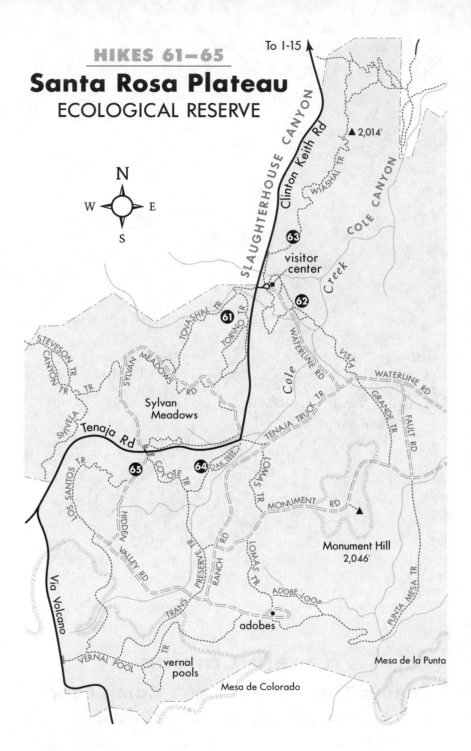

To I-15

SLAUGHTERHOUSE CANYON

Clinton Keith Rd

WIASHAL TR

▲ 2,014'

COLE CANYON

Creek

N
W — E
S

63

visitor
center

TOVASHAL TR

61

TORINO TR

62

WATERLINE RD

Cole

VISTA

WATERLINE RD

STEVESON TR

CANYON TR

TR

SYLVAN

MEADOWS

RD

Sylvan
Meadows

GRANDE TR

FAULT RD

SHVELA

Tenaja Rd

TENAJA TRUCK TR

65

COYOTE TR

64

OAK TREE

LOMAS TR

LOS SANTOS TR

HIDDEN VALLEY RD

PRESERVE TR

RANCH RD

LOMAS TR

MONUMENT RD

▲

Monument Hill
2,046'

PUNTA MESA TR

Via Volcano

TRANS

ADOBE LOOP

adobes

VERNAL POOL

TR

vernal
pools

Mesa de Colorado

Mesa de la Punta

61. Tovashal Trail—
Sylvan Meadows Loop

SANTA ROSA PLATEAU ECOLOGICAL RESERVE

Hiking distance: 2.1-mile loop
Hiking time: 1 hour
Configuration: loop
Elevation gain: 100 feet
Difficulty: easy
Exposure: exposed plateau grasslands with pockets of trees
Dogs: not allowed
Maps: U.S.G.S. Wildomar · Santa Rosa Plateau Ecological Reserve map

The Santa Rosa Plateau in Riverside County marks the southern end of the Santa Ana Mountains near the San Diego—Orange County line. A 9,000-acre ecological reserve spreads across the plateau and former ranchland. The rolling topography includes several basalt-capped mesas that rise to over 2,000 feet in elevation. The reserve provides a habitat for threatened and endangered wildlife. It also protects three rare southern California plant communities of Engelmann oak woodlands, a vernal pool ecosystem, and bunchgrass prairie (an endangered native grassland). This gentle loop begins at the visitor center and strolls through the rolling grasslands of Sylvan Meadows.

To the trailhead

39400 CLINTON KEITH ROAD · MURRIETA   33.543446, -117.271069

From the I-15 (Temecula Valley) Freeway in Wildomar, just north of Murrieta, take the Clinton Keith Road exit. Drive 4.2 miles south to the posted Santa Rosa Plateau Ecological Reserve Visitor Center on the left. Park in the lot on the left. A day-use fee is required.

The hike

From the visitor center parking lot, cross Clinton Keith Road to the posted Tovashal Trail by the white fence. Climb up and over the small hill, winding through an oak grove to a bridge at 0.1 mile. Cross the bridge and walk 20 yards to a posted trail split. Begin the loop to the right, staying on the Tovashal Trail. Stroll through grasslands and oak groves over small dips and rises. At 0.9 miles the trail ends at a T-junction with Sylvan Meadows Road in a vast meadow with twisted oaks and rock outcroppings. Take the narrow, unpaved road to the left 0.4 miles to the posted junction with the Torino Trail. Bear left through the scrub brush and curve left, looping around the oak-covered hillside. Complete the loop by the bridge, and return to the visitor center. ■

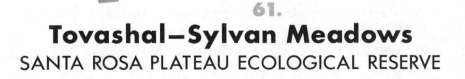

61.
Tovashal–Sylvan Meadows
SANTA ROSA PLATEAU ECOLOGICAL RESERVE

62. Granite—Vista Grande— Waterline Loop
SANTA ROSA PLATEAU ECOLOGICAL RESERVE

Hiking distance: 2.7-mile double loop
Hiking time: 1.5 hours
Configuration: figure-8 loop
Elevation gain: 100 feet
Difficulty: easy
Exposure: exposed grassland plateau with pockets of trees
Dogs: not allowed
Maps: U.S.G.S. Wildomar · Santa Rosa Plateau Ecological Reserve map

The Santa Rosa Plateau lies adjacent to the city of Murrieta and is accessed south of town through Slaughterhouse Canyon. The canyon emerges from the top of the plateau, where this trail begins. The hike explores the vast cross-section of habitats within the plateau reserve. The trails circle the visitor center through native chaparral with beautiful rock outcroppings, bunchgrass prairie meadows, oak woodlands, overlooks with vistas of the reserve, and streamside riparian habitats. Along the creek are *tenajas*, pools in the basalt-lined creekbeds that contain water throughout the dry summer.

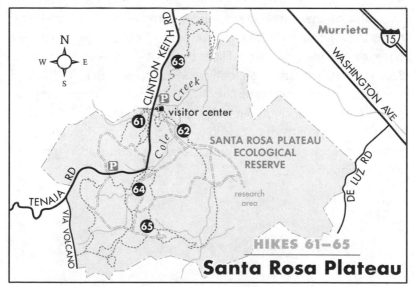

To the trailhead

From the I-15 (Temecula Valley) Freeway in Wildomar, just north of Murrieta, take the Clinton Keith Road exit. Drive 4.2 miles south to the posted Santa Rosa Plateau Ecological Reserve Visitor Center on the left. Park in the lot on the left. A day-use fee is required.

The hike

From the south side of the parking lot, take the posted Granite Loop Trail past the visitor center through native scrub and rock outcroppings. Climb over a small hill to vistas of the reserve, oak woodlands, and beautiful rock formations. Descend to the grassland meadows and oak groves. Cross a footbridge over the seasonal creek, a tributary of Cole Creek. Traverse the small hills from meadow to meadow, passing majestic, twisted oaks. Cross a second footbridge over an ephemeral stream to a junction at Waterline Road. To the left, the dirt road leads 0.2 miles back to the visitor center. Stay on the path straight ahead for 50 yards to another junction. The Granite Loop continues straight.

For now, bear right on the Vista Grande Trail along the east side of the waterway, the beginning of the second loop. Cross a bridge over the wetland. Detour 25 yards to the right to an overlook of the creekside pools. Return to the main trail, and climb the hill to a meadow surrounded by oaks. Follow the east edge of the meadow to a T-junction with the Waterline Road. Bear right 100 yards to a junction with Tenaja Truck Trail. Go to the right, staying on Waterline Road 0.6 miles, completing the second loop. Bear right, back on the Granite Loop Trail. Head up the hill past granite outcroppings. Wind through the tall scrub, looping back to the north side of the trailhead parking lot and visitor center. ■

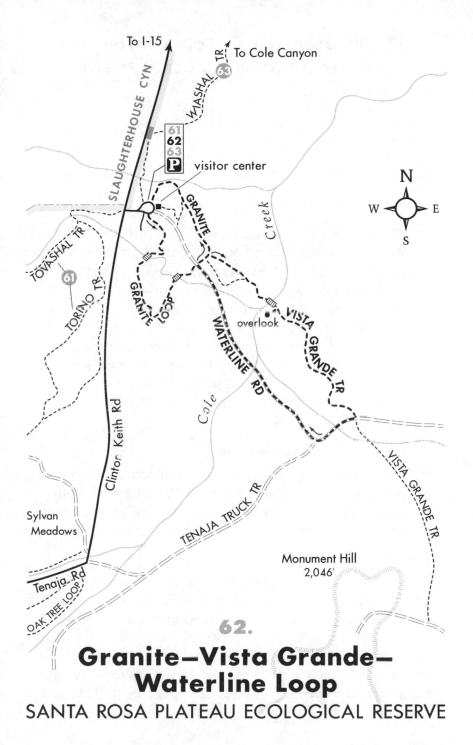

To I-15

To Cole Canyon

SLAUGHTERHOUSE CYN

WIASHAL TR

63

61
62
63
Ⓟ visitor center

N
W ⚬ E
S

GRANITE

Creek

TOVASHAL TR

61

TORINO TR

GRANITE LOOP

overlook

VISTA GRANDE TR

WATERLINE RD

Cole

Clinton Keith Rd

VISTA GRANDE TR

Sylvan
Meadows

TENAJA TRUCK TR

Monument Hill
2,046'

Tenaja Rd

OAK TREE LOOP

62.
Granite–Vista Grande–
Waterline Loop
SANTA ROSA PLATEAU ECOLOGICAL RESERVE

63. Wiashal Trail to Cole Canyon
SANTA ROSA PLATEAU ECOLOGICAL RESERVE

Hiking distance: 6 miles round trip
Hiking time: 3.5 hours
Configuration: lollipop, with trail spur to Cole Canyon
Elevation gain: 1,000 feet
Difficulty: strenuous
Exposure: exposed rocky ridgeline with segment of wooded canyon
Dogs: not allowed
Maps: U.S.G.S. Wildomar · Santa Rosa Plateau Ecological Reserve map

Cole Canyon is a short, narrow canyon with 800-foot walls. The stream-fed canyon is located at the edge of Temecula Valley by Murrieta and east of Slaughterhouse Canyon. Access to the canyon from the Santa Rosa Plateau is via the Wiashal Trail, a demanding hike that follows the ridge straddling Slaughterhouse and Cole canyons. The trail begins at the visitor center and climbs along the spine of the mountain from summit to summit, with frequent elevation gains and losses. From the ridge are panoramic views of the Santa Anas and the Santa Margaritas. The route descends from the arid ridge into riparian, oak-filled Cole Canyon.

To the trailhead

39400 CLINTON KEITH ROAD · MURRIETA   33.543446, -117.271069

From the I-15 (Temecula Valley) Freeway in Wildomar, just north of Murrieta, take the Clinton Keith Road exit. Drive 4.2 miles south to the posted Santa Rosa Plateau Ecological Reserve Visitor Center on the left. Park in the lot on the left. A day-use fee is required.

The hike

From the upper end of the parking lot, next to Clinton Keith Road, take the posted Wiashal Trail north, parallel to the road. Cross a footbridge over a drainage to a roadside trailhead. Head up the hill and away from the road, passing giant granite boulders to the top of a knoll. Continue across the hills, roughly following the ridge from summit to summit and valley to valley. Just before the prominent 2,014-foot summit is a posted junction.

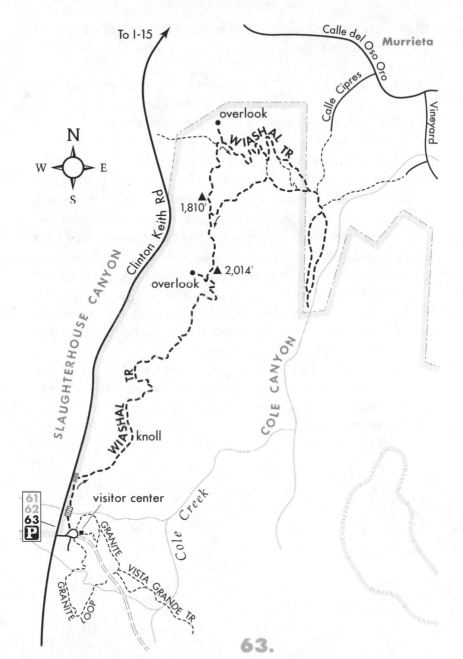

To I-15

Calle del Oso Oro **Murrieta**

Calle Cipres

Vineyard

overlook

WIASHAL TR

N
W E
S

Clinton Keith Rd

1,810'

2,014'

overlook

SLAUGHTERHOUSE CANYON

WIASHAL TR

COLE CANYON

knoll

visitor center

61
62
63
P

GRANITE

Cole Creek

VISTA GRANDE TR

GRANITE LOOP

63.
Wiashal Trail to Cole Canyon
SANTA ROSA PLATEAU ECOLOGICAL RESERVE

Detour 0.1 mile left to the overlook on a finger of land, with vistas of Murrieta, the Santa Ana Range, and the Santa Margarita Mountains.

Return to the Wiashal Trail and continue north, curving around the west side of the summit. Follow the ridge across the saddle toward the 1,810-foot peak. In the saddle is a trail on the right—the return route. At this point, stay on the ridge between Slaughterhouse Canyon and Cole Canyon, climbing to the peak while overlooking Temecula Valley. Just beyond the summit is another junction. Detour a short distance to the left, passing huge boulders to an overlook of the distant San Bernardino and San Jacinto Mountains. Return and descend on the east-facing slope, zigzagging down towards the mouth of Cole Canyon. On a left switchback, 250 feet above the canyon floor, a trail veers off to the right. This is the return route. For now, continue to the canyon bottom through an oak woodland. Bear right along the base of the canyon's west wall. Several parallel paths weave into the canyon. Explore along your own route.

Head back up the hillside to the return trail. Take the sandy path and weave up the draw between the two peaks, completing the loop in the saddle on the ridge. Return to the left (south) along the same trail. ▪

64. Coyote Trail—Oak Tree Loop

SANTA ROSA PLATEAU ECOLOGICAL RESERVE

Hiking distance: 2.2 miles round trip
Hiking time: 1 hour
Configuration: lollipop
Elevation gain: 100 feet
Difficulty: easy
Exposure: mostly open grassland plateau
Dogs: not allowed
Maps: U.S.G.S. Wildomar · Santa Rosa Plateau Ecological Reserve map

The Santa Rosa Plateau was a hunting ground and acorn gathering area for the Luiseno Indians for more than 2,000 years. Indian mortar holes can be found in the granite outcrops. This short loop hike meanders through the rolling hill country, weaving through bunchgrass prairie, rare Engelmann oak woodlands, rock outcroppings, and streamside riparian habitat.

To the trailhead

22113 TENAJA ROAD · MURRIETA   33.527389, –117.284212

From the I-15 (Temecula Valley) Freeway in Wildomar, just north of Murrieta, take the Clinton Keith Road exit. Drive 5.9 miles south to the posted Hidden Valley Trailhead on the left. (The turnoff is located 1.7 miles past the Santa Rosa Plateau Reserve Visitor Center.) A day-use fee is required.

The hike

At the trailhead, the right fork follows Hidden Valley Road, an old ranch road to Mesa de Colorado (Hike 65). Take the left fork on the Coyote Trail. Wind up the hillside to vistas of the surrounding terrain. Traverse the hillside across rolling grasslands and oak woodlands. Curve right and descend to a junction with the Trans Preserve Trail at a half mile. The right fork leads 1.3 miles to historic adobes, early ranch buildings from 1846 (Hike 65).

Bear left and curve downhill through the oak-dotted meadows to a trail split with the Oak Tree Trail. Veer left, hiking the loop clockwise. Meander through oak groves strewn with multicolored rocks to the former Oak Tree trailhead, located at the junction of Clinton Keith Road and Tenaja Road. Just before reaching the road, veer sharply to the right to Cole Creek. Parallel the seasonal creek through oaks and sycamores, completing the loop. Bear left, retracing your steps back to the trailhead. ■

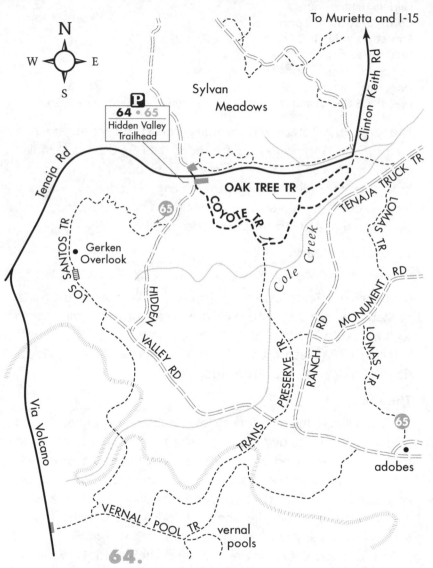

Coyote Trail—Oak Tree Loop
SANTA ROSA PLATEAU ECOLOGICAL RESERVE

65. Vernal Pools and Historic Adobes Loop

SANTA ROSA PLATEAU ECOLOGICAL RESERVE

Hiking distance: 6.5-mile loop
Hiking time: 3 hours
Configuration: loop
Elevation gain: 250 feet
Difficulty: easy to moderate
Exposure: open grassland plateau
Dogs: not allowed
Maps: U.S.G.S. Wildomar · Santa Rosa Plateau Ecological Reserve map

Atop Mesa de Colorado on the Santa Rosa Plateau are four shallow depressions formed from ancient lava flows. Water collects in the basalt rock depressions, creating pools. As the pools evaporate, concentric rings of multi-colored wildflowers grow along the moist, receding shoreline. The springtime pools along this trail are among the largest vernal pools in the state and act as a seasonal wetland for waterfowl.

Below the mesa on the valley floor are two ranch structures known as the Moreno and Machado Adobes. They are original buildings from the 47,815-acre Rancho Santa Rosa, dating back to 1846. These are the oldest surviving buildings in Riverside County. A majestic pecan grove by the adobes was planted in the early 1900s.

This hike forms a loop—visiting both the vernal pools and the historic adobes—on old ranch roads and trails in the southwest section of the reserve.

To the trailhead

22113 TENAJA ROAD · MURRIETA   33.527389, -117.284212

From the I-15 (Temecula Valley) Freeway in Wildomar, just north of Murrieta, take the Clinton Keith Road exit. Drive 5.9 miles south to the posted Hidden Valley Trailhead on the left. (The turnoff is located 1.7 miles past the Santa Rosa Plateau Reserve Visitor Center.) A day-use fee is required.

The hike

From the trailhead, the Coyote Trail (Hike 64) bears left. Take the right fork, straight ahead, on the Hidden Valley Road. Cross the open rolling grasslands on the old ranch road. At the crest of the first hill is a trail. Bear right on the Los Santos Trail, and weave up, down, and around the oak-dotted hills to a cluster of oaks on the ridge overlooking the De Luz Creek drainage to the west. Follow the ridge south to a bench on the Gerken Overlook, with views across the reserve basin to the Mesa De Burro Research Area. Drop into a small valley and cross a footbridge over a transient stream. Follow the drainage to a posted junction at 1.4 miles. Bear right, staying on the Los Santos Trail through the oak-studded hills on the west ridge of the valley. Descend and cross a canyon to Mesa De Colorado and a T-junction at 2.6 miles. To the right is the Vernal Pool Trailhead on Via Volcano.

Bear left and follow the mesa east 0.7 miles to an interpretive panel describing the life cycle of the pools, granite, and volcanic rock. Ahead is a four-way junction. Take either of the two right forks, looping through the vernal pool area on a boardwalk, and return to the junction. Continue on the main trail, steadily dropping from the mesa to the valley floor. At 4.3 miles, the trail ends on Ranch Road. Go 0.1 mile to the right towards the barn by the adobes and explore the area.

From the end of the road, the Punta Mesa Trail heads east. Instead, take the Lomas Trail north from the barn, up the hillside. Cross the oak savanna 0.7 miles to Monument Road, and bear left to Ranch Road. Cross the road and follow the footpath to the Trans Preserve Trail. Bear right and descend to the oak-filled canyon floor. Cross Cole Creek two times to a trail split. Bear left on the Coyote Trail, returning to the trailhead a half mile ahead. ■

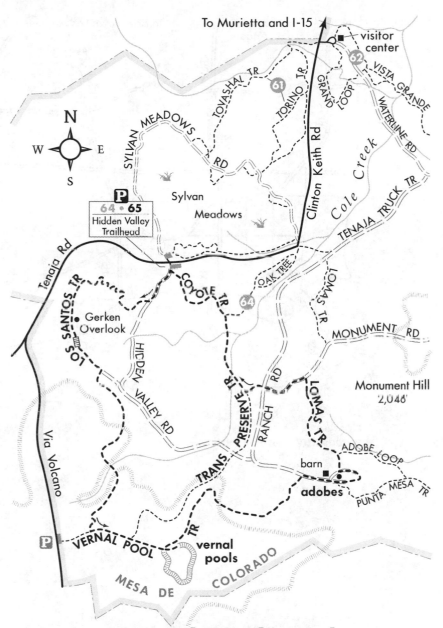

To Murietta and I-15

visitor center

62

VISTA GRANDE

TOYASHAL TR

61

TORINO TR

GRAND LOOP

WATERLINE RD

Clinton Keith Rd

Cole Creek

TENAJA TRUCK TR

N
W • E
S

SYLVAN MEADOWS RD

Sylvan Meadows

P
64 • 65
Hidden Valley Trailhead

Tenaja Rd

LOS SANTOS TR

Gerken Overlook

COYOTE TR

OAK TREE

64

LOMAS TR

MONUMENT RD

Monument Hill
2,048'

HIDDEN VALLEY RD

TRANS. PRESERVE TR

RANCH RD

LOMAS TR

ADOBE LOOP

barn

adobes

PUNTA MESA TR

Via Volcano

P
VERNAL POOL TR

vernal pools

MESA DE COLORADO

65. **Vernal Pools and Historic Adobes Loop**
SANTA ROSA PLATEAU ECOLOGICAL RESERVE

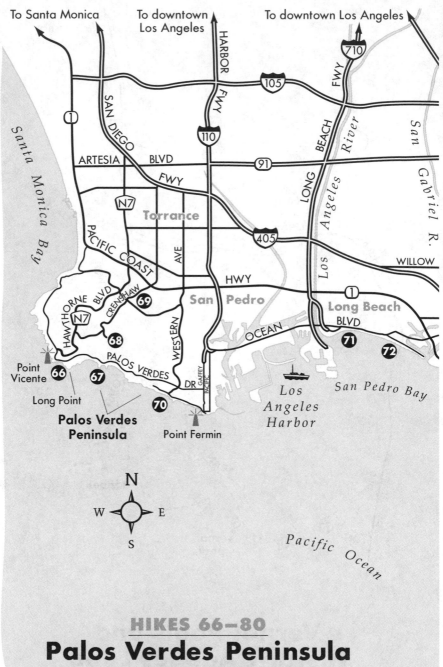

To Santa Monica

To downtown Los Angeles

To downtown Los Angeles

HARBOR FWY

105

710

I-710 FWY

SAN DIEGO FWY

1

San Gabriel R.

BEACH

Los Angeles River

San

ARTESIA BLVD

FWY

91

LONG

Angeles

N7

Torrance

405

PACIFIC COAST BLVD

AVE

Los

WILLOW

HAWTHORNE BLVD

CRENSHAW

69

HWY

San Pedro

N7

WESTERN

68

OCEAN

Long Beach

BLVD

71

72

PALOS VERDES

Point Vicente 66

67

DR

GAFFEY

PACIFIC

Long Point

70

Los Angeles Harbor

San Pedro Bay

Palos Verdes Peninsula

Point Fermin

N

W — E

S

Pacific Ocean

HIKES 66–80

Palos Verdes Peninsula to Corona Del Mar

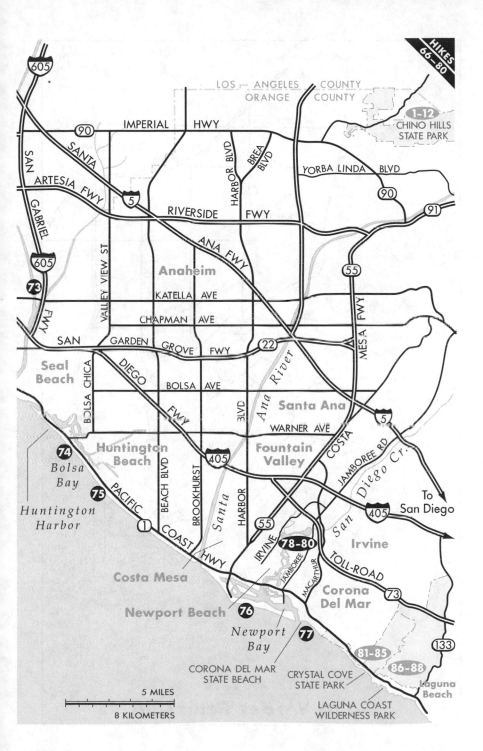

HIKES 66–80

LOS ANGELES COUNTY
ORANGE COUNTY

1-12
CHINO HILLS
STATE PARK

IMPERIAL HWY

90

SANTA

ARTESIA FWY

SAN GABRIEL FWY

605

73

5

RIVERSIDE FWY

HARBOR BLVD

BREA BLVD

YORBA LINDA BLVD

90

91

ANA FWY

Anaheim

VALLEY VIEW ST

KATELLA AVE

CHAPMAN AVE

SAN GARDEN GROVE FWY

22

55

MESA FWY

Seal Beach

BOLSA CHICA

SAN DIEGO FWY

BOLSA AVE

Ana River

Santa Ana

5

74

Bolsa Bay

75

Huntington Beach

PACIFIC COAST HWY

1

BEACH BLVD

BROOKHURST

BLVD

Santa Harbor

WARNER AVE

405

COSTA

Fountain Valley

JAMBOREE RD

San Diego Cr.

To San Diego

405

Huntington Harbor

Costa Mesa

55

Irvine

78–80

JAMBOREE

San

Irvine

TOLL-ROAD

73

Corona Del Mar

133

Newport Beach

76

MACARTHUR

Newport Bay

77

81–85

86–88

Laguna Beach

CORONA DEL MAR
STATE BEACH

CRYSTAL COVE
STATE PARK

LAGUNA COAST
WILDERNESS PARK

5 MILES

8 KILOMETERS

225

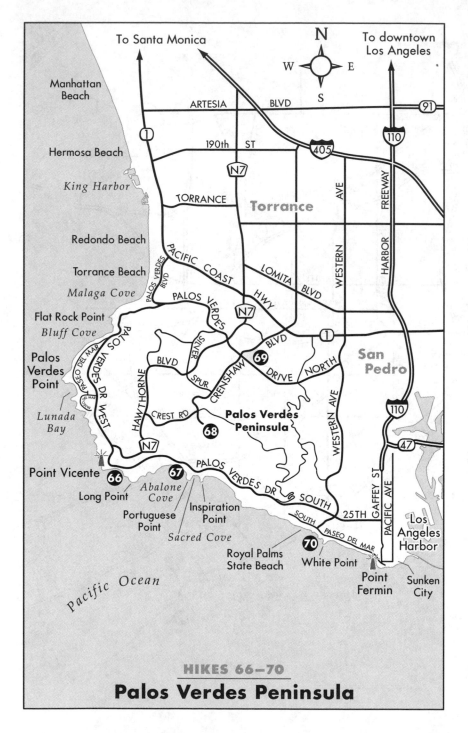

HIKES 66–70
Palos Verdes Peninsula

66. Point Vicente
FISHING ACCESS TRAIL

Hiking distance: 1.5 miles round trip
Hiking time: 1 hour
Configuration: out-and-back
Elevation gain: 140 feet
Exposure: exposed coastline
Difficulty: easy
Dogs: allowed
Maps: U.S.G.S. Redondo Beach

Point Vicente is situated on the southwest point of the Palos Verdes Peninsula. Perched on the cliffs high above the shore is the historic 67-foot Point Vicente Lighthouse, built in 1926. The lighthouse warned ships of the rocky shoals in the Catalina Channel. From the 140-foot scalloped bluffs are vistas of the lighthouse, Santa Catalina Island, and Long Point on the southeast end of the bay. This is a premier spot to observe migrating gray whales from mid-December through March.

The Point Vicente Fishing Access Trail descends the eroding cliffs to the rounded cobblestone beach beneath Point Vicente and Long Point, where the tidepools are teeming with marine life. The crescent-shaped bay with large offshore rocks is a popular site for scuba divers, surfers, and anglers.

To the trailhead

6400 Palos Verdes Drive South · Rancho Palos Verdes
33.741539, -118.402509

From the Pacific Coast Highway (Highway 1) at the south end of Torrance, take Hawthorne Boulevard south 7.3 miles to its terminus at the coast. Turn left on Palos Verdes Drive South, and drive 0.8 miles to the posted fishing access. Park in the lot on the right.

The hike

Walk to the west (upper) end of the parking lot. Take the well-defined dirt path, just beyond the restrooms. Descend the cliffs on an easy grade towards the prominent Point Vicente Lighthouse. Halfway down the slope, switchback left, dropping down to the rocky cobblestone shoreline. The beach pocket is bordered on the west by steep cliffs and a natural rock jetty. On the south end, the beach ends near Long Point, where the cliffs drop 100 feet into the sea near the offshore rock outcroppings. ■

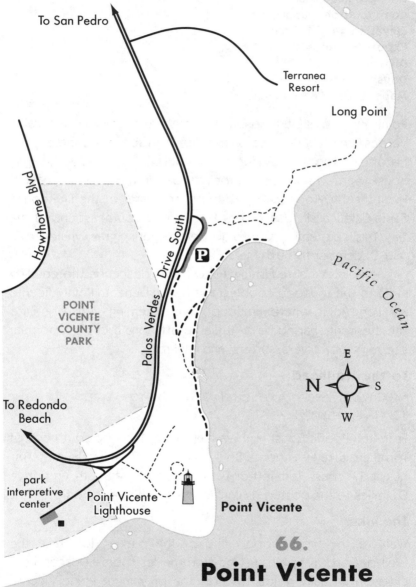

66.
Point Vicente
FISHING ACCESS TRAIL

67. Abalone Cove and Portuguese Point
PALOS VERDES PENINSULA

Hiking distance: 2 miles round trip
Hiking time: 1 hour
Configuration: two loops
Elevation gain: 150 feet
Exposure: exposed coastline
Difficulty: easy
Dogs: allowed
Maps: U.S.G.S. Redondo Beach and San Pedro

Abalone Cove Shoreline Park and Ecological Preserve is a federal reserve where grassy 180-foot bluffs offer easy access to the rocky shoreline. The 80-acre preserve extends from Abalone Cove to Portuguese Point and Sacred Cove (also known as Smugglers Cove). Sacred Cove is bordered by tidepools at both points. From Portuguese Point are magnificent views of Abalone Cove, Long Point, Sacred Cove, Inspiration Point, White Point, Point Fermin, and Catalina Island. The oceanfront park sits at the foot of the unstable and actively slipping Portuguese Bend landslide area.

To the trailhead

5970 PALOS VERDES DRIVE SOUTH · RANCHO PALOS VERDES
33.744121, -118.381392

From the Pacific Coast Highway/Highway 1 at the south end of Torrance, take Hawthorne Boulevard south 7.3 miles to its terminus at the coast. Turn left on Palos Verdes Drive South, and drive 2.2 miles to the posted Abalone Cove Shoreline Park entrance. Turn right and park in the lot. A parking fee is required.

The hike

From the east end of the parking lot, cross the grassy picnic area onto a wide gravel path. Continue to a vehicle-restricted road. Bear left and wind up the hillside on the restricted road to Palos Verdes Drive. Bear to the left on the narrow path, parallel to the highway, for 0.2 miles to the Portuguese Point access. Walk up the curving, gated road to the north edge of the peninsula and a trail split. First, take the left fork out to Portuguese Point, which stays atop the peninsula and loops around the perimeter.

After enjoying the awesome coastal views from the point, return to the trail split Take the left fork down to the beach and tidepools near an old rock enclosure. The trail to the left leads to the base of the cliffs at Portuguese Point. To return, follow the shoreline trail back along Abalone Cove for 0.4 miles to Upper Beach, a raised, man-made sandy beach and lifeguard station just above the rocky shore. Curve right and take the old paved road to a trail junction. The footpath to the left ascends the cliffs through the dense brush, back to the parking lot. ■

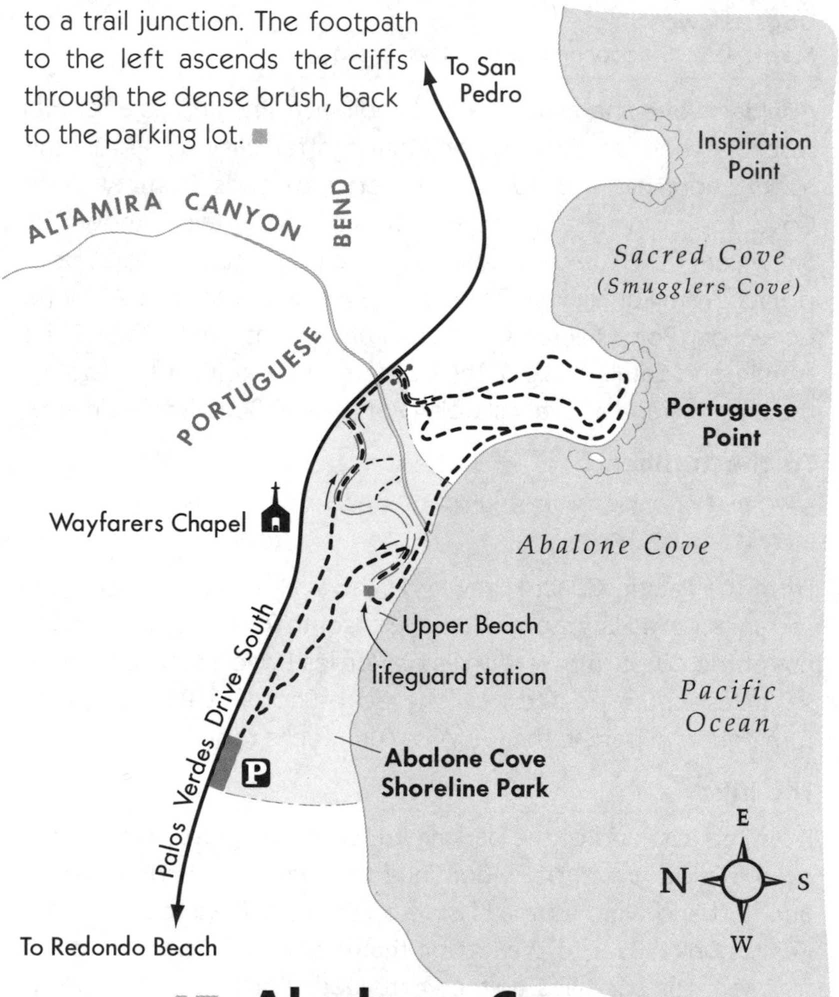

To San Pedro

ALTAMIRA CANYON

BEND

Inspiration Point

Sacred Cove
(Smugglers Cove)

PORTUGUESE

Portuguese Point

Wayfarers Chapel

Abalone Cove

Upper Beach

lifeguard station

Pacific Ocean

Palos Verdes Drive South

P

Abalone Cove Shoreline Park

E

N ◆ S

W

To Redondo Beach

67. Abalone Cove Portuguese Point

68. Portuguese Bend Overlook
Crenshaw Extension Trail from Del Cerro Park

PALOS VERDES PENINSULA

Hiking distance: 2.8 miles round trip
Hiking time: 1.5 hours
Configuration: out-and-back with loop
Elevation gain: 500 feet
Exposure: exposed with shaded pockets
Difficulty: easy to moderate
Dogs: allowed
Maps: U.S.G.S. Torrance

This hike begins in Del Cerro Park in Rancho Palos Verdes, which sits atop the Palos Verdes Peninsula at more than 1,100 feet. From the park overlook are spectacular southern views of the 13 distinct marine terraces that make up the peninsula and the massive 270-acre landslide area of Portuguese Bend. The Crenshaw Extension Trail descends from Del Cerro Park into the precarious bowl-shaped canyon, still active with faults and shifting ground. A trail system winds through the rolling green hills and ancient wave-cut terraces to the shady Portuguese Bend Overlook, perched high above Portuguese Bend, Portuguese Point, and Inspiration Point (Hike 67).

To the trailhead

2 PARK PLACE · RANCHO PALOS VERDES   33.757170, -118.368810

From the Pacific Coast Highway/Highway 1 at the south end of Torrance, take Crenshaw Boulevard south 3.9 miles to the trailhead at the end of the road.

The hike

Before starting down the trail, walk 30 yards up the road, and bear left into Del Cerro Park for a bird's-eye view of the surrounding hills, coastline, and the trails that you are about to hike. Return to the metal trailhead gate, and take the unpaved road, passing a few hilltop homes. Descend into the unspoiled open space overlooking layers of rolling hills, the magnificent Palos

Verdes coastline, and the island of Catalina. At just under a half mile is a three-way trail split by a water tank on the left. Follow the main road, curving to the right a quarter mile to an unsigned footpath on the left. Detour left to the distinctive 950-foot knoll dotted with pine trees. From the overlook are sweeping coastal views, including Point Vicente, Portuguese Point, Inspiration Point, and Catalina Island.

Return from the overlook to the main trail. Continue downhill, curving left on a wide horseshoe bend. Just beyond the bend, a road veers off to the right, leading to Narcissa Drive. Twelve yards past this road split is a distinct footpath on the left. Leave the road and take this path through a forest of feathery sweet fennel plants. The path curves left, overlooking Portuguese Canyon. A switchback cuts back to the west and climbs the hillside to a ridge at a T-junction. The right fork follows the ridge uphill to the summit again, completing a loop on the pine-covered knoll. Descend from the knoll to the main trail (the same route hiked earlier). Bear right, returning to the trailhead. ■

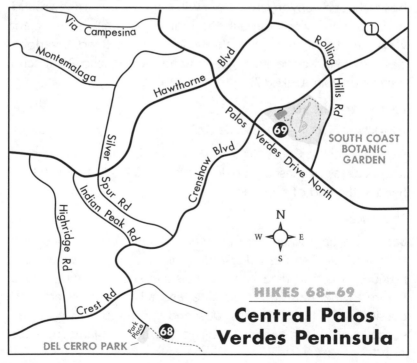

HIKES 68–69
**Central Palos
Verdes Peninsula**

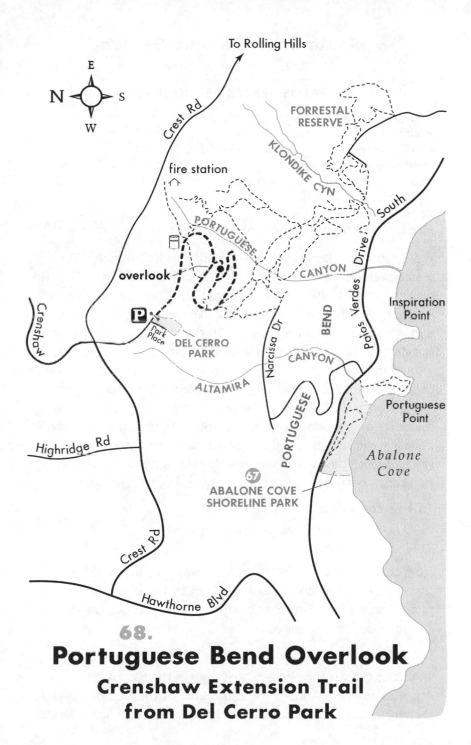

68.
Portuguese Bend Overlook
Crenshaw Extension Trail
from Del Cerro Park

69. South Coast Botanic Garden

Open daily 9 a.m.—5 p.m.

PALOS VERDES PENINSULA

Hiking distance: 1—2 miles round trip
Hiking time: 1—2 hours
Configuration: many inter-connecting paths
Elevation gain: 100 feet
Exposure: mixed sun and shade gardens
Difficulty: very easy
Dogs: not allowed
Maps: U.S.G.S. Torrance · South Coast Botanic Garden map

The South Coast Botanic Garden, owned by Los Angeles County, was developed on a sanitary landfill site in 1959. The 87-acre garden includes plant collections that represent southern Africa, Australia, and the Mediterranean. Within this impressive garden is a rose garden with more than 1,600 hybrids that circles a large fountain, a children's garden with a miniature enchanted house, a gazebo, an arched bridge over a fish pond, a succulent and cactus garden, herb and vegetable gardens, a fuchsia garden, and a water-wise garden. A large man-made lake with an island supports an abundant bird population. A canyon with a channel of water winds through riparian and marshland habitats, a woodland of pines and junipers, coastal redwoods, flowering fruit trees, palm trees, and over 50 species of eucalyptus trees.

To the trailhead

26300 CRENSHAW BLVD · PALOS VERDES PENINSULA
33.783524, -118.349045

From the Pacific Coast Highway/Highway 1 at the south end of Torrance, take Crenshaw Boulevard south 1 mile to the posted turnoff on the left. Turn left and drive 0.2 miles to the parking lot. An entrance fee is required.

The hike

Walk past the gift shop to a hub of trails at the top of the garden. A paved road/trail circles the perimeter of the botanic garden. Numerous unpaved roads and trails weave through the tiered landscape leading to the lake. Let your interests lead you through the gardens along your own route. ■

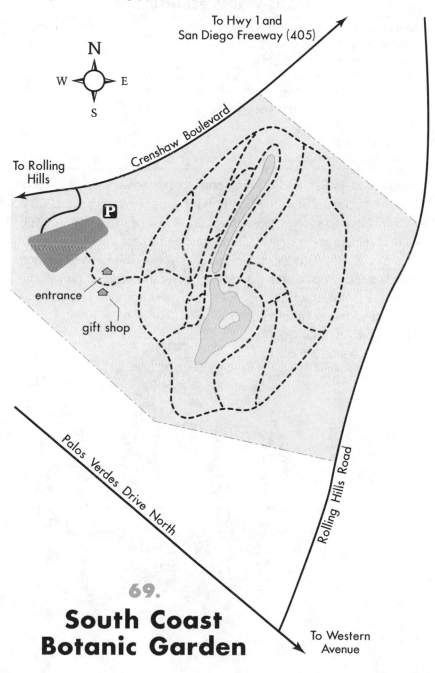

To Hwy 1 and
San Diego Freeway (405)

N
W ← ⊕ → E
S

Crenshaw Boulevard

To Rolling
Hills

P

entrance

gift shop

Palos Verdes Drive North

Rolling Hills Road

To Western
Avenue

69.

South Coast Botanic Garden

70. White Point and Point Fermin Park
PALOS VERDES PENINSULA

Hiking distance: 4 miles round trip
Hiking time: 2 hours
Configuration: out-and-back
(or return along South Paseo Del Mar for a loop)
Elevation gain: 100 feet
Exposure: exposed coastline and shady blufftop park
Difficulty: easy
Dogs: allowed
Maps: U.S.G.S. San Pedro

White Point in San Pedro was home to the Royal Palms Hotel, a booming spa resort with hot sulphur pools predating the 1920s. Falling victim to storms, pounding surf, and an earthquake in 1933, all that remain are majestic palms, garden terraces, and remnants of the concrete foundation. To the east of the point is White Point Beach, a rocky cove with tidepools below the sedimentary cliffs. From the point, the trail continues two miles to Point Fermin Park, located at the southernmost tip in Los Angeles County. The long coastal park sits

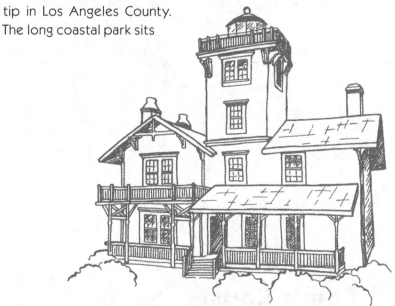

The Point Fermin Lighthouse was build in 1874.

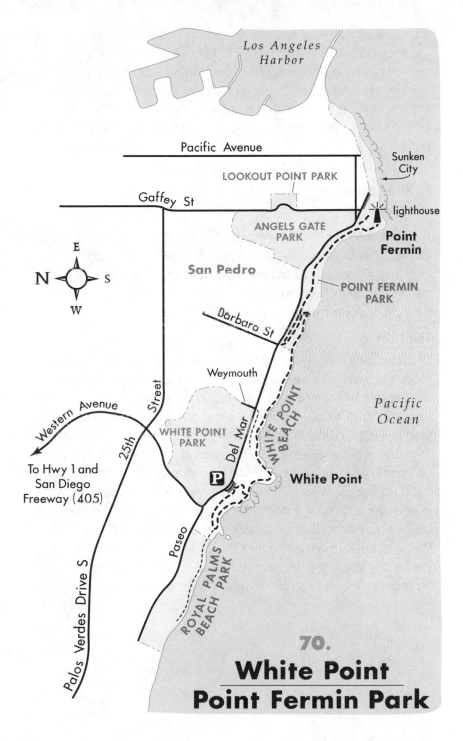

Los Angeles Harbor

Pacific Avenue

LOOKOUT POINT PARK

Sunken City

Gaffey St

lighthouse

ANGELS GATE PARK

Point Fermin

San Pedro

E

N ✦ S

W

POINT FERMIN PARK

Darbara St

Weymouth

Western Avenue

Street

WHITE POINT PARK

Del Mar

WHITE POINT BEACH

Pacific Ocean

25th

To Hwy 1 and San Diego Freeway (405)

P

White Point

Paseo

ROYAL PALMS BEACH PARK

Palos Verdes Drive S

70.

White Point
Point Fermin Park

atop grassy tree-shaded bluffs that jut prominently out to sea. The scenic 37-acre park has flower gardens, mature fig trees, and curving pathways that lead from the bluffs to the rocky shoreline.

Point Fermin Lighthouse is an historic Victorian structure that sits on the edge of the vertical cliffs. It was built in 1874 with lumber and bricks shipped around Cape Horn. The lighthouse was in use for nearly a century. It is now a museum and open for tours (Tuesday through Sunday).

To the trailhead

1700 WEST PASEO DEL MAR · SAN PEDRO   33.716462, -118.317981

From the intersection of Western Avenue and 25th Street in San Pedro, drive 0.5 miles south to the end of Western Avenue at the coastline. Curve left onto Paseo Del Mar, and drive 0.1 mile to the White Point Bluff Park parking lot on the right. Park in the lot for a fee or alongside the road for free.

The hike

Descend the cliffs on the dirt path or walk west down the paved road to Royal Palms Beach Park. Head east and follow the coastline around White Point, crossing over small boulders and slabs of rock. Stroll along the rocky shore of White Point Beach below the ruins of the Royal Palms Hotel. Continue following the shoreline past a group of old homes at the base of the sheer 120-foot cliffs. At 1.2 miles, take the distinct path on the left, and head up the cliffs to the west. Half way up, the path becomes paved. Wind through a palm tree grove and up to the top of the bluffs across from Barbara Street, at the west end of Point Fermin Park. Continue east for one mile through the narrow, tree-shaded park along the edge of the grassy bluffs to Point Fermin and the lighthouse. This is the turn-around point. Return along the same path. ▪

71. Long Beach Oceanfront Trail to Belmont Pier

LONG BEACH CITY BEACH

Hiking distance: 7 miles round trip
Hiking time: 3.5 hours
Configuration: out-and-back; optional side trip out onto Belmont Pier
Elevation gain: level
Exposure: exposed beach coastline
Difficulty: easy to moderate
Dogs: not allowed
Maps: U.S.G.S. Long Beach

The Long Beach Oceanfront Trail is a paved walking and biking path along the San Pedro Bay coastline in Long Beach. Long Beach is the southernmost coastal city in Los Angeles County. Long Beach City Beach, which fronts the path, extends four miles from the Long Beach Harbor to the Alamitos Peninsula and San Gabriel River on the Orange County line.

This hike begins at the mouth of the Los Angeles River in Queensway Bay by Shoreline Village, a tourist attraction with shops and restaurants. The path follows the coastline along Long Beach City Beach to Belmont Pier. En route is Bluff Park, an elevated grassy park above the wide, sandy beach overlooking San Pedro Bay. Bluff Park backs the beach and runs parallel to Ocean Boulevard. Offshore from the beach and path are four artificial tropical islands with postcard-perfect fronts. They are actually landscaped oil drilling platforms.

Belmont Pier—the destination for the hike—is a 1,600-foot T-shaped pier that bisects Long Beach City Beach. The pier was built in 1968 at the foot of 39th Place in Belmont Shore, a charming seaside community filled with shops and eateries. After Belmont Pier, the path continues along the shoreline to Alamitos Bay—Hike 72.

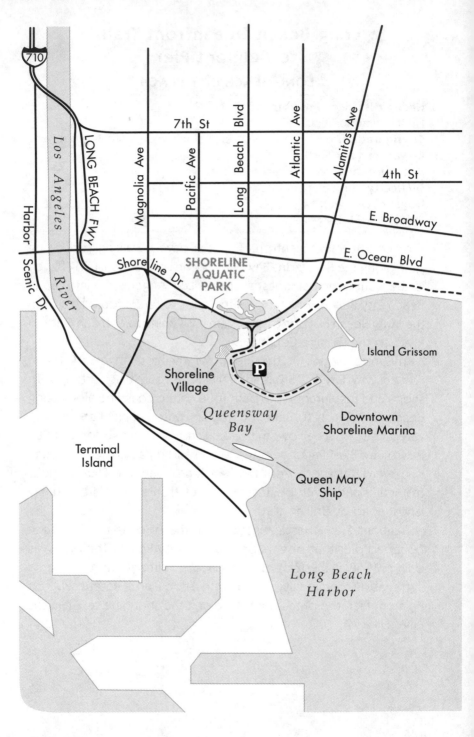

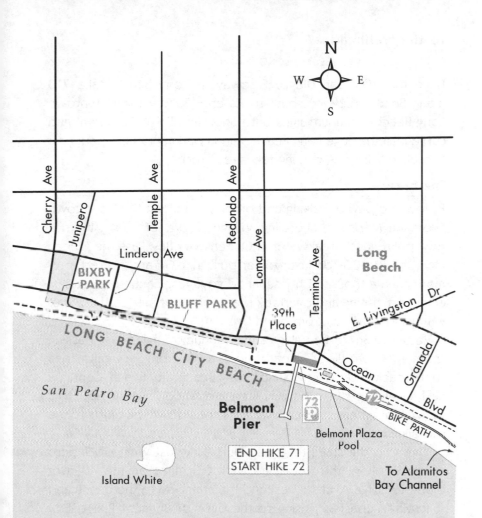

Cherry Ave

Junipero

Temple Ave

Lindero Ave

Redondo Ave

Loma Ave

Termino Ave

Long Beach

BIXBY PARK

BLUFF PARK

39th Place

E. Livingston Dr

LONG BEACH CITY BEACH

Granada

San Pedro Bay

Ocean

Blvd

Belmont Pier

72 P

Belmont Plaza Pool

72

BIKE PATH

END HIKE 71
START HIKE 72

Island White

To Alamitos Bay Channel

Island Freeman

Island Chaffe

71.
Long Beach Oceanfront Trail to Belmont Pier

LONG BEACH CITY BEACH

To the trailhead

435 SHORELINE VILLAGE DR · LONG BEACH   33.759564, -118.191222

From the 405 (San Diego) Freeway in Long Beach, take 710 (Long Beach Freeway) south to its end. Follow the Downtown Long Beach/Aquarium signs onto Shoreline Drive. Turn right and curve into the huge Long Beach Marina parking lot and park near Shoreline Village. A parking fee is required.

The hike

Follow the paved walking and biking path along the Downtown Shoreline Marina to Shoreline Village. Curve left along the narrow, palm-lined breakwater in Queensway Bay. Pass the Queen Mary, an 81,000-ton luxury liner built in 1934 and retired after more than a thousand transatlantic voyages. Continue past several short fishing and overlook piers for a half mile to the breakwater's end, across from Island Grissom.

Return to Shoreline Village and continue 0.5 miles east, passing the marina boat slips. The path curves away from the small marina to the back end of wide, sandy Long Beach City Beach. Continue east, curving past the historic lifeguard station built in 1938, to a parking lot where Junipero Avenue winds down the bluffs to the shoreline parking lot.

Climb up the stairs to grassy Bluff Park, just west of Lindero Avenue. Follow the tree-filled park 0.8 miles on the 40-foot bluffs to Loma Avenue. Descend the stairway to the beach and follow the coastline, rising to the base of Belmont Pier off of 39th Place in Belmont Shore. This is the turn-around spot.

For an optional side trip, The Belmont Pier extends 1,600 feet into the bay. The long pier is a popular site for fishing and strolling.

The oceanfront trail continues along the sandy coastline for another two miles to Alamitos Peninsula—Hike 72. ▩

72. Belmont Pier
to Alamitos Peninsula and Bay
LONG BEACH CITY BEACH

Hiking distance: 4 miles round trip
Hiking time: 2 hours
Configuration: out-and-back with loop around peninsula
Elevation gain: level
Exposure: exposed beach coastline
Difficulty: easy
Dogs: allowed
Maps: U.S.G.S. Long Beach and Seal Beach

Long Beach City Beach stretches over four miles, from the port of Long Beach to the Alamitos Bay entrance channel at the Orange County border. This hike begins at Belmont Pier near the middle of the coastal beach. The 1,620-foot-long, T shaped pier extends from the foot of 39th Place. The hike explores both shores of the narrow Alamitos Peninsula to the mouth of Alamitos Bay. The route follows the Seaside Walk (a wooden boardwalk) and Bay Shore Walk (a paved walkway) along the San Pedro Bay coastline. From Belmont Pier, the hike can be extended west on the Long Beach Oceanfront Trail—Hike 71.

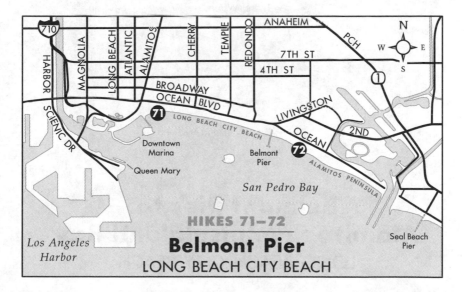

243

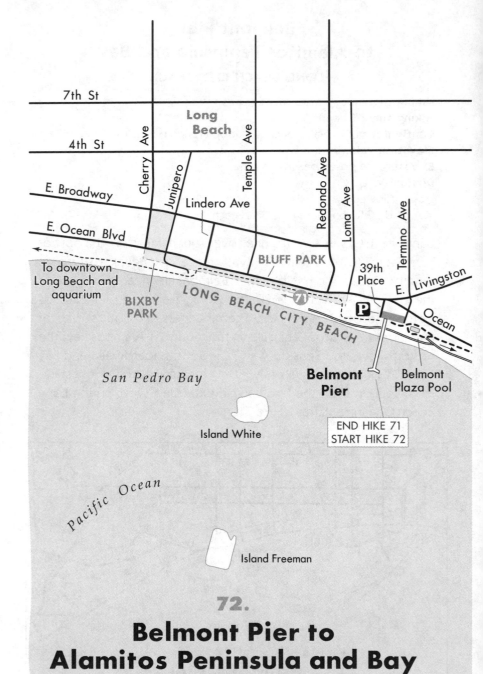

7th St

Long Beach

4th St

E. Broadway

Cherry Ave

Junipero

Temple Ave

Redondo Ave

Loma Ave

Termino Ave

Lindero Ave

E. Ocean Blvd

To downtown Long Beach and aquarium

BIXBY PARK

LONG BEACH CITY BEACH

BLUFF PARK

39th Place

E. Livingston

Ocean

San Pedro Bay

Island White

Belmont Pier

Belmont Plaza Pool

END HIKE 71
START HIKE 72

Pacific Ocean

Island Freeman

72.
Belmont Pier to Alamitos Peninsula and Bay
LONG BEACH CITY BEACH

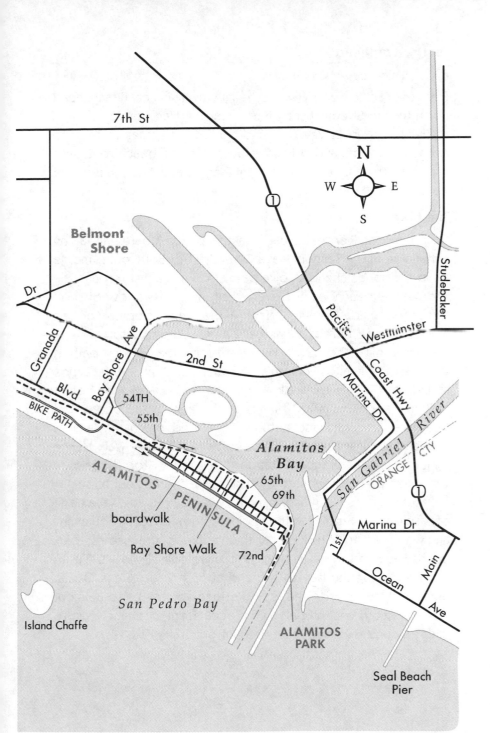

7th St

N
W E
S

Belmont
Shore

Dr

Granada

Blvd

Bay Shore Ave

BIKE PATH

2nd St

54TH

55th

Pacific

Westminster

Marina Dr

Coast Hwy

San Gabriel River

ORANGE CITY

Studebaker

*Alamitos
Bay*

ALAMITOS

PENINSULA

65th

69th

boardwalk

Bay Shore Walk

72nd

San Pedro Bay

Island Chaffe

Marina Dr

1st

Ocean

Main

Ave

ALAMITOS
PARK

Seal Beach
Pier

To the trailhead

30 S. TERMINO AVE · LONG BEACH   33.758806, -118.146193

From the Pacific Coast Highway (Highway 1) in Seal Beach, head north to 2nd Street in Long Beach. Turn left and drive 1.7 miles to Livingston Drive. Veer left and continue 0.4 miles to Termino Avenue. Turn left and drive 2 blocks into the beachfront parking lot on the east side of Belmont Pier, adjacent to the Belmont Plaza Olympic Pool.

The hike

From Belmont Pier, head east on the paved boardwalk along either side of the Belmont Plaza Olympic Pool. Both routes merge a short distance ahead. A bike path also winds east through the wide sandy beach. At just over a half mile, pass a row of palm trees by Granada Avenue. Offshore, the scenic, tropical-looking islands with palm trees are actually disguised oil platforms.

At one mile, the paved bike path joins the walking path at the head of Alamitos Peninsula by 54th Place. Walk on the sandy strand to the Seaside Walk, a wooden boardwalk that begins at 55th Place. Continue 0.7 miles to the end of the oceanfront boardwalk at 69th Place. Return to the sand, reaching Alamitos Park and the Alamitos Bay Channel by 72nd Place. Walk to the right, passing the lifeguard station to the jetty. Atop the jetty, a rock-lined path, frequented by fisherman, extends out to sea.

Return to the small grassy park. A paved path follows the edge of Alamitos Bay, ending at the marina. Return to Ocean Boulevard and walk west to 65th Place. At the north end of the street, pick up the Bay Shore Walk, a paved public walkway. Follow the path 0.4 miles along the bay to the end at 55th Place. Cross Ocean Boulevard, completing the loop. Retrace your steps to Belmont Pier. To extend your hike along the oceanfront, continue west to Bluff Park and the Long Beach Oceanfront Trail—Hike 71. ▪

73. El Dorado Nature Center

EL DORADO PARK

Open Tuesday—Sunday

Hiking distance: 2-mile loop
Hiking time: 1 hour
Configuration: loop (with optional cut-across for a 1-mile loop)
Elevation gain: level
Exposure: shade with some exposed pathways
Difficulty: easy
Dogs: not allowed
Maps: U.S.G.S. Los Alamitos · El Dorado Nature Center Trail Map

El Dorado Park is a 450-acre parkland in Long Beach just west of the Los Angeles–Orange County line. The park includes fishing lakes, tree groves, picnic shelters, a petting zoo, 4.5 miles of paved biking trails, and a nature center. The park is divided into an east section and a west section. The developed west section has a golf course and athletic fields. The west section has interconnecting roads and paved walkways.

This hike makes a loop through the least developed section of the park in the southwest corner. The pastoral 105-acre area is known as the El Dorado Nature Center. An interpretive trail loops around two lakes and meanders through the sanctuary along rolling hills, tree-lined meadows, chaparral communities, oak woodlands, and a stream connecting the two lakes. An interpretive trail pamphlet is available at the museum.

To the trailhead

7550 E. SPRING STREET · LONG BEACH   33.810086, -118.085569

From the 405 (San Diego) Freeway in Long Beach, take the Studebaker Road exit. Drive 1.4 miles north to Spring Street and turn right. Continue 0.8 miles to the park entrance on the right. Park just beyond the entrance station, near the posted trailhead on the right. A parking fee is required.

The hike

Enter the lush, forested parkland on the paved path to the bridge. Cross the bridge to the nature center building, perched on an island in North Lake. After visiting the center, loop clockwise to the backside of the buildings. Cross another bridge, leaving the island to a three-way junction. The two trails on the right comprise a paved quarter-mile, handicapped-accessible loop. Take the unpaved left fork along the west edge of North Lake to a junction.

Begin the One-Mile Trail and Two-Mile Trail loops to the right. Parallel North Lake's outlet stream, and zigzag up the chaparral-covered hillside, passing the observation tower on the right, the highest point in the preserve. Descend and cross the bridges

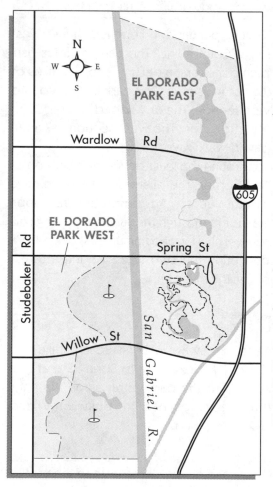

over the stream two times. Wind through eucalyptus and oak groves, and cross another bridge over the stream to a junction. The One-Mile Trail continues to the left for a shorter loop. Stay to the right on the Two-Mile Trail, and descend to the north shore of South Lake. Follow the west edge of the lake to the inlet stream. Cross a bridge and return to the south end of the lake. The meandering path returns to the north, completing the loop at North Lake. Return to the right. ■

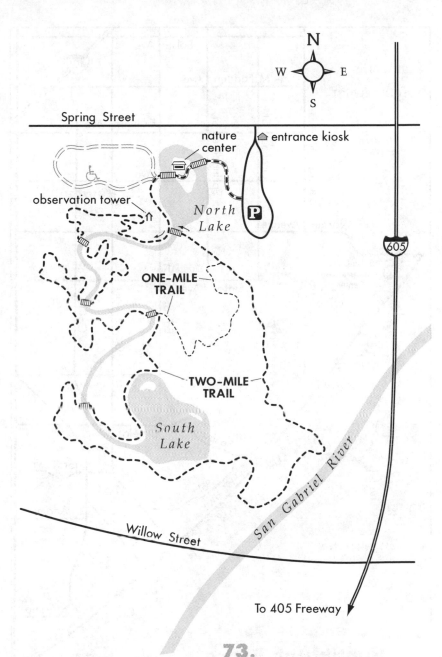

N
W E
S

Spring Street

nature center

🏠 entrance kiosk

observation tower

North Lake

P

ONE-MILE TRAIL

TWO-MILE TRAIL

South Lake

San Gabriel River

Willow Street

605

To 405 Freeway ↓

73.

El Dorado Nature Center
EL DORADO PARK

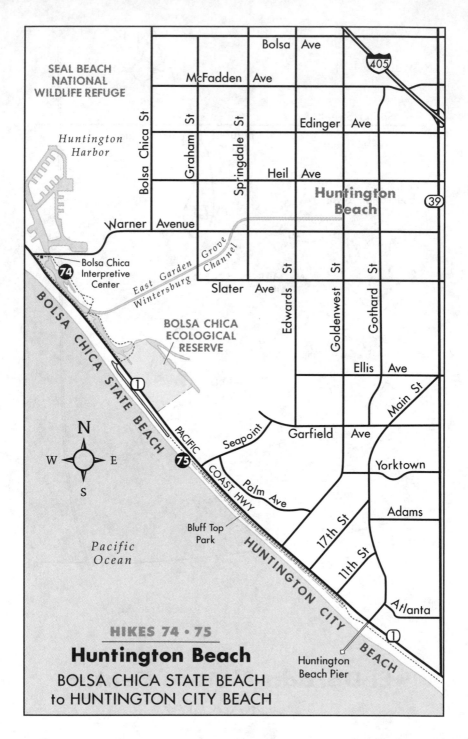

SEAL BEACH
NATIONAL
WILDLIFE REFUGE

*Huntington
Harbor*

Bolsa Chica St

Graham St

Springdale St

McFadden Ave

Bolsa Ave

Edinger Ave

Heil Ave

**Huntington
Beach**

405

39

Warner Avenue

Bolsa Chica
Interpretive
Center

74

East Garden Grove
Wintersburg Channel

Slater Ave

Edwards St

Goldenwest St

Gothard St

**BOLSA CHICA
ECOLOGICAL
RESERVE**

1

Ellis Ave

BOLSA CHICA STATE BEACH

PACIFIC

Seapoint

Garfield Ave

Main St

75

COAST HWY

Palm Ave

Yorktown

Adams

N
W   E
S

17th St

11th St

Bluff Top
Park

*Pacific
Ocean*

HUNTINGTON CITY

Atlanta

1

BEACH

HIKES 74 • 75

Huntington Beach

BOLSA CHICA STATE BEACH
to HUNTINGTON CITY BEACH

Huntington
Beach Pier

74. Bolsa Chica Ecological Reserve

Hiking distance: 3-mile loop
Hiking time: 1.5 hours
Configuration: loop (with optional cut-across path)
Elevation gain: 20 feet
Difficulty: easy
Exposure: exposed coastal wetlands
Dogs: not allowed
Maps: U.S.G.S. Seal Beach

The Bolsa Chica tidal basin encompasses 1,300 wetland acres and 300 mesa acres between Seal Beach and Huntington Beach along the Pacific coast at the northwest end of Orange County. The Bolsa Chica Ecological Reserve is a 557-acre protected wildlife habitat within the Bolsa Bay wetlands, which runs parallel to Bolsa Chica State Beach. The preserve, established in 1973, has inter-tidal mudflats, salt flats, salt marsh communities, ponds, grasslands, lowland dunes, two bird nesting islands, and flood control channels. The area is located along the Pacific Flyway, a 2,000-mile migratory bird route between Alaska and Latin America.

This hike begins near the Outer Bay and loops around the slough, passing interpretive panels and overlooks with benches for wildlife viewing. The route makes a long loop parallel to Highway 1. Directly across the highway is the state beach.

To the trailhead

3842 WARNER AVE · HUNTINGTON BEACH   33.711431, -118.061486

NORTHERN TRAILHEAD: From the 405 (San Diego) Freeway in Fountain Valley, take the Warner Avenue West exit. Drive 5.5 miles west to the well-signed trailhead parking lot and interpretive center on the left. The parking lot is located after crossing the bridge over the Bolsa Bay Channel and before the Pacific Coast Highway.

SOUTHERN TRAILHEAD: The southern trailhead access is located on the Pacific Coast Highway, 1.4 miles south of Warner Avenue.

The hike

From the interpretive center at the north trailhead, walk east, past the trailhead kiosks. Continue to the edge of the Bolsa Bay tidal waters. Bear left and cross the bridge over Warner Avenue on the shoulder of the road. Pick up the trail to the right. Follow the 15-foot-high mesa terrace on the west edge of the grassy open expanse on the inland bank of the water channel. Just shy of a palm tree grove is a trail split. Stay to the right, on the levee along the slough. Both paths rejoin at an overlook of the coastline and the entire wetland. In clear conditions, the views extend to Palos Verdes, Catalina Island, and the San Gabriel Mountains. Continue south and cross the flood control channel on the tidegate. Curve around the south end of the reserve to a wooden footbridge spanning the lagoon. Cross the bridge to the southern trailhead at a parking lot off of the Pacific Coast Highway, opposite of Bolsa Chica State Beach. Return on the footpath sandwiched between the west bank of the bay and the PCH. ▪

75. Huntington Beach • Bluff Top Park
BOLSA CHICA STATE BEACH to HUNTINGTON PIER

Hiking distance: 5.6 miles round trip
Hiking time: 3 hours
Configuration: out-and-back along parallel paths
Elevation gain: 30 feet
Difficulty: easy to moderate
Exposure: open coastal bluffs and low dunes
Dogs: on paved trail only (not allowed on sand). However, Dog Beach at the end of Goldenwest Street allows off-leash dogs.
Maps: U.S.G.S. Seal Beach

Huntington City Beach is a 3.5-mile strand of wide, sandy shoreline between Bolsa Chica State Beach and Huntington State Beach. Huntington Beach, known as Surf City, is one of Orange County's most popular surfing beaches. This hike follows the 30-foot bluffs of Bluff Top Park, from the south end of Bolsa

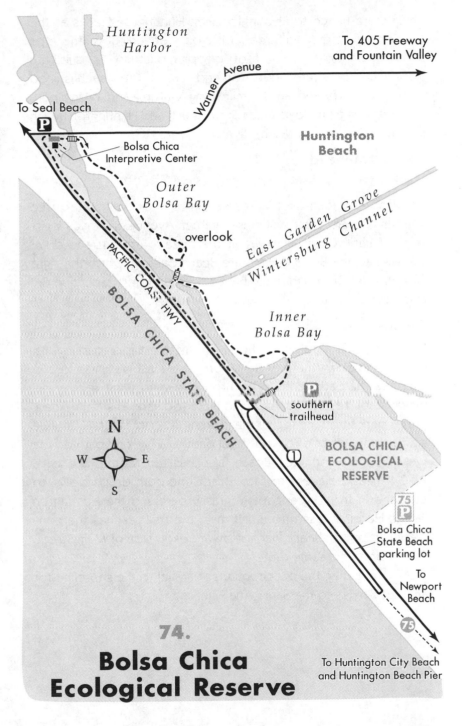

Huntington
Harbor

To 405 Freeway
and Fountain Valley

Warner Avenue

To Seal Beach

P

Bolsa Chica
Interpretive Center

**Huntington
Beach**

*Outer
Bolsa Bay*

East Garden Grove
Wintersburg Channel

overlook

PACIFIC COAST HWY

BOLSA CHICA STATE BEACH

*Inner
Bolsa Bay*

P

southern
trailhead

1

N
W — E
S

**BOLSA CHICA
ECOLOGICAL
RESERVE**

75
P

Bolsa Chica
State Beach
parking lot

To
Newport
Beach

75

74.

Bolsa Chica
Ecological Reserve

To Huntington City Beach
and Huntington Beach Pier

Chica State Beach to Huntington Pier. Huntington Pier is at the foot of the city's Main Street. It is a busy beach hub with shops and restaurants. The 1,850-foot-long pier, built in 1914, is lit with floodlights for after-dark fishing and surfing. The beach is lined with low bluffs and an 8.5-mile-long walking and biking path that extends from Bolsa Chica State Beach and Huntington Beach southward to the Santa Ana River.

To the trailhead

18333 PACIFIC COAST HWY · HUNTINGTON BCH   33.695023, -118.046631

From the 405 (San Diego) Freeway in Fountain Valley, take the Warner Avenue West exit. Take Warner Avenue 5.6 miles west to the Pacific Coast Highway at the ocean. Turn left and drive 1.5 miles to the Bolsa Chica State Beach parking lot on the right (ocean side). Turn right into the lot and curve left. Continue 0.9 miles and park at the south end of the long lot.

The hike

From the south end of the Bolsa Chica State Beach parking lot, head south along the low dunes on the paved walking and biking path. The path gently rises through low-growing vegetation, which stabilizes the dunes, up to Bluff Top Park. The palm-lined, grassy park sits at the top of the eroding 30-foot bluffs. Continue south along either of two parallel paths—a walking path on the west or the Huntington Beach Bike Trail ten feet to the east. At 2.4 miles, adjacent to 11th Street, the path drops down to the sand in front of a sloping, grassy park and the Huntington Pacific Hotel. In less than a half mile, the trail reaches the concrete Huntington Beach Pier, a seaward extension of Main Street. Return along the same route.

After the pier, the path continues parallel to the shoreline for another 3 miles to the Santa Ana River. ▥

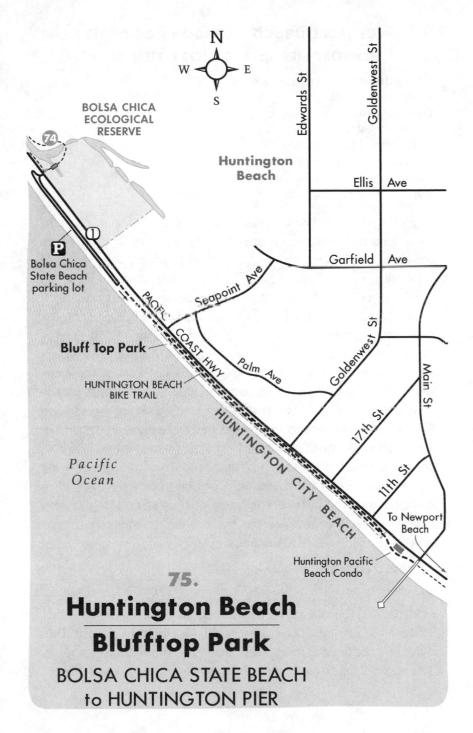

75.
Huntington Beach
Blufftop Park
BOLSA CHICA STATE BEACH
to HUNTINGTON PIER

76. Newport Beach • Balboa Peninsula
NEWPORT PIER to WEST JETTY VIEW PARK

Hiking distance: 5.6 miles round trip
Hiking time: 3 hours
Configuration: out-and-back
Elevation gain: level
Difficulty: easy to moderate
Exposure: exposed beachfront
Dogs: on paved trail only (not allowed on sand)
Maps: U.S.G.S. Newport Beach • Franko's Map of Newport Harbor

Newport Beach and Balboa Beach are broad, white sand beaches on Balboa Peninsula, a four-mile long finger of land between the Newport Bay Harbor and the Pacific Ocean. The peninsula is populated with homes along its north (inland) side while the sandy beach stretches along the entire south (ocean) side.

This hike strolls along the length of the Balboa Peninsula on the oceanfront promenade, from the Newport Pier to West Jetty View Park at the mouth of the bay. Newport Beach and Newport Pier—where the hike begins—are at the west end of the peninsula. The public fishing pier, built in 1888, is the oldest pier in southern California. A long boardwalk leads to Balboa Beach and Balboa Pier. Adjacent to the pier is Peninsula Park, an expansive grassland with palm trees, ball fields, and picnic areas. The hike continues to the peninsula's tip by the mouth of the harbor. West Jetty View Park and The Wedge, a popular body surfing area in the elbow of the jetty, are located at the far end of the hike. From the park are views across the channel to the rock formations and beach coves in Corona Del Mar (Hike 77).

To the trailhead

100 21ST PLACE • NEWPORT BEACH   33.608218, -117.928856

From the 405 (San Diego) Freeway in Costa Mesa, take the Harbor Boulevard south exit. Drive 3.2 miles to Newport Boulevard. Turn right and continue 2 miles south towards the Balboa Peninsula. Just after 23rd Street, veer right towards the signed "Beach

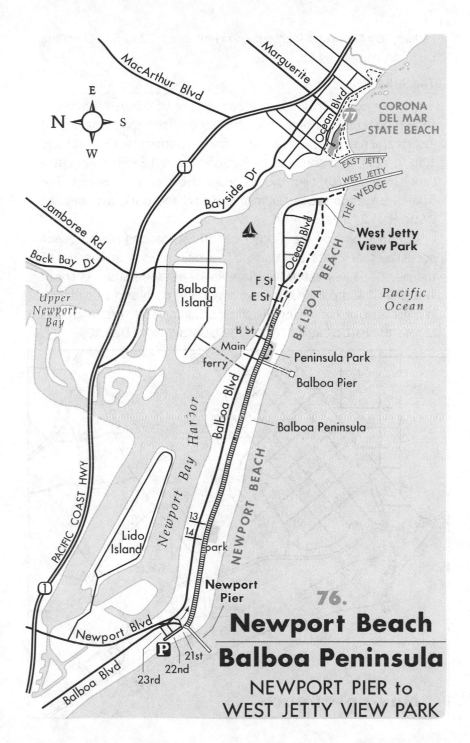

MacArthur Blvd

Marguerite

E
N—S
W

1

CORONA
DEL MAR
STATE BEACH

Ocean Blvd

77

EAST JETTY

WEST JETTY

THE WEDGE

Bayside Dr

Jamboree Rd

Back Bay Dr

Upper
Newport
Bay

Balboa
Island

F St
E St

B St

Main
ferry

Ocean Blvd

BALBOA BEACH

West Jetty
View Park

Pacific
Ocean

Peninsula Park

Balboa Pier

Balboa Peninsula

Newport Bay Harbor

Balboa Blvd

NEWPORT BEACH

PACIFIC COAST HWY

Lido
Island

13
14
park

1

Newport
Pier

Newport Blvd

P
21st
22nd
23rd

Balboa Blvd

76.

Newport Beach

Balboa Peninsula

NEWPORT PIER to
WEST JETTY VIEW PARK

Parking" by Newport Pier, curving right onto 22nd Street to the oceanfront parking lot.

The hike

From Newport Pier, head southeast on the boardwalk. Stroll between beachfront homes and the back of the sandy beach. At just over a half mile, pass a wide, grassy park between 14th and 13th Streets, and continue to Balboa Pier at 1.8 miles. Peninsula Park stretches for two blocks from the pier to B Street. The boardwalk ends a quarter mile beyond the park, just east of E Street at 2.1 miles.

Continue east on the sandy beachfront, passing paved beach accesses that cross the dunes. The beach ends at the tip of the peninsula in West Jetty View Park near the harbor channel. The palm-lined park has a paved walking path and benches. It is a great spot for observing the boats and rock outcroppings across the harbor. Return along the boardwalk or beach. ■

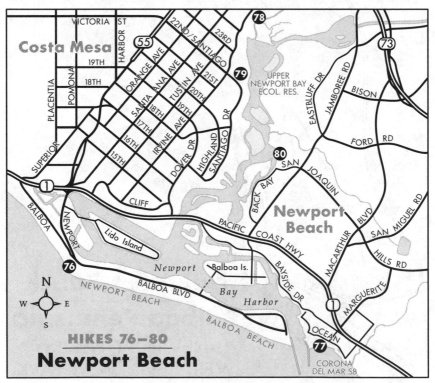

HIKES 76–80
Newport Beach

77. Corona Del Mar State Beach

Hiking distance: 1.5-mile loop
Hiking time: 1 hour
Configuration: loop, with short spur trail to the beach
Elevation gain: 50 feet
Difficulty: easy
Exposure: exposed sandy beach
Dogs: not allowed between 9 a.m. and 5 p.m.
Maps: U.S.G.S. Newport Beach and Laguna Beach
Franko's Map of Newport Harbor

Corona Del Mar, meaning "Crown of the Sea," is a small blufftop community on the east side of Newport Harbor. It is located at the start of the scenic oceanfront cliffs that extend south to San Clemente and San Onofre. The beach, which sits at the mouth of the harbor, is a triangular wedge of land with gorgeous white sand coves beneath 80-foot bluffs. The state beach has tide-pools and offshore rock formations. To the south, a stream-fed canyon drains through Little Corona Del Mar Beach, a seclud-ed cove with lush riparian vegetation in the Robert E. Badham Marine Life Refuge. This hike begins at the east jetty of Newport Harbor and explores the beaches and marine refuges, making a loop from the palisades to the sandy beaches.

To the trailhead

100 BREAKERS DRIVE · CORONA DEL MAR   33.594442, -117.876417

From the 405 (San Diego) Freeway in Irvine, take the Jamboree Road exit. Drive 1.6 miles south to MacArthur Boulevard and turn left. Continue 4 miles to the Pacific Coast Highway and turn left. Drive 0.6 miles to Marguerite Avenue and turn right. Go two blocks to Ocean Boulevard and turn right. In one block, veer left and descend to the posted beach parking. Park near the north end of the parking lot.

The hike

Walk west to the jagged rock formations at the Newport Bay Harbor Channel. Explore the rocks, caves, and sandy beach pocket. To the south, a path follows the seawall along the edge of the channel to the rock jetty. To the north, atop the rock formation, a footpath leads to Lookout Point, a blufftop park that overlooks the harbor and Balboa Peninsula. From the lookout, stroll southeast along the bluffs. Parallel Ocean Boulevard to Inspiration Point, a small park at the foot of Orchid Avenue that overlooks Corona Del Mar Beach and the offshore rock formations. The walkway leading down the cliffs is the return route.

For now, continue east to an overlook with a bench by Poppy Avenue. Descend on the paved path into Little Corona Del Mar Beach, a beach pocket tucked between vertical rock cliffs with tidepools and scenic offshore rocks carved by wind and surf.

Return to Inspiration Point on the bluffs. Descend on the walkway down the cliffs past an overlook extending off the rocky knob. Cross the sandy beach, returning to the parking lot. ◼

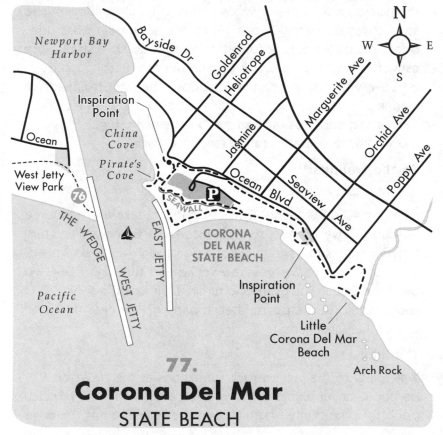

77.
Corona Del Mar
STATE BEACH

78. Upper Newport Bay Ecological Reserve

NORTH CORRIDOR from INTERPRETIVE CENTER

Hiking distance: 3.5 miles round trip
Hiking time: 2 hours
Configuration: loop and out-and-back
Elevation gain: 50 feet
Difficulty: easy
Exposure: open estuary hillside
Dogs: allowed
Maps: U.S.G.S. Newport Beach and Tustin
Franko's Map of Newport Bay

Upper Newport Bay Ecological Reserve is renowned as one of the finest birding sites in North America. The shallow coastal bay, where fresh river water mixes with salty seawater, is on the Pacific Flyway, the migratory route from Mexico to Alaska. The estuary is a vital feeding, resting, and nesting habitat for up to 30,000 migrating shorebirds and waterfowl. The varied habitats include open waters, salt marshes, mud flats, dunes, sandy

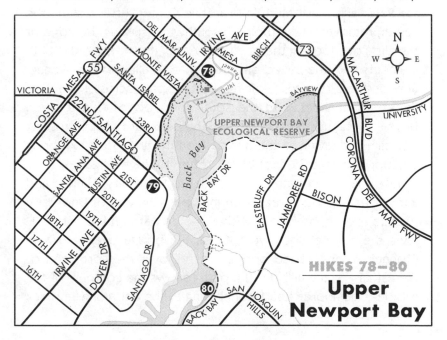

HIKES 78–80

Upper
Newport Bay

beaches, bluffs, riparian woodlands, and ponds. Hiking, biking, and equestrian trails weave through the preserve on bluffs covered with coastal sage scrub and native grasslands.

This hike begins from the Peter and Mary Muth Interpretive Center, an earth-sheltered structure built on the bluffs overlooking Back Bay. The center has interactive exhibits, classrooms, a gift shop, and volunteer naturalists.

To the trailhead

2301 UNIVERSITY DRIVE · NEWPORT BEACH   33.654902, -117.885740

From the 405 (San Diego) Freeway on the Costa Mesa/Irvine border, take the MacArthur Boulevard exit. Drive 0.7 miles south to Campus Drive and turn right. Continue 1.8 miles to University Drive and turn left. (Campus Drive becomes Irvine Avenue after crossing the 73 Freeway.) Quickly turn right into the Muth Interpretive Center parking lot on the southeast corner of University Drive and Irvine Avenue.

The hike

From the parking lot, a paved path winds southeast down to the Peter and Mary Muth Interpretive Center. After visiting the center, return and take the path southwest, skirting the edge of the cliffs overlooking the preserve. Along the way, the dirt path connects with the paved bike path that parallels Irvine Avenue. Stay on the dirt path, rejoining the bike path across from 23rd Street. To connect with the south loop off of Constellation Drive—the nature preserve—take the bike path south, crossing a stream-fed ravine to the dirt path on the left. After exploring the loop atop the 75-foot bluffs, return to the trailhead.

Take the paved path east, parallel to University Avenue and a row of eucalyptus trees. Continue past the end of University Avenue and descend to a bridge. A side path on the right follows the channel southwest. Cross the bridge over the Delhi Channel. A long, raised bridge crosses over the north end of the estuary to the hillside. The path follows the contours of the hillside to Jamboree Road, connecting to the trail along Bay Back Drive (Hike 80). ▦

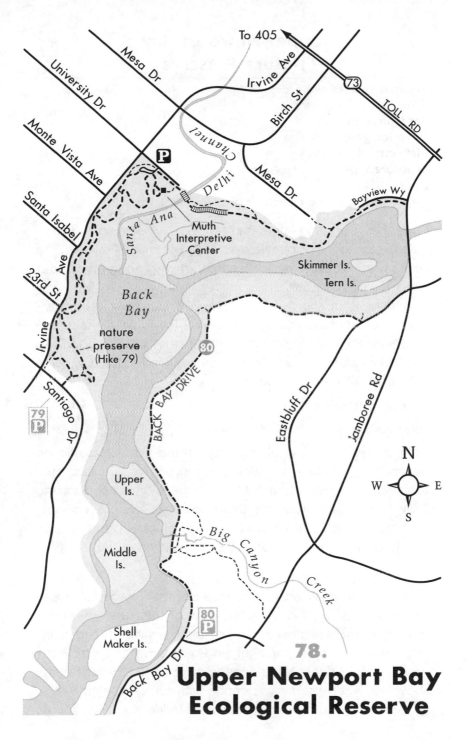

To 405

University Dr
Mesa Dr
Irvine Ave
Birch St
73
TOLL RD

Monte Vista Ave
Channel
Mesa Dr
Bayview Wy

Santa Isabel
P
Delhi

Santa Ana
Muth
Interpretive
Center
Skimmer Is.
Tern Is.

23rd St
Ave

*Back
Bay*

Irvine

nature
preserve
(Hike 79)
80

79
P

Santiago Dr

BACK BAY DRIVE

Eastbluff Dr

Jamboree Rd

N
W ✦ E
S

Upper
Is.

Big Canyon

Middle
Is.

Creek

80
P

Shell
Maker Is.

Back Bay Dr

**78.
Upper Newport Bay
Ecological Reserve**

79. Upper Newport Bay Nature Preserve

Hiking distance: 1-mile loop
Hiking time: 30 minutes
Configuration: loop
Elevation gain: 50 feet
Difficulty: very easy
Exposure: open estuary hillside
Dogs: allowed
Maps: U.S.G.S. Newport Beach · Franko's Map of Newport Bay

Upper Newport Bay Nature Preserve is a 142-acre upland habitat adjacent to the Upper Newport Bay Ecological Preserve. The nature preserve is on the north and northwest end of the upper bay, known as Back Bay.

This hike is the short version of Hike 78, exploring just the upper west end of the ecological reserve. The route makes a small loop atop 75-foot bluffs on the west bank of the upper bay. The trail includes a great view of the wetland sanctuary, home to nearly 200 species of birds.

To the trailhead

2000 CONSTELLATION DR · NEWPORT BEACH   33.641235, -117.893018

From the 405 (San Diego) Freeway on the Costa Mesa/Irvine border, take the MacArthur Boulevard exit. Drive 0.7 miles south to Campus Drive and turn right. Continue 2.9 miles to Santiago Drive and turn left. (Campus Drive becomes Irvine Avenue after crossing the 73 Freeway.) Drive one block and turn left on Constellation Drive. Park alongside the dead-end road.

The hike

Walk past the trailhead gate, and descend 40 yards to a trail split. From this junction is a great view of the massive wetland reserve, the sedimentary cliffs, and the bay's islands and channels. Begin the loop to the right, and head down the hillside towards the bay. Curve left along the edge of the 25-foot bluffs above the wetlands. The serpentine path curves along the edge of the eroding bluffs. As the path nears Irvine Avenue, a couple

of trails branch left. The right fork continues on a paved hiking/
biking path, paralleling Irvine Avenue, to University Drive by the
Peter and Mary Muth Interpretive Center (Hike 78). For this hike,
veer left on the loop. Wind through the native vegetation on the
upper flat, overlooking the estuary, the San Joaquin Hills, and
the Santa Ana Mountains in the distance. Complete the loop and
return to the trailhead on the right. ▪

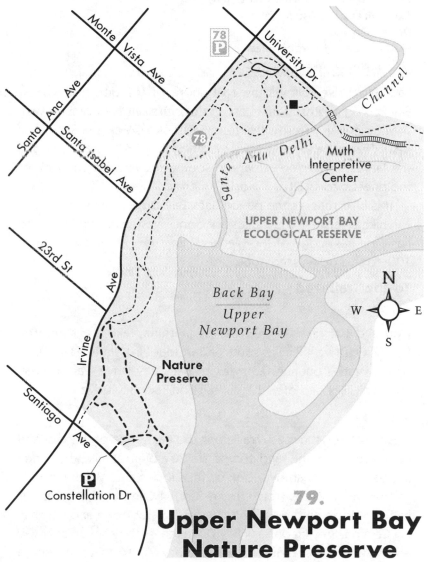

79.
Upper Newport Bay
Nature Preserve

80. Back Bay Drive

UPPER NEWPORT BAY ECOLOGICAL RESERVE

Hiking distance: 4.6 miles round trip
Hiking time: 2 hours
Configuration: out-and-back
Elevation gain: 100 feet
Difficulty: easy to slightly moderate
Exposure: open estuary bluffs
Dogs: allowed
Maps: U.S.G.S. Newport Beach and Tustin
Franko's Map of Newport Bay

Back Bay Drive follows the east shore of the Upper Newport Bay Ecological Reserve, where the ocean's salt water mixes with the nutrient-rich freshwater from San Diego Creek, the Santa Ana Delhi Channel, and various side streams. The 752-acre wetland is the largest remaining estuary in southern California and one of the finest birding sites in North America.

This hike follows the paved Back Bay Drive, a multi-use road for hikers, bikers, and occasional one-way vehicles. The road hugs the east edge of the wetland sanctuary along the base of 100-foot eroding sandstone cliffs.

To the trailhead

2498 BACK BAY DRIVE · NEWPORT BEACH   33.625329, –117.884584

From the 405 (San Diego) Freeway in Irvine, take the Jamboree Road exit. Drive 4.2 miles south to San Joaquin Hills Road and turn right (west). Continue 0.3 miles to Back Bay Drive. Park on San Joaquin Hills Road or in the pullouts on Back Bay Drive.

The hike

Head north on the road/trail along the east edge of the wetland preserve below the sandstone cliffs. At a quarter mile, the winding path reaches an overlook of the Upper and Middle Islands to the west, across from stream-fed Big Canyon to the east. A half-mile loop on the right tours a freshwater pond and marsh in Big Canyon. Staying on Back Bay Drive, cross the canyon spillway and follow the contours of the estuary. At 1.5 miles, ascend a gentle rise to a gravel walkway and overlook with interpretive panels that describe the waterfowl. At just over 2 miles, climb the 100-foot cliffs to the blufftop at Eastbluff Drive. On the left is an overlook of the estuary. Return along the same trail. ■

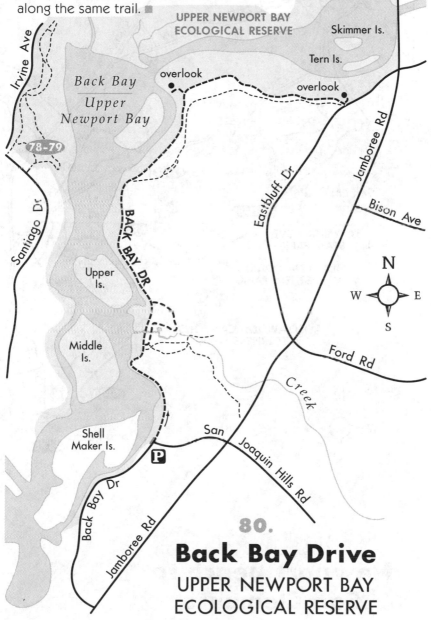

80.

Back Bay Drive
UPPER NEWPORT BAY ECOLOGICAL RESERVE

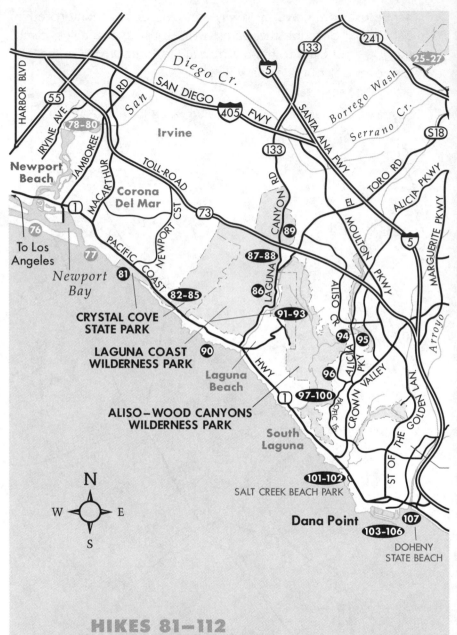

CRYSTAL COVE
STATE PARK

LAGUNA COAST
WILDERNESS PARK

ALISO–WOOD CANYONS
WILDERNESS PARK

SALT CREEK BEACH PARK

DOHENY
STATE BEACH

Newport Beach to San Clemente

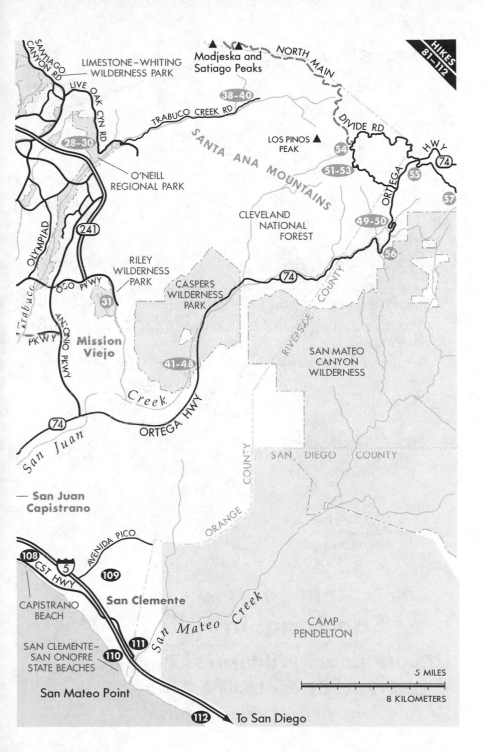

SANTIAGO CANYON RD

LIMESTONE-WHITING WILDERNESS PARK

▲ Modjeska and Satiago Peaks

NORTH MAIN

LIVE OAK CYN RD

TRABUCO CREEK RD

38-40

DIVIDE RD

28-30

SANTA ANA MOUNTAINS

LOS PINOS PEAK ▲

54

51-53

HWY

74

55

O'NEILL REGIONAL PARK

ORTEGA

57

241

CLEVELAND NATIONAL FOREST

49-50

56

OLYMPIAD

RILEY WILDERNESS PARK

CASPERS WILDERNESS PARK

74

Trabuco

OSO PKWY

31

ANTONIO PKWY

Mission Viejo

41-48

RIVERSIDE COUNTY

SAN MATEO CANYON WILDERNESS

PKWY

Creek

ORTEGA HWY

74

San Juan

— San Juan Capistrano

SAN DIEGO COUNTY

ORANGE COUNTY

AVENIDA PICO

108

CST HWY

5

109

San Clemente

CAPISTRANO BEACH

San Mateo Creek

CAMP PENDELTON

SAN CLEMENTE– SAN ONOFRE STATE BEACHES

111

110

5 MILES

San Mateo Point

8 KILOMETERS

112 ➤ To San Diego

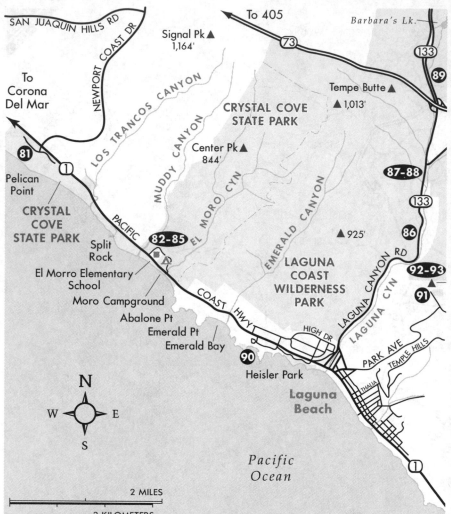

San Juaquin Hills Rd

To 405

Barbara's Lk.

Signal Pk ▲
1,164'

73

133

89

To
Corona
Del Mar

NEWPORT COAST DR

LOS TRANCOS CANYON

MUDDY CANYON

Tempe Butte ▲
▲ 1,013'

CRYSTAL COVE
STATE PARK

Center Pk ▲
844'

81

1

Pelican
Point

CRYSTAL
COVE
STATE PARK

PACIFIC

EL MORO CYN

87-88

133

▲ 925'

86

82-85

Split
Rock

El Morro Elementary
School

Moro Campground

Abalone Pt

Emerald Pt

Emerald Bay

COAST HWY

EMERALD CANYON

LAGUNA
COAST
WILDERNESS
PARK

LAGUNA CANYON RD

92-93

91

HIGH DR

LAGUNA CYN

PARK AVE

TEMPLE HILLS

THALIA

90

Heisler Park

Laguna
Beach

1

N
W E
S

Pacific
Ocean

2 MILES

3 KILOMETERS

HIKES 81–100
San Juaquin Hills
South Coast Wilderness Parks:
Crystal Cove • Laguna Coast
Aliso and Wood Canyons

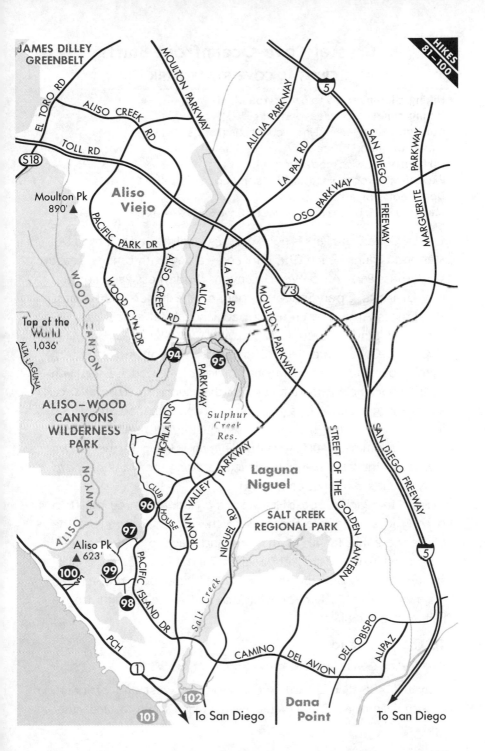

JAMES DILLEY
GREENBELT

EL TORO RD

ALISO CREEK RD

TOLL RD

S18

MOULTON PARKWAY

ALICIA PARKWAY

LA PAZ RD

SAN DIEGO FREEWAY

5

MARGUERITE PARKWAY

Moulton Pk
890' ▲

Aliso
Viejo

PACIFIC PARK DR

OSO PARKWAY

73

WOOD CANYON

ALISO CREEK RD

WOOD CYN DR

ALICIA

LA PAZ RD

MOULTON PARKWAY

Top of the
World
1,036'

ALTA LAGUNA

94

95

ALISO-WOOD
CANYONS
WILDERNESS
PARK

ALISO CANYON

HIGHLANDS

PARKWAY

Sulphur
Creek
Res.

Laguna
Niguel

STREET OF THE GOLDEN LANTERN

SAN DIEGO FREEWAY

CLUB HOUSE

CROWN VALLEY PARKWAY

NIGUEL RD

SALT CREEK
REGIONAL PARK

5

96

97

Aliso Pk
▲ 623'

100

99

98

PACIFIC ISLAND DR

Salt Creek

PCH

1

CAMINO DEL AVION

DEL OBISPO

ALIPAZ

102

101

To San Diego

Dana
Point

To San Diego

81. Crystal Cove Oceanfront Bluffs
CRYSTAL COVE STATE PARK

Hiking distance: 0.5 to 6 miles round trip
Hiking time: 15 minutes to 3 hours
Configuration: several inter-connecting loops
Elevation gain: 100 feet
Difficulty: easy to moderate
Exposure: exposed coastal bluffs and open beachfront
Dogs: not allowed
Maps: U.S.G.S. Laguna Beach · Crystal Cove State Park map

Crystal Cove State Park is a 2,791-acre park between Corona Del Mar and Laguna Beach. The parkland—along with Laguna Coast Wilderness Park, Aliso-Wood Canyons Wilderness Park, and the City of Irvine Open Space—is part of the larger South Coast Wilderness Area. The undeveloped lands total almost 20,000 acres along the southern Orange County coastline.

Crystal Cove State Park offers 3.25 miles of unobstructed, scenic coastline. The oceanfront portion of the park is lined with an 80-foot ancient marine terrace that supports coastal sage scrub and grasses. A designated underwater marine life refuge lies adjacent to the shoreline. The beach is a premier destination for swimming, surfing, snorkeling, and diving. Farther down the coast, the parkland spreads inland along the sides of Moro Canyon and up rugged coastal ridges.

From the Pacific Coast Highway, the park has three blufftop parking lots and eight accesses to the beach. Trails cross the bluffs the entire length of the park and lead down to the scalloped coastline and pocket beaches. This hike explores the cliff-sheltered sandy beach with rocky coves, tidepools, reefs. There are a variety of bluff-to-beach loops that range in length from a half mile to six miles.

To the trailhead

EAST PACIFIC COAST HWY · NEWPORT BEACH   33.582924, -117.848856

From the 405 (San Diego) Freeway on the west end of Irvine, take the Jamboree Road exit. Drive 1.6 miles south to Macarthur

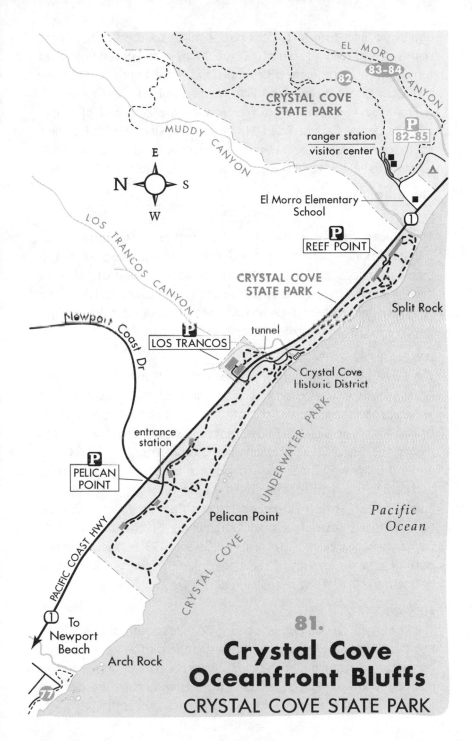

EL MORO CANYON

83-84

82

CRYSTAL COVE
STATE PARK

ranger station
visitor center

P
82-85

MUDDY CANYON

E

N S

W

El Morro Elementary
School

1

LOS TRANCOS CANYON

P
REEF POINT

CRYSTAL COVE
STATE PARK

Split Rock

Newport Coast Dr

P
LOS TRANCOS

tunnel

Crystal Cove
Historic District

UNDERWATER PARK

entrance
station

P
PELICAN
POINT

Pelican Point

Pacific
Ocean

CRYSTAL COVE

PACIFIC COAST HWY

1 To
Newport
Beach

Arch Rock

77

81.

**Crystal Cove
Oceanfront Bluffs**

CRYSTAL COVE STATE PARK

Boulevard and turn left. Continue 4 miles to the Pacific Coast Highway and turn left (south). Drive 2.1 miles to Pelican Point and turn right into the signed Crystal Cove State Park (across from Newport Coast Drive). A parking fee is required.

From the 405 (San Diego) Freeway on the east end of Irvine, take the Laguna Canyon Road (Highway 133) exit and drive 8.2 miles south to the Pacific Coast Highway. Turn right (north) and continue 4.7 miles to Pelican Point Drive. Turn left into Crystal Cove State Park.

The hike

PELICAN POINT

The Pelican Point parking lot is the northernmost entrance of the state park. Paved and meandering natural paths parallel the crenulated coastal bluffs. There are expansive views of offshore rocks, Catalina Island, Newport Beach, Long Beach, and Abalone Point. A concrete ramp leads down the sedimentary cliffs to the beach and tidepools off Pelican Point.

LOS TRANCOS

The Los Trancos parking lot is located a half mile south of the Pelican Point entrance on the inland side of the PCH. A paved walking road leads in two directions from the southeast corner of the lot, dropping into Los Trancos Canyon. The two routes merge near the PCH at a beach access tunnel built in 1932. Cross under the highway, emerging in a grove of eucalyptus, sycamores, and palms. The right fork climbs up to the bluffs towards Pelican Point. The left fork follows Los Trancos Canyon into the Crystal Cove Historic District, a small community of charming wood-frame cottages built in the late 1920s and 1930s. Just past the cottages, at the mouth of the canyon, is the sandy beachfront beneath the 100-foot sandstone cliffs.

REEF POINT

The Reef Point parking lot is located 1.6 miles south of the Pelican Point entrance. A paved path runs atop the bluffs. Various natural paths meander along the cliff's edge, reconnecting with the main path. Paved ramps descend from each end of the parking lot to the seashore near tidepools and rock outcroppings. ■

82. West Wall of El Moro Canyon
No Name Ridge—Ticketron—Red Tail Ridge Loop
CRYSTAL COVE STATE PARK

Hiking distance: 9.5-mile loop
Hiking time: 5 hours
Configuration: loop
Elevation gain: 900 feet
Difficulty: strenuous
Exposure: mostly exposed ridgeline
Dogs: not allowed
Maps: U.S.G.S. Laguna Beach · Crystal Cove State Park map

Crystal Cove State Park is an undeveloped coastal parkland in the San Joaquin Hills. The coastal portion of the parkland stretches between Highway 1 and the shore (Hike 81). However, the majority of the park—2,200 acres—spreads across wooded canyons and high ridges along the El Moro Canyon drainage. In this section of the park, the rugged hills rise to just over 1,000 feet at the head of El Moro Canyon and up to 1,164 feet atop Signal Peak at the head of Los Trancos Canyon. Hikes 82—85 explore the rugged upland geography of the park.

This hike climbs the west canyon wall above Muddy Canyon, Deer Canyon, and El Moro Canyon to a 950-foot ridge east of Signal Peak. At the summit are 360-degree vistas of the surrounding hills, canyons, and the Orange County coastline. The hike travels along old ranch roads from the park's former life as part of the Irvine Ranch.

To the trailhead

8681 N. PACIFIC COAST HWY · LAGUNA BEACH   33.564205, -117.825967

From the 405 (San Diego) Freeway on the west end of Irvine, take the Jamboree Road exit. Drive 1.6 miles south to Macarthur Boulevard and turn left. Continue 4 miles to the Pacific Coast Highway and turn left (south). Drive 4 miles to El Moro Canyon. Turn left, then curve left on the frontage road past the school. Turn right, curving a quarter mile into the Crystal Cove State Park parking lot and ranger station. A parking fee is required.

From the 405 (San Diego) Freeway on the east end of Irvine, take the Laguna Canyon Road (Highway 133) exit, and drive 8.2 miles south to the Pacific Coast Highway. Turn right (north) and continue 2.8 miles to El Moro Canyon. Turn right, then curve left on the frontage road past the school. Turn right, curving a quarter mile into the Crystal Cove State Park parking lot and ranger station.

The hike

Pass the ranger station to the upper (north) end of the parking lot. Take the unpaved No Dogs Road, and climb the sloping chaparral-covered hillside on the west canyon wall. At one mile is a junction with the Poles Trail on the right. Bear left on the No Name Ridge Trail, quickly topping out on a level, grassy stretch. Curve left and follow the dips and rises along the ridge between El Moro Canyon and Muddy Canyon. Continue to a junction with the West Cut-Across Trail in a saddle at 1.3 miles. Stay left along the fenced west boundary to a junction. Bear right on the Ticketron Trail and descend into Deer Canyon, with sculpted sandstone formations and caves. Pass the Deer Canyon Campground to the left at 3 miles. From the canyon floor, ascend the east canyon wall to the ridge and a junction.

Take a sharp right on the Red Tail Ridge Trail. Follow the ridge between Deer Canyon and El Moro Canyon. Cross a large, grassy knoll to a T-junction. Go to the right on a wide, sweeping S-curve to the canyon floor. Ascend the west canyon wall on an easy grade to a T-junction with the West Cut-Across Trail. Stay to the left, dropping to the floor of El Moro Canyon. Bear right and head down canyon for 1.4 miles to the trailhead parking lot. ▪

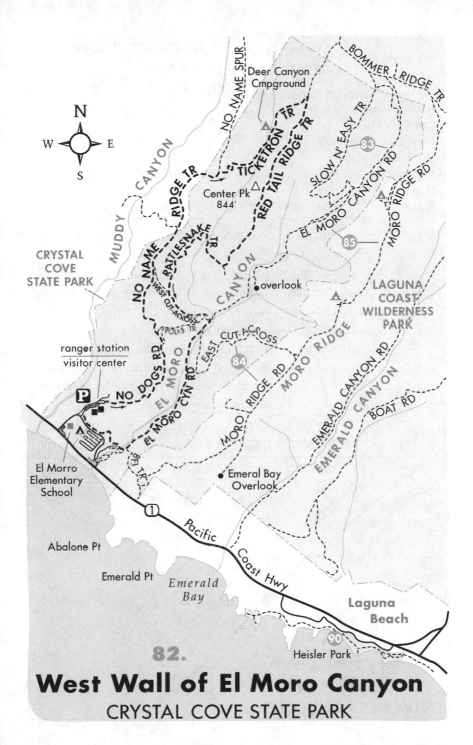

N
W E
S

NO NAME SPUR

BOMMER RIDGE TR

Deer Canyon
Cmpground

MUDDY CANYON

RIDGE TR

TICKETRON TR

RED TAIL RIDGE TR

SLOW N' EASY TR

83

MORO CANYON RD

MORO RIDGE RD

Center Pk
844'

CRYSTAL
COVE
STATE PARK

NO NAME

RATTLESNAKE TR

WEST CUT-ACROSS

?POLES TR

CANYON

EL MORO CANYON RD

85

overlook

LAGUNA
COAST
WILDERNESS
PARK

ranger station
visitor center

EL MORO CYN RD

NO DOGS RD

P

EAST CUT-ACROSS

84

MORO RIDGE RD

MORO RIDGE

EMERALD CANYON RD

EMERALD CANYON

EMERALD BOAT RD

El Morro
Elementary
School

BFI TR

EL MORO CYN RD

MORO RIDGE RD

Emeral Bay
Overlook

1

Pacific

Coast Hwy

Laguna
Beach

Abalone Pt

Emerald Pt

Emerald
Bay

90

82.

Heisler Park

West Wall of El Moro Canyon
CRYSTAL COVE STATE PARK

83. El Moro Canyon to Bommer Ridge
CRYSTAL COVE STATE PARK

Hiking distance: 8.5 miles round trip
Hiking time: 4.5 hours
Configuration: lollipop
Elevation gain: 900 feet
Difficulty: strenuous
Exposure: mostly exposed with some shady riparian vegetation
Dogs: not allowed
Maps: U.S.G.S. Laguna Beach · Crystal Cove State Park map

Crystal Cove State Park encompasses 2,200 inland acres of riparian woodland, chaparral, and scrub hillsides. The trails are old ranch roads from the former Irvine Ranch, which wind up deep canyons, traverse hillsides, and follow ridges. The roads and footpaths form a network of hiking, biking, and equestrian trails that loop through the state park.

This hike climbs up El Moro Canyon, which drains through the center of the park on its course to the ocean. At the upper reaches of the canyon, the route makes a loop up to Bommer Ridge, then returns back along the canyon floor. From the ridge are excellent vistas of the Orange County coast and the ridges and canyons across the San Joaquin Hills.

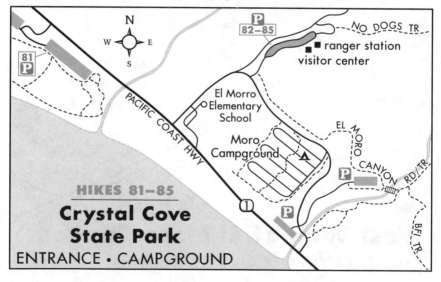

HIKES 81–85
**Crystal Cove
State Park**
ENTRANCE · CAMPGROUND

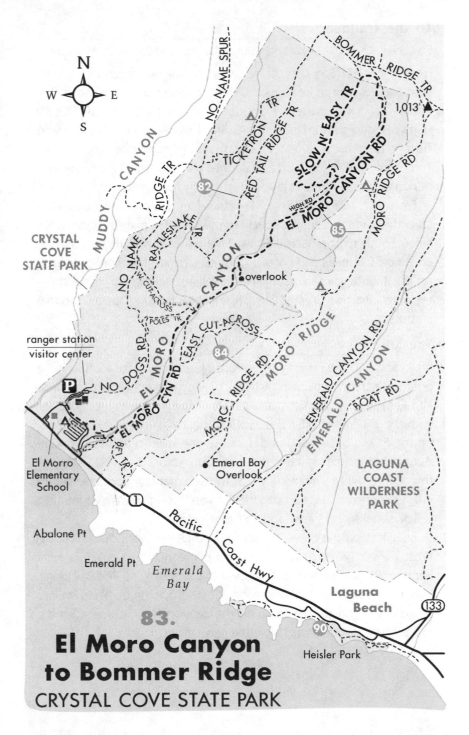

N
W · E
S

MUDDY CANYON

NO NAME SPUR

RIDGE TR

BOMMER RIDGE TR

1,013'

TICKETRON TR

RED TAIL RIDGE TR

SLOW N' EASY TR

EL MORO CANYON RD

MORO RIDGE RD

82

85

HIGH RD

CRYSTAL
COVE
STATE PARK

NO NAME

RATTLESNAKE TR

CANYON

CUT-ACROSS

overlook

POLES TR

EAST CUT-ACROSS

MORO RIDGE

ranger station
visitor center

NO DOGS RD

EL MORO CYN RD

84

MORO RIDGE RD

EMERALD CANYON RD

EMERALD CANYON

BOAT RD

P

EL MORO

BFI TR

El Morro
Elementary
School

Emeral Bay
Overlook

LAGUNA
COAST
WILDERNESS
PARK

Abalone Pt

Emerald Pt

Emerald
Bay

Pacific Coast Hwy

1

Laguna
Beach

133

83.

**El Moro Canyon
to Bommer Ridge**

Heisler Park

90

CRYSTAL COVE STATE PARK

To the trailhead

8681 N. PACIFIC COAST HWY · LAGUNA BEACH   33.564205, –117.825967

From the 405 (San Diego) Freeway on the west end of Irvine, take the Jamboree Road exit. Drive 1.6 miles south to Macarthur Boulevard and turn left. Continue 4 miles to the Pacific Coast Highway and turn left (south). Drive 4 miles to El Moro Canyon. Turn left, then curve left on the frontage road past the school. Turn right, curving a quarter mile into the Crystal Cove State Park parking lot and ranger station. A parking fee is required.

From the 405 (San Diego) Freeway on the east end of Irvine, take the Laguna Canyon Road (Highway 133) exit, and drive 8.2 miles south to the Pacific Coast Highway. Turn right (north) and continue 2.8 miles to El Moro Canyon. Turn right, then curve left on the frontage road past the school. Turn right, curving a quarter mile into the Crystal Cove State Park parking lot and ranger station.

The hike

Walk down to the parking lot entrance, and bear left (south) on the posted fire road/trail. Skirt the back of Moro Campground, and drop into El Moro Canyon. Cross the seasonal stream to a signed junction with the BFI Trail at 0.5 miles. Go left, heading up the canyon floor on the El Moro Canyon Road/Trail. At one mile, pass the East Cut-Across Trail on the right and the West Cut-Across Trail 100 yards farther. Curve right to an overlook of the sedimentary rock formations in a side canyon. Descend into the canyon through dense vegetation, willows, oaks, and sycamores to a posted junction.

Bear left on the Slow N' Easy Trail to begin the loop. Climb the west canyon wall to the ridge, and curve north to a Y-fork near Bommer Ridge. The left fork follows the fenceline to Red Tail Ridge. Stay to the right and make a wide loop, dropping back down into El Moro Canyon. Return south on the canyon floor, completing the loop. Retrace your steps down the canyon. ▪

84. Emerald Bay Overlook

CRYSTAL COVE STATE PARK

Hiking distance: 5-mile loop
Hiking time: 2.5 hours
Configuration: loop
Elevation gain: 600 feet
Difficulty: moderate
Exposure: mostly exposed canyon slopes
Dogs: not allowed
Maps: U.S.G.S. Laguna Beach · Crystal Cove State Park map

The Emerald Bay Overlook sits at the southeast corner of Crystal Cove State Park, 600 feet above Abalone Point, Emerald Point, and Emerald Bay. From the overlook are dramatic coastal vistas of Dana Point, Laguna Beach, and Newport Bay. On clear days, the views extend to San Clemente Island, Catalina Island, and Palos Verdes. This loop route to the overlook follows the lower end of El Moro Canyon, climbing the east canyon wall to Moro Ridge.

To the trailhead

8681 N. PACIFIC COAST HWY · LAGUNA BEACH   33.564205, -117.825967

From the 405 (San Diego) Freeway on the west end of Irvine, take the Jamboree Road exit. Drive 1.6 miles south to Macarthur Boulevard and turn left. Continue 4 miles to the Pacific Coast Highway and turn left (south). Drive 4 miles to El Moro Canyon. Turn left, then curve left on the frontage road past the school. Turn right, curving a quarter mile into the Crystal Cove State Park parking lot and ranger station. A parking fee is required.

From the 405 (San Diego) Freeway on the east end of Irvine, take the Laguna Canyon Road (Highway 133) exit, and drive 8.2 miles south to the Pacific Coast Highway. Turn right (north) and continue 2.8 miles to El Moro Canyon. Turn right, then curve left on the frontage road past the school. Turn right, curving a quarter mile into the Crystal Cove State Park parking lot and ranger station.

The hike

Walk down to the parking lot entrance, and bear left (south) on the posted fire road/trail. Skirt the back of Moro Campground, and drop into El Moro Canyon. Cross the seasonal stream to a signed junction with the BFI Trail on the right at 0.5 miles. Begin the loop to the left. Head up the canyon floor another mile to a junction with the East Cut-Across Trail. Bear right and wind 500 feet up the east canyon wall, reaching Moro Ridge at 2.5 miles.

Take the right fork on the Moro Ridge Road/Trail. Head south atop the ridge for 0.6 miles, crossing under power poles to a Y-fork with the BFI Trail. The BFI Trail—on the right—is the return route. For now, stay left, following the ridge past the junction on the partially paved path. The short spur trail leads to the Emerald Bay Overlook on a circular flat by a radio transmitter. From the overlook are sweeping coastal vistas, including Abalone Point, Emerald Point, and Emerald Bay, directly below. Return to the BFI Trail, and wind downhill on the old service road. The road curves right on a footpath and completes the loop in El Moro Canyon. ▦

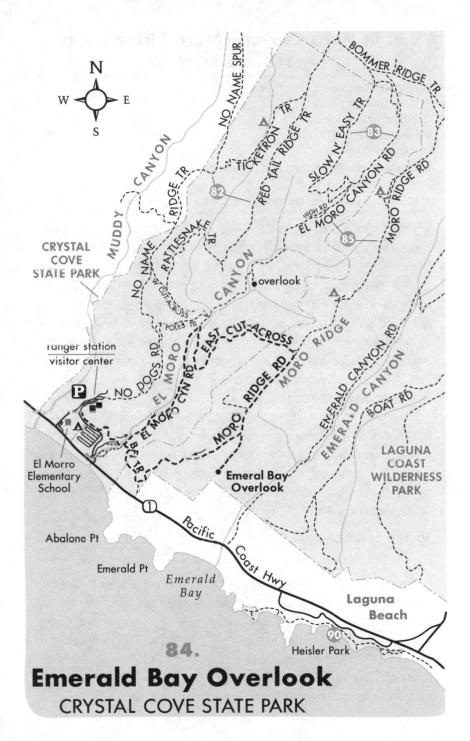

N
W · E
S

BOMMER RIDGE TR

NO NAME SPUR

TICKETRON TR

RED TAIL RIDGE TR

SLOW N' EASY TR

83

82

MORO RIDGE RD

MUDDY CANYON

RIDGE TR

HIGH RD

EL MORO CANYON RD

85

NO NAME

RATTLESNAKE TR

CANYON

overlook

CRYSTAL COVE STATE PARK

W CUT-ACROSS

POLES TR

EAST CUT-ACROSS

NO DOGS RD

EL MORO

EL MORO CYN RD

MORO RIDGE RD

MORO RIDGE

EMERALD CANYON RD

EMERALD CANYON

BOAT RD

ranger station
visitor center

P

MORO

EL MORO CYN RD

BFI TR

LAGUNA COAST WILDERNESS PARK

El Morro Elementary School

Emeral Bay Overlook

1

Pacific

Coast Hwy

Abalone Pt

Emerald Pt

Emerald Bay

Laguna Beach

90

Heisler Park

84.

Emerald Bay Overlook
CRYSTAL COVE STATE PARK

85. El Moro Canyon—Moro Ridge Loop

CRYSTAL COVE STATE PARK

Hiking distance: 9.5-mile loop
Hiking time: 5 hours
Configuration: loop
Elevation gain: 900 feet
Difficulty: strenuous
Exposure: mostly exposed ridges and grasslands
Dogs: not allowed
Maps: U.S.G.S. Laguna Beach · Crystal Cove State Park map

Crystal Cove State Park is a 2,791-acre oceanfront park between Laguna Beach and Corona Del Mar. The state park includes 2,200 inland acres in the San Joaquin Hills, rising 1,100 feet from the coastal plain to the ridge in only three miles. The undeveloped backcountry has hiking, biking, and equestrian trails that lead up wooded canyons and across 1,000-foot ridges. Crystal Cove State Park is part of the South Coast Wilderness Area, along with Aliso-Wood Canyons and the adjacent Laguna Coast Wilderness Park. The park encompasses the El Moro Canyon watershed and all the adjoining drainages.

This long loop begins in Crystal Cove State Park and ascends El Moro Canyon through riparian woodlands with sycamores, willows, and live oaks. It returns along Moro Ridge in Laguna Coast Wilderness Park. The return trail—an old ranch road—travels through chaparral, coastal sage scrub, and grasslands while facing the Pacific Ocean.

To the trailhead

8681 N. PACIFIC COAST HWY · LAGUNA BEACH   33.564205, -117.825967

From the 405 (San Diego) Freeway on the west end of Irvine, take the Jamboree Road exit. Drive 1.6 miles south to Macarthur Boulevard and turn left. Continue 4 miles to the Pacific Coast Highway and turn left (south). Drive 4 miles to El Moro Canyon. Turn left, then curve left on the frontage road past the school. Turn right, curving a quarter mile into the Crystal Cove State Park parking lot and ranger station. A parking fee is required.

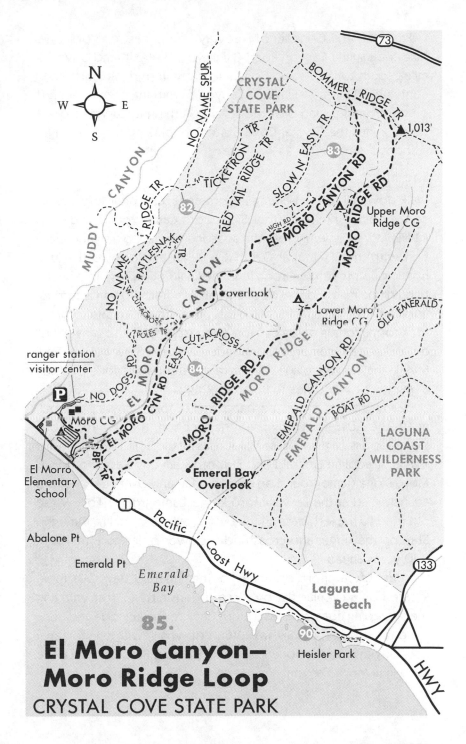

N
W ◆ E
S

73

CRYSTAL
COVE
STATE PARK

NO NAME SPUR

BOMMER RIDGE TR

▲ 1,013'

TICKETRON TR

RED TAIL RIDGE TR

SLOW N' EASY TR

83

EL MORO CANYON RD

MORO RIDGE RD

Upper Moro
Ridge CG

82

HIGH RD

MUDDY CANYON

RIDGE TR

NO NAME

RATTLESNAKE TR

W. CUT-ACROSS

CANYON

▲ overlook

POLES TR

EAST CUT-ACROSS

CUT-ACROSS

Lower Moro
Ridge CG

OLD EMERALD

ranger station
visitor center

NO DOGS RD

EL MORO CYN RD

84

MORO RIDGE RD

MORO RIDGE

EMERALD CANYON RD

EMERALD CANYON

BOAT RD

P

Moro CG

EL MORO

LAGUNA
COAST
WILDERNESS
PARK

BFI TR

El Morro
Elementary
School

● Emeral Bay
Overlook

1

Pacific

Abalone Pt

Coast Hwy

Emerald Pt

Emerald
Bay

Laguna
Beach

133

85.

90

El Moro Canyon–
Moro Ridge Loop

Heisler Park

HWY

CRYSTAL COVE STATE PARK

From the 405 (San Diego) Freeway on the east end of Irvine, take the Laguna Canyon Road (Highway 133) exit, and drive 8.2 miles south to the Pacific Coast Highway. Turn right (north) and continue 2.8 miles to El Moro Canyon. Turn right, then curve left on the frontage road past the school. Turn right, curving a quarter mile into the Crystal Cove State Park parking lot and ranger station.

The hike

Walk downhill to the parking lot entrance, and bear left (south) on the posted fire road/trail. Skirt Moro Campground, and drop into El Moro Canyon. Cross the seasonal stream to a signed junction with the BFI Trail at 0.5 miles. Begin the loop to the left, heading up the canyon floor. Pass the East Cut-Across Trail on the right in one mile and the West Cut-Across Trail 100 yards farther. Curve up the west-facing hillside to an overlook of sedimentary rock formations in a side canyon. Drop down into the canyon under oaks and sycamores to a junction with the Slow N' Easy Trail. Stay in the canyon to a Y-split. Take the steep right fork, climbing along the power poles to Bommer Ridge.

Bear right and cross the head of El Moro Canyon, just beneath the 1,013-foot ridge. At the junction, the left fork continues across Laguna Coast Wilderness Park. Bear right on Moro Ridge, straddling Emerald and El Moro Canyons. Pass the Upper Moro Ridge Campground on a grassy flat, and continue to an old asphalt road at the Lower Moro Ridge Campground. Follow the old road to the left, passing the East Cut-Across Trail to the right. Stay on the ridge, and cross under power poles to a trail fork 200 yards ahead.

Veer left a short distance to the Emerald Bay Overlook, located on a circular flat by a radio transmitter. After enjoying the sweeping coastal vistas, return back to the junction and continue the loop on the BFI Trail. Wind downhill, with phenomenal coastal views of Abalone Point and Emerald Bay. Complete the loop in El Moro Canyon. ▓

86. Bommer Ridge—Laguna Ridge Loop from Laguna Canyon

LAGUNA COAST WILDERNESS PARK

trails open 7:00 a.m. to sunset · parking lots 8:00 a.m. to 5:00 p.m.

Hiking distance: 3.2-mile loop
Hiking time: 1.5 hours
Configuration: loop
Elevation gain: 750 feet
Difficulty: moderate to strenuous
Exposure: mostly open hillsides
Dogs: not allowed
Maps: U.S.G.S. Laguna Beach · Laguna Coast Wilderness Park map

Laguna Coast Wilderness Park is a diverse 7,000-acre natural parkland between Laguna Canyon and Crystal Cove State Park, stretching inland from Laguna Beach to Irvine. Once a working cattle ranch, it is now a protected natural landscape and a part of the 20,000-acre South Coast Wilderness Area. The park has 40 miles of multi-use hiking, biking, and equestrian trails.

This loop hike offers a broad cross-section of habitats in the upper reaches of the park. The trail begins in Laguna Canyon and climbs up the Big Bend Trail, named for a wide curve of Laguna Canyon. The trail continues up a sage-covered hillside to Bommer Ridge. From the 900-foot ridge are views of Crystal Cove State Park, Aliso and Wood Canyons Wilderness Park, the Laguna coastline, and the oak woodlands in Emerald Canyon. The trail returns to the canyon bottom along a rocky footpath.

To the trailhead

20000 Laguna Canyon Rd · Laguna Beach   33.566658, -117.764081

From the 405 (San Diego) Freeway in Irvine, take the Laguna Canyon Road (Highway 133) exit. Drive 6 miles south to the Big Bend Equestrian Staging Area parking lot on the right. The parking lot is located one mile south of the Laguna Coast Wilderness Park main entrance. A parking fee is required

From the Pacific Coast Highway in downtown Laguna Beach, head 2.3 miles north on Broadway (which becomes Laguna Canyon Road/Highway 133) to the posted trailhead on the left.

The hike

From the parking lot, a trail to the right (north) leads to the main park entrance by Willow Canyon. Instead, take the posted Big Bend Trail to the left. Parallel Laguna Canyon Road at the base of the hills. Climb the hillside toward the canyon's Big Bend. At the bend is a posted junction with the Laguna Ridge Trail—the return route. Begin the loop to the right, steeply climbing the scrub- and sage-covered hillside on the Big Bend Trail. The ridge temporarily levels out, with views of the West Ridge Trail across the canyon (Hikes 92—93), Modjeska Peak and Santiago Peak (which form prominent Old Saddleback), the San Gabriel Mountains, and the ocean at Laguna Beach. Steeply ascend the spine of the hillside, then drop down and curve left along the ridge. Cross the head of the canyon to a T-junction on Bommer Ridge at 1.6 miles. The right fork leads to the head of Willow Canyon.

Bear left and head south, overlooking Emerald Canyon. Pass the Old Emerald Trail along the rolling ridge. Make a 90-degree left bend, and climb a hill to a posted junction with Boat Road on the right. Continue 35 yards along the ridge to the Laguna Ridge Trail on the left by signpost 16 at 2.4 miles.

Leave Bommer Ridge and cross over a knoll. Descend on the eroded path with natural rock steps. Steadily descend for nearly a mile. The footpath ends by Laguna Canyon Road at the south end of Big Bend. Bear left, walk parallel to the road, and climb the base of the hill. Traverse the cliff-edge path above the road, and descend to the base of the hill by a towering eucalyptus tree. Return to the junction with the Big Bend Trail, completing the loop. Return downhill to the right. ■

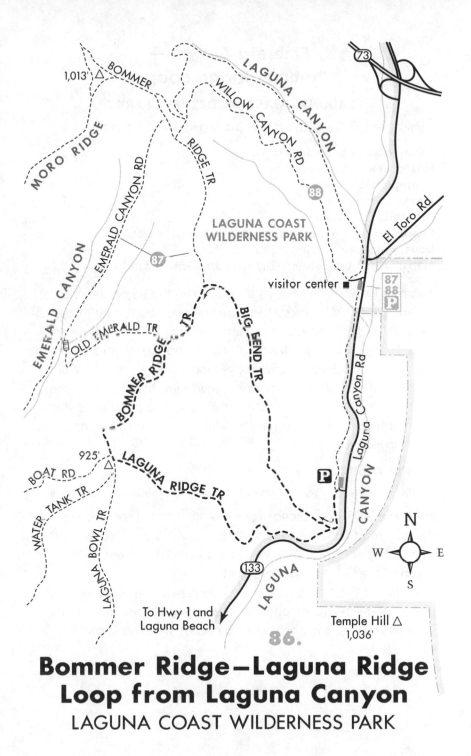

86.

Bommer Ridge–Laguna Ridge
Loop from Laguna Canyon
LAGUNA COAST WILDERNESS PARK

87. Emerald Canyon—
Bommer Ridge Loop

LAGUNA COAST WILDERNESS PARK

trails open 7:00 a.m. to sunset · parking lots 8:00 a.m. to 5:00 p.m.

Hiking distance: 6.5 miles round trip
Hiking time: 3.5 hours
Configuration: lollipop
Elevation gain: 1,400 feet
Difficulty: strenuous
Exposure: a mix of open ridgelines and riparian vegetation
Dogs: not allowed
Maps: U.S.G.S. Laguna Beach · Laguna Coast Wilderness Park map

This hike begins from the visitor center in the upper reaches of Laguna Coast Wilderness Park. The hike loops through coastal canyons and high open ridges in the heart of the park. The strenuous route travels up Willow Canyon and down into Emerald Canyon, then up to Bommer Ridge and back down into Willow Canyon on the return. En route are shady groves of trees, meadows, and weather-carved rock formations. The panoramic views from atop the ridge span across the ocean, coastline, and San Joaquin Hills.

To the trailhead

20050 LAGUNA CANYON RD · LAGUNA BCH   33.580080, -117.762080

From the 405 (San Diego) Freeway in Irvine, take the Laguna Canyon Road (Highway 133) exit, and drive 5 miles south to the signed Laguna Coast Wilderness parking lot on the right, just south of the El Toro Road intersection.

From the Pacific Coast Highway in downtown Laguna Beach, head 3.2 miles north on Broadway (which becomes Laguna Canyon Road) to the posted Laguna Coast Wilderness parking lot on the left.

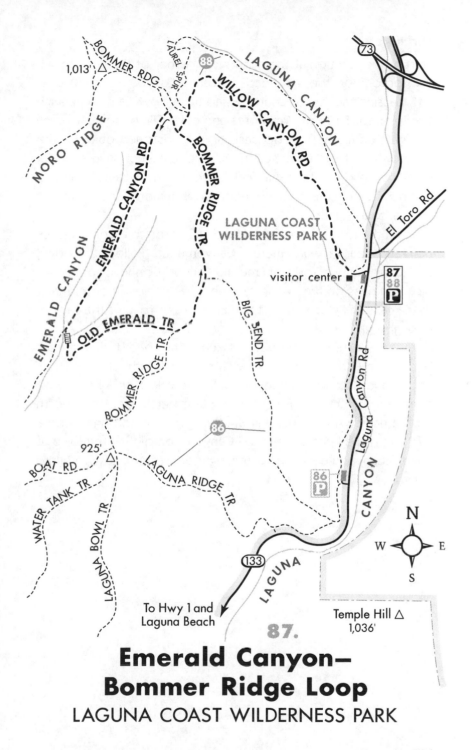

87.
Emerald Canyon–
Bommer Ridge Loop
LAGUNA COAST WILDERNESS PARK

The hike

Start at the junction at the northwest corner of the parking lot. The footpath to the right leads to Laurel Canyon (Hike 88). Bear left, passing the visitor center. Head up Willow Canyon, leaving the coveted shade of sycamores and oaks. Climb the south canyon wall on a steep grade past large sandstone boulders. The path levels out and traverses the hillside to a junction in a saddle on Willow Ridge. The right fork descends into Laurel Canyon; another trail on the right connects to Bommer Ridge. Continue straight to a T-junction.

Begin the loop to the right. Head 150 yards to a posted junction, and bear left on Emerald Canyon Road. Follow the ridge, straddling the two forks of Emerald Canyon. Continue south over dips and rises on the gentle downhill grade, slowly descending to the canyon floor. Stay on the main trail as it follows the canyon through a grassy oak woodland.

At an oak tree by signpost 14, leave the road/trail and veer left on the Old Emerald Trail, a narrow footpath. Cross a footbridge and ascend the canyon wall. Curve left on a horseshoe bend, and climb to a T-junction on Bommer Ridge. Head north on the narrow ridge, passing Big Bend Trail on the right. Curve left across the head of Emerald Canyon, completing the loop at Willow Canyon Road. Go to the right and return down Willow Canyon. ■

88. Laurel Canyon—Willow Canyon Loop

LAGUNA COAST WILDERNESS PARK

trails open 7:00 a.m. to sunset · parking lots 8:00 a.m. to 5:00 p.m.

Hiking distance: 3.5-mile loop
Hiking time: 2 hours
Configuration: loop
Elevation gain: 600 feet
Difficulty: moderate
Exposure: exposed slope and shady canyon
Dogs: not allowed
Maps: U.S.G.S. Laguna Beach · Laguna Coast Wilderness Park map

The Irvine Ranch occupied this land for over a century. In the late 1980s, landowners and the adjacent communities worked together to preserve a large parcel of the ranchland from development, opening the Laguna Coast Wilderness Park in 1993.

This picturesque loop explores the upper reaches of the park through Laurel and Willow Canyons. The two adjacent canyons, filled with oaks and sycamores, run parallel to each other, divided by Willow Ridge. The scenic ridge overlooks the San Joaquin Hills, the coastal canyons, and the Pacific Ocean. Laurel Canyon is a hiking-only, stream-fed riparian corridor with large, weather-sculpted sandstone formations.

To the trailhead

20050 LAGUNA CANYON RD · LAGUNA BCH   33.580080, -117.762080

From the 405 (San Diego) Freeway in Irvine, take the Laguna Canyon Road (Highway 133) exit, and drive 5 miles south to the signed Laguna Coast Wilderness parking lot on the right, just south of the El Toro Road intersection.

From the Pacific Coast Highway in downtown Laguna Beach, head 3.2 miles north on Broadway (which becomes Laguna Canyon Road) to the posted Laguna Coast Wilderness parking lot on the left.

The hike

From the northwest corner of the parking lot, the left fork leads to the visitor center and Willow Canyon (the return route). Take the Laurel Canyon Trail to the right, passing massive sandstone outcroppings with sculpted caves and arches. Climb up and over the rise to the mouth of Laurel Canyon, adjacent to El Toro Road. Head up the forested canyon floor. Parallel the seasonal stream under the shade of oaks and sycamores. Cross the streambed and steadily climb the north wall of the narrow canyon. Recross the streambed at the brink of a 40-foot ephemeral waterfall. The footpath ends at an unpaved park road.

Bear left, curving up the road/trail to a T-junction on Willow Ridge in a saddle. Detour to the right to Bommer Ridge for a spectacular view of the mountains and ocean. After enjoying the views, return back down the Willow Canyon Trail. Traverse the south canyon wall while walking steadily downhill, overlooking the inland valley and the Santa Ana Mountains. Pass more sandstone boulders and drop into a shady oak and sycamore woodland to the visitor center near the trailhead. ▧

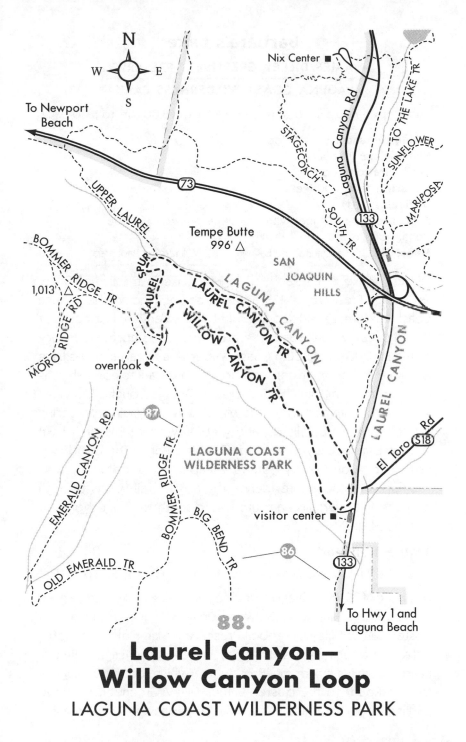

88.

Laurel Canyon–
Willow Canyon Loop

LAGUNA COAST WILDERNESS PARK

89. Barbara's Lake

JAMES DILLEY GREENBELT PRESERVE

LAGUNA COAST WILDERNESS PARK

trails open 7:00 a.m. to sunset · parking lots 8:00 a.m. to 5:00 p.m.

Hiking distance: 2.7-mile loop
Hiking time: 1.5 hours
Configuration: loop
Elevation gain: 300 feet
Difficulty: easy
Exposure: open hillsides with occasional pockets of shade
Dogs: not allowed
Maps: U.S.G.S. Laguna Beach · Laguna Coast Wilderness Park map

Barbara's Lake is a 12-acre spring-fed lake in the James Dilley Greenbelt Preserve, a 173-acre parcel of land in the Laguna Coast Wilderness Park. Located in Laguna Canyon, just north of the Highway 73 toll road, the area forms the north boundary of the 20,000-acre South Coast Wilderness Area. Barbara's Lake is named in honor of conservationist Barbara Rabinowitsh. It is one of three remaining natural lakes in Orange County. The year-round lake is rimmed with willows, cattails, and bulrush, offering habitat for coots, mallards, and grebes. West of Barbara's Lake (across Laguna Canyon Road) is Bubble's Pond. The pond was named for Lion County Safari's escaped hippopotamus, who took up a temporary residence there. The trail winds through canyons and over hills en route to the south and east shores of Barbara's Lake.

To the trailhead

19000 LAGUNA CANYON RD · LAGUNA BEACH   33.595295, -117.760210

From the 405 (San Diego) Freeway in Irvine, take the Laguna Canyon Road (Highway 133) exit. Drive 3.9 miles south to the posted James Dilley Greenbelt Preserve parking lot on the left.

From the Pacific Coast Highway in downtown Laguna Beach, head 4.3 miles north on Broadway (which becomes Laguna Canyon Road) to the posted James Dilley Greenbelt Preserve parking lot on the right, just north of the Highway 73 toll road.

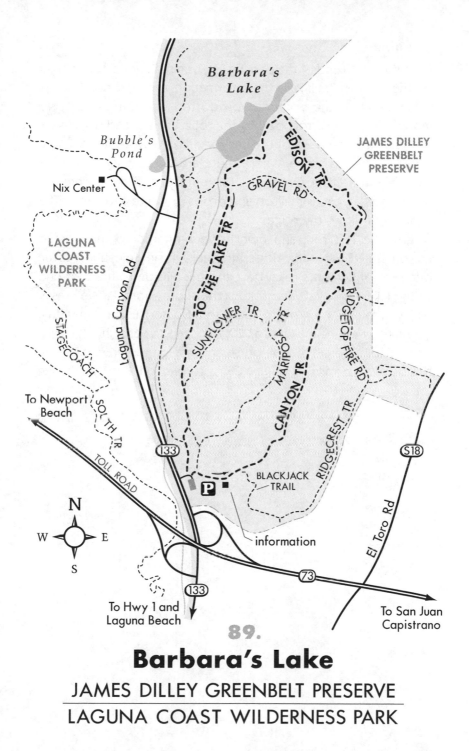

Barbara's Lake

Bubble's Pond

Nix Center

JAMES DILLEY GREENBELT PRESERVE

EDISON TR

GRAVEL RD

LAGUNA COAST WILDERNESS PARK

Canyon Rd

Laguna Canyon Rd

STAGECOACH

SOUTH TR

TO THE LAKE TR

SUNFLOWER TR

MARIPOSA TR

CANYON TR

RIDGETOP FIRE RD

RIDGECREST TR

To Newport Beach

TOLL ROAD

133

BLACKJACK TRAIL

P

information

El Toro Rd

S18

N
W E
S

To Hwy 1 and Laguna Beach

133

73

To San Juan Capistrano

89.
Barbara's Lake
JAMES DILLEY GREENBELT PRESERVE
LAGUNA COAST WILDERNESS PARK

The hike

From the north end of the parking lot, begin the loop to the right on the Canyon Trail. Pass the information cart and head north, meandering up the open canyon dotted with oaks and sycamores. The path, surrounded by the rolling hills, steadily gains elevation. Near the head of the canyon, make a sweeping S-curve through a cactus grove, where there are views back down the canyon to the Pacific Ocean. A short but steep climb reaches the ridge on a flat, circular hilltop and drops down to a trail fork. The right fork follows the ridge.

Take the left fork and quickly veer right onto the posted Edison Trail. Follow the ridge, gradually losing elevation to an overlook of Barbara's Lake. Descend the hillside to the east end of the lake. Curve left and follow the south shore. Pass a grassy picnic area under a grove of oaks to a posted T-junction with a gravel road. Go to the left for 20 yards, and veer right at a signpost. Stroll through the tall brush and grasslands, traversing the hillside. Walk parallel to Laguna Canyon Road, back to the parking lot. ■

90. Laguna Beach Bluffs and Heisler Park

CRESCENT BAY POINT PARK to MAIN BEACH

Hiking distance: 1.8 miles round trip
Hiking time: 1 hour
Configuration: out-and-back
Elevation gain: 80 feet
Difficulty: easy
Exposure: open coastline
Dogs: allowed
Maps: U.S.G.S. Laguna Beach

Heisler Park is a beautifully landscaped park on the cliffs above the ocean in the heart of Laguna Beach. The park sits at the base of the San Joaquin Hills, 80 feet above the scalloped coastline. The Laguna Beach Marine Life Refuge, a protected marine park with tidepools, stretches along the coast beneath Heisler Park. It is a popular area for snorkeling and diving.

This hike begins in Crescent Bay Point Park overlooking the coast, with views of Seal Rock, the rocky coastline, Catalina Island, and San Clemente Island. A paved path along the palisades offers views of the magnificent seascape, passing a series of craggy points and sheltered sandy coves. Paths and stairways descend to the protected coves that are surrounded by steep cliffs, rock formations, and pockets of tidepools.

To the trailhead

1300 CLIFF DRIVE · LAGUNA BEACH   33.547648, -117.800852

From the 405 (San Diego) Freeway in Irvine, take the Laguna Canyon Road (Highway 133) exit, and drive 8.2 miles south to the Pacific Coast Highway in downtown Laguna Beach. Turn right and drive 0.7 miles to the second Cliff Drive intersection. Turn left and park along the bluffs (metered parking).

The hike

Walk to the west towards Crescent Bay Point Park on the northwest end of the bay. From the park are great views of the bay and offshore rocks. Return southeast along the bluffs, passing Twin Points, Shaw's Cove, Fisherman's Cove, and Diver's Cove. (Stairs descend to the sandy beaches in Crescent Bay and Fisherman's Cove.) Enter Heisler Park and follow the crenulated coastline under pines and palms. Continue past Picnic Beach, Recreation Point, and Rockpile Beach. Stairways lead down the eroded cliffs to the off-shore rocks at the point and beach. At the west end of Cliff Drive is a cliff-edge gazebo that overlooks the ocean and Bird Rock. A path on the right winds through dense foliage and rejoins the main path. Descend from the east end of the bluffs on a sloping grade and down steps to Main Beach, a sandy beach at the south end of Broadway. A wooden boardwalk snakes along the coastline be-tween the beachfront and the grassy park in downtown Laguna Beach, ending at Forest Avenue. Return by retracing your steps. ▪

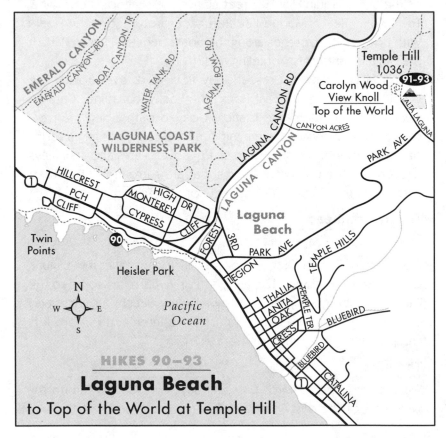

HIKES 90–93

Laguna Beach

to Top of the World at Temple Hill

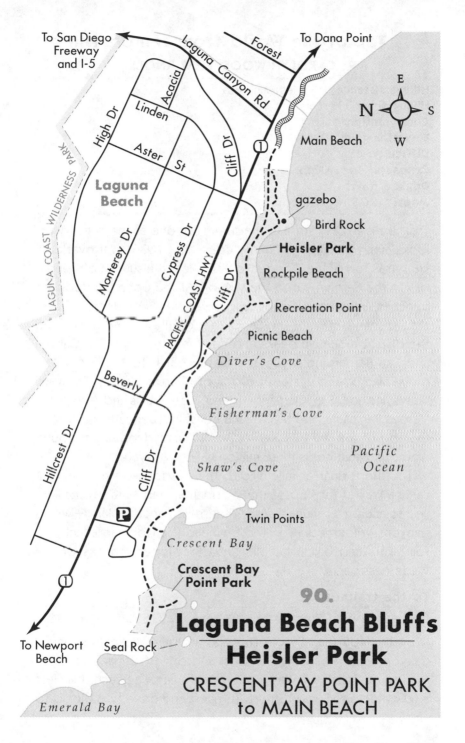

To San Diego Freeway and I-5

Laguna Canyon Rd

Forest

To Dana Point

Acacia

Linden

High Dr

Aster

St

Cliff Dr

Main Beach

E

N — S

W

Laguna Beach

LAGUNA COAST WILDERNESS PARK

gazebo

Bird Rock

Monterey Dr

Cypress Dr

PACIFIC COAST HWY

Cliff Dr

Heisler Park

Rockpile Beach

Recreation Point

Picnic Beach

Diver's Cove

Beverly

Fisherman's Cove

Hillcrest Dr

Cliff Dr

Shaw's Cove

Pacific Ocean

P

Twin Points

Crescent Bay

Crescent Bay Point Park

To Newport Beach

Seal Rock

Emerald Bay

90.

Laguna Beach Bluffs
Heisler Park

CRESCENT BAY POINT PARK to MAIN BEACH

91. Top of the World from Temple Hill
CAROLYN WOOD VIEW KNOLL

Hiking distance: 0.5 miles round trip
Hiking time: 30 minutes
Configuration: lollipop
Elevation gain: 40 feet
Difficulty: easy
Exposure: open hilltop
Dogs: allowed
Maps: U.S.G.S. Laguna Beach

This hike is an easy stroll to the summit of one of the finest over-looks along the Orange County coast. The 1,036-foot overlook, known as Top of the World, is located near the summit of Temple Hill on the Carolyn Wood View Knoll. At the open overlook are benches, interpretive maps, and sweeping 360-degree vistas. Map displays identify the Saddleback Valley communities and the distant mountain peaks and canyons, from the San Gabriel and San Bernardino Mountains in the north to the Santa Ana Mountains on the eastern border of Orange County. Seaward views include San Clemente Island, Catalina Island, the Palos Verdes Peninsula, and the Laguna coastline. Beneath the knoll is the Top of the World Reservoir, an 18-foot-deep underground water tank that holds three million gallons of water.

The short, quarter-mile hike to the overlook starts from Alta Laguna Park at the Top of the World Trailhead. Alta Laguna Park lies adjacent to Laguna Coast Wilderness Park and Aliso—Wood Canyons Wilderness Park. The trailhead is a popular launch site for hikers and bikers heading into the upper reaches of the wilderness parks.

To the trailhead

3325 ALTA LAGUNA BLVD · LAGUNA BEACH   33.555329, -117.759634

From the 405 (San Diego) Freeway in Irvine, take the Laguna Canyon Road (Highway 133) exit, and drive 8.2 miles south to the Pacific Coast Highway in downtown Laguna Beach. Turn left a few blocks to Legion Street. Turn left and drive two blocks to

Park Avenue. Veer right onto Park Avenue, and wind 1.7 miles up the hill to Alta Laguna Boulevard at the end of the road. Turn left and continue 0.2 miles to Alta Laguna Park. Turn right and park.

The hike

From the north end of Alta Laguna Boulevard, adjacent to Alta Laguna Park, walk up the wide dirt path to the trail information board and junction. The right fork follows the West Ridge Trail into the heart of Aliso and Wood Canyons Wilderness Park (Hikes 92–92). Stay to the left. Follow the ridge through scrub oak, overlooking the Pacific Ocean and Laguna Canyon to the left and Wood Canyon to the right. Loop up the knoll to the summit, where there are display maps, benches, and world-class panoramas. Several paths connect to perimeter trails that spiral around the knoll. ■

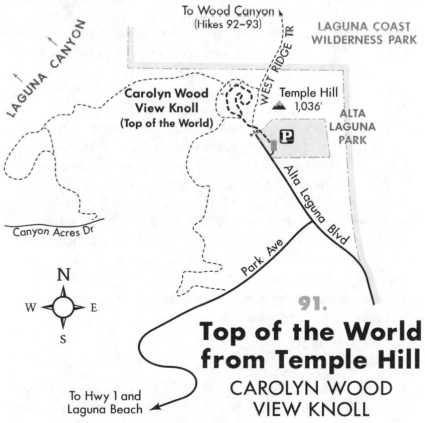

91.

Top of the World from Temple Hill

CAROLYN WOOD
VIEW KNOLL

92. Lower West Ridge—
Wood Canyon—Mathis Canyon Loop

LAGUNA COAST WILDERNESS PARK

ALISO and WOOD CANYONS WILDERNESS PARK

Hiking distance: 5.5 miles round trip
Hiking time: 4 hours
Configuration: lollipop
Elevation gain: 850 feet
Difficulty: moderate to strenuous
Exposure: mostly open hillsides with woodlands along creek
Dogs: not allowed
Maps: U.S.G.S. Laguna Beach and San Juan Capistrano
Aliso and Wood Canyons Wilderness Park map

From Laguna Beach, the San Joaquin Hills rise abruptly from the sea to an elevation over 1,000 feet. Spread across the hills are large undeveloped tracts of land that have been preserved as public parks and wilderness areas. An extensive network of hiking, mountain biking, and equestrian trails crisscross the parkland.

One of these treasures, Aliso and Wood Canyons Wilderness Park, spreads across 4,000 acres and includes more than 30 miles of trails. The park has massive sandstone formations, several forested canyons, two year-round streams, lush riparian vegetation, oaks, elderberries, sycamores, and native grasslands.

This hike begins from the Top of the World trailhead on Temple Hill, the highest point in the park at 1,036 feet. The amazing bird's-eye views extend across the Pacific Ocean and into Laguna and Wood Canyons. From Temple Hill, the undulating path follows a ridge separating the canyons, then drops into the upper end of Wood Canyon. The trail follows a stream amongst ancient oaks and sycamores before climbing out of the canyon and back up to Temple Hill.

To the trailhead

3325 ALTA LAGUNA BLVD · LAGUNA BEACH   33.555329, -117.759634

From the 405 (San Diego) Freeway in Irvine, take the Laguna Canyon Road exit (Highway 133), and drive 8.2 miles south to

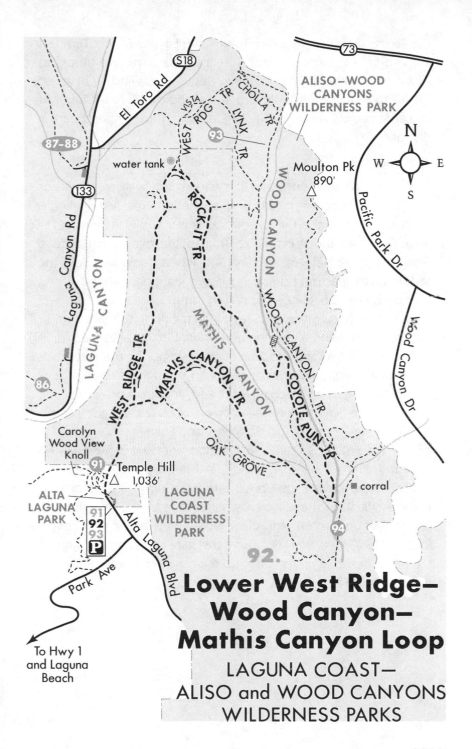

ALISO–WOOD
CANYONS
WILDERNESS PARK

S18

73

87-88

133

86

El Toro Rd

VISTA

WEST RDG TR

CHOLLA TR

LYNX TR

93

water tank

ROCK-IT TR

WOOD CANYON

Moulton Pk
890'

Pacific Park Dr

Wood Canyon Dr

N
W   E
S

Laguna Canyon Rd

LAGUNA CANYON

WEST RIDGE TR

MATHIS CANYON TR

MATHIS CANYON

WOOD CANYON

COYOTE RUN TR

Carolyn
Wood View
Knoll

OAK GROVE

corral

91

Temple Hill
△ 1,036'

ALTA
LAGUNA
PARK

91
92
93
P

Alta Laguna Blvd

LAGUNA
COAST
WILDERNESS
PARK

94

92.

Park Ave

To Hwy 1
and Laguna
Beach

Lower West Ridge– Wood Canyon– Mathis Canyon Loop

LAGUNA COAST– ALISO and WOOD CANYONS WILDERNESS PARKS

the Pacific Coast Highway in downtown Laguna Beach. Turn left a few blocks to Legion Street. Turn left and drive two blocks to Park Avenue. Veer right onto Park Avenue, and wind 1.7 miles up the hill to Alta Laguna Boulevard at the end of the road. Turn left and continue 0.2 miles to Alta Laguna Park. Turn right and park in the lot.

The hike

From the northwest corner of the parking lot, walk up the steps to a trail information board and a junction. The left fork is a short walk up to the Carolyn Wood View Knoll on Temple Hill (Hike 91). Take the West Ridge Trail to the right and descend along the spine between Laguna and Wood Canyons. Cross the saddle on the narrow ridge to a posted junction with the Mathis Canyon Trail at 0.6 miles—the return route.

Begin the loop to the left, staying on the ridge to a large water tank on the left and a junction on the right at 1.5 miles. Bear right on the Rock-It Trail and descend a minor ridge. The trail descends on an easy grade, then becomes steep through a slab rock section of trail. Make a sweeping left bend, and drop down into the canyon at the Coyote Run Trail at three miles. Curve right through an oak grove to the Wood Canyon floor. Follow the west edge of the creek to a streamside junction with the signed Mathis Canyon Trail.

Bear right, leaving the creek, and head uphill. Curve around the west flank of the hillside by sandstone caves. Pass the Oak Grove Trail on the left, and climb up a steep grade to an overlook of Oak Grove. Walk through a trail gate and steeply climb up the ridge, completing the loop on the ridge. Bear left and return to Alta Laguna Park. ■

93. Upper West Ridge—
Upper Wood Canyon Loop

LAGUNA COAST WILDERNESS PARK

ALISO and WOOD CANYONS WILDERNESS PARK

Hiking distance: 7.6 miles round trip
Hiking time: 4 hours
Configuration: lollipop
Elevation gain: 850 feet
Difficulty: strenuous
Exposure: exposed ridgelines and riparian woodlands
Dogs: not allowed
Maps: U.S.G.S. Laguna Beach and San Juan Capistrano
Aliso and Wood Canyons Wilderness Park map

The South Coast Wilderness Area (also known as the Laguna Greenbelt) includes a contiguous series of parks, open spaces, wilderness areas, and marine preserves that cover 20,000 acres in the low-rolling San Juaquin Hills. This hike loops through the upper reaches of Aliso and Wood Canyons Wilderness Park, a 4,000-acre park on the southeast end of the Laguna Greenbelt. The hike begins at the Top of the World trailhead on a 1,000-foot ridge known as Temple Hill, located between Laguna Canyon and Wood Canyon. Sweeping views span across the Pacific coastline, north to the San Gabriel Mountains, and southeast to the Santa Ana Range. The route follows the east crest of Laguna Canyon, vegetated with chaparral and coastal sage scrub. The loop drops into the forested streamside vegetation of upper Wood Canyon, then climbs back up to the West Ridge Trail along the hillcrest.

To the trailhead

3325 ALTA LAGUNA BLVD · LAGUNA BEACH   33.555329, -117.759634

From the 405 (San Diego) Freeway in Irvine, take the Laguna Canyon Road (Highway 133) exit, and drive 8.2 miles south to the Pacific Coast Highway in downtown Laguna Beach. Turn left a few blocks to Legion Street. Turn left and drive two blocks to

Park Avenue. Veer right onto Park Avenue, and wind 1.7 miles up the hill to Alta Laguna Boulevard at the end of the road. Turn left and continue 0.2 miles to Alta Laguna Park. Turn right and park in the lot.

The hike

From the northwest corner of the parking lot, walk up the steps to a trail information board and a junction. The left fork is a short walk up to the Carolyn Wood View Knoll on Temple Hill (Hike 91). Take the wide West Ridge Trail to the right, overlooking the Saddleback Valley, San Joaquin Hills, and the Santa Ana Mountains. Descend along the spine between Laguna Canyon and Wood Canyon, crossing a saddle on the narrow ridge. Pass the Mathis Canyon Trail on the right, viewing layers of minor ridges and canyons. At 1.5 miles is a large water tank on the left and a junction with the Rock-It Trail on the right—the return route.

Begin the loop to the left, staying on the ridge. Pass the Lynx Trail to the gated park boundary. Take the signed Cholla Trail to the right, and wind down the serpentine path to the shady floor of Wood Canyon. Bear right, heading down Wood Canyon under oaks and sycamores. One mile down canyon, take the posted Coyote Run Trail on the right. Cross a wooden footbridge over the creek to a T-junction a quarter mile ahead. The Coyote Run Trail heads left.

Take the Rock-It Trail to the right and leave the canyon floor. Ascend the hillside while steadily climbing the minor ridge to the West Ridge Trail, completing the loop. Return to the trailhead, 1.5 miles to the left. ∎

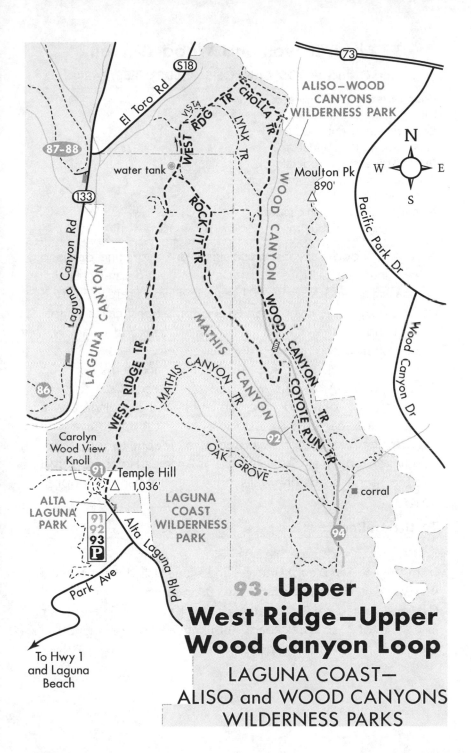

S18

73

ALISO–WOOD
CANYONS
WILDERNESS PARK

El Toro Rd

VISTA

WEST RDG TR

CHOLLA TR

LYNX TR

87-88

water tank

Moulton Pk
890'

N
W · E
S

133

Pacific Park Dr

ROCK-IT TR

WOOD CANYON

Laguna Canyon Rd

LAGUNA CANYON

Wood Canyon Dr

86

MATHIS

WOOD CANYON

COYOTE RUN TR

WEST RIDGE TR

MATHIS CANYON TR

MATHIS CANYON

92

Carolyn
Wood View
Knoll

OAK GROVE

94

91

Temple Hill
△ 1,036'

corral

ALTA
LAGUNA
PARK

LAGUNA
COAST
WILDERNESS
PARK

91
92
93
P

Alta Laguna Blvd

Park Ave

To Hwy 1
and Laguna
Beach

**93. Upper
West Ridge–Upper
Wood Canyon Loop**

LAGUNA COAST–
ALISO and WOOD CANYONS
WILDERNESS PARKS

94. Aliso Canyon and Wood Canyon
ALISO and WOOD CANYONS WILDERNESS PARK

Hiking distance: 5.7 miles round trip
Hiking time: 3 hours
Configuration: out-and-back
Elevation gain: 150 feet
Difficulty: easy to moderate
Exposure: mostly open grasslands
Dogs: not allowed
Maps: U.S.G.S. San Juan Capistrano
Aliso and Wood Canyons Wilderness Park map

Aliso and Wood Canyons Wilderness Park is pristine parkland tucked into the hillsides and valleys between Laguna Beach, Laguna Niguel, and Aliso Viejo. The undeveloped refuge has two major stream-fed canyons, sandstone formations, caves sculpted by wind and water, aged groves of live oaks and sycamores, and an extensive hiking and biking trail system.

This hike travels west into Aliso Canyon and turns north up Wood Canyon. Along the way, the trail passes Cave Rock, a 26-million-year-old sandstone formation, and Dripping Cave, a historic water-carved cave also known as Robber's Cave. The overhanging rock shelter was used as a hideout to rob stagecoaches en route from San Diego to Los Angeles. Holes are bored into the interior sandstone walls, once used for hanging supplies on pegs.

To the trailhead

28373 ALICIA PARKWAY · LAGUNA NIGUEL   33.551501, -117.719978

From the I-5 (San Diego) Freeway in Laguna Hills, take the Alicia Parkway exit. Head 4 miles south to the posted Aliso and Wood Canyons Wilderness Park on the right. (The turnoff is a quarter mile south of Aliso Creek Road.) Turn right and park in the lot on the left. A parking fee is required.

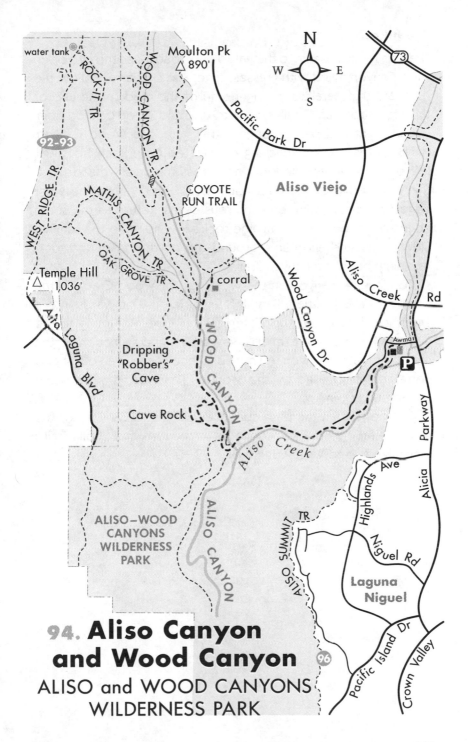

water tank

ROCK-IT TR

WOOD CANYON TR

Moulton Pk
△ 890'

N
W   E
S

73

Pacific Park Dr

92-93

WEST RIDGE TR

MATHIS CANYON TR

OAK GROVE TR

COYOTE
RUN TRAIL

Aliso Viejo

Temple Hill
△ 1,036'

corral

Aliso Creek Rd

Wood Canyon Dr

Alto Laguna Blvd

Dripping
"Robber's"
Cave

WOOD CANYON

Awma

P

Cave Rock

Aliso Creek

Parkway

Highlands Ave

Alicia

ALISO–WOOD
CANYONS
WILDERNESS
PARK

ALISO CANYON

SUMMIT TR

ALISO

Niguel Rd

Laguna
Niguel

**94. Aliso Canyon
and Wood Canyon**
ALISO and WOOD CANYONS
WILDERNESS PARK

96

Pacific Island Dr

Crown Valley

The hike

Walk past the museum to the gated park road. Descend into open Aliso Canyon, filled with grasses, sage, and chaparral. Follow the footpath that parallels the right side of the road to the end of the access road at 1.5 miles, where Aliso and Wood Canyons join.

Bear right and pass through a trail gate into Wood Canyon. Head up the canyon, reaching the posted Cave Rock Trail. Bear left on the quarter-mile loop, and cross the grassy meadow to the south edge of the enormous rock. Detour along the west edge of the formation by numerous caves. Return to the south edge and follow the trail up the rock's low spine to the summit. Slowly descend and curve around the north end of the rock, rejoining the Wood Canyon Trail.

Continue up canyon on the west side of Wood Creek to the Dripping Cave junction. Bear left and detour 350 yards into a shady oak grove and the water-carved cave. Returning to the main trail, cross a stream spillway to a signed junction at the mouth of Mathis Canyon. A short distance ahead is an old sheep corral, originally used by the Moulton Ranch family. This is the turn-around point.

To hike farther, the path continues up Wood Canyon. At the canyon's far end, the trail connects to the Lynx and Cholla Trails, which lead up to West Ridge (Hikes 92—93). ▪

95. Sulphur Creek Reservoir

LAGUNA NIGUEL REGIONAL PARK

28241 La Paz Road · Laguna Niguel

Hiking distance: 1.6-mile loop
Hiking time: 1 hour
Configuration: loop
Elevation gain: 20 feet
Difficulty: very easy
Exposure: open parkland with pockets of trees
Dogs: allowed
Maps: U.S.G.S. San Juan Capistrano · Laguna Niguel Regional Park map

Laguna Niguel Regional Park is comprised of 236 acres of rolling terrain with hiking, biking, and equestrian trails. Within the

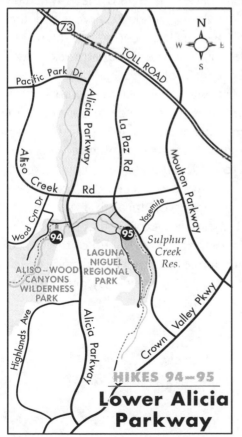

park are eucalyptus, sycamore, white alder, and acacia woodlands. The centerpiece of the park is Sulphur Creek Reservoir, a creek-fed, 44-acre lake. The picturesque lake is a popular recreational site for fishing and boating, as well as a wildlife sanctuary for ducks, geese, and other waterfowl. This hike loops around the lake on a level hiking path, crossing a bridge over Sulphur Creek and passing shady picnic areas.

To the trailhead

28241 LA PAZ ROAD · LAGUNA NIGUEL   33.552420, -117.709851

From I-5 (San Diego Freeway) in Laguna Hills, take the La Paz Road exit. Head 3.9 miles south to the posted park entrance on the right. After entering the park, turn left and continue 0.2 miles to the parking lot on the right by picnic shelter 7.

From I-5 (San Diego Freeway) in Laguna Niguel, take the Crown Valley Parkway exit, and head 4.2 miles south to La Paz Road. Turn right and drive 1.4 miles to the park entrance on left. After entering the park, turn left and continue 0.2 miles to the parking lot on the right by picnic shelter 7.

The hike

Follow the park road uphill. Curve left toward the fish hatchery to an overlook of the Sulphur Creek Reservoir and the tree-covered hillside. Continue along the west side of the reservoir to a footpath on the left, just before the boat dock. Leave the road and descend to the lake. Stroll through a shoreline fishing area that is often teeming with ducks. At the south end of the lake, the waterway narrows to a creek near a trail split and a bridge. The right fork continues south along Sulphur Creek to Crown Valley Community Park and the Niguel Botanical Preserve.

Take the left fork and cross the bridge over Sulphur Creek, walking through a grove of willows and eucalyptus trees. Head north on the east side of the reservoir through a grassy flat, following the contours of the cattail-lined lake that sits 80 feet below La Paz Road. Near the dam at the north end of the lake, a tunnel on the right crosses under La Paz Road to Yosemite Road. Continue past the dam and drop down to a grassy, tree-dotted parkland. Curve left, completing the loop. ▧

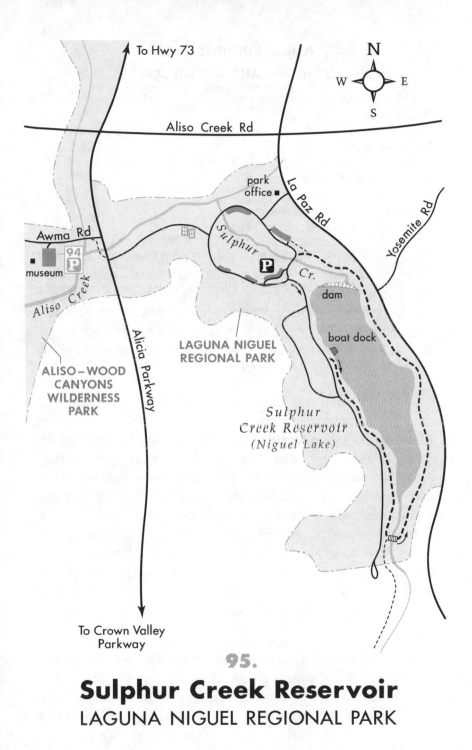

95.

Sulphur Creek Reservoir
LAGUNA NIGUEL REGIONAL PARK

96. Aliso Summit Trail

ALISO and WOOD CANYONS WILDERNESS PARK

Hiking distance: 4 miles round trip
Hiking time: 2 hours
Configuration: out-and-back with optional return loop on street
Elevation gain: 200 feet
Difficulty: easy
Exposure: open cliffside pathway
Dogs: allowed
Maps: U.S.G.S. San Juan Capistrano
       Aliso and Wood Canyons Wilderness Park map

The Aliso Summit Trail is a little known gem discretely perched on the steep cliffs of Aliso Canyon. It is tucked behind the gated community of Coronado Pointe in Laguna Niguel and borders the east boundary of Aliso and Wood Canyons Wilderness Park. The serpentine trail follows 800-foot-high cliffs on the east rim of the canyon. Throughout the hike are views of the stream-fed Aliso Canyon and the Pacific Ocean.

To the trailhead

30775 PACIFIC ISLAND DR · LAGUNA NIGUEL   33.516261, -117.727263

From I-5 (San Diego Freeway) in Laguna Niguel, take the Crown Valley Parkway exit. Head 5.7 miles south to Pacific Island Drive. Turn right (west) and drive 1.8 miles to La Brise. Park along the curb on either side of Pacific Island Drive. The posted trailhead is on the west side of the road, across from La Brise.

From the Pacific Coast Highway, drive 0.8 miles north on Crown Valley Parkway to Pacific Island Drive on the left. Turn left (west) and drive 1.8 miles to La Brise. Park along the curb on either side of Pacific Island Drive. The posted trailhead is on the west side of the road, across from La Brise.

The hike

Walk past the posted trailhead gate, and follow the paved path on the east lip of Aliso Canyon. Continue on the wide gravel path, landscaped with ponderosa pines, eucalyptus, willows, palms, and tall oleander hedges. The winding path meanders

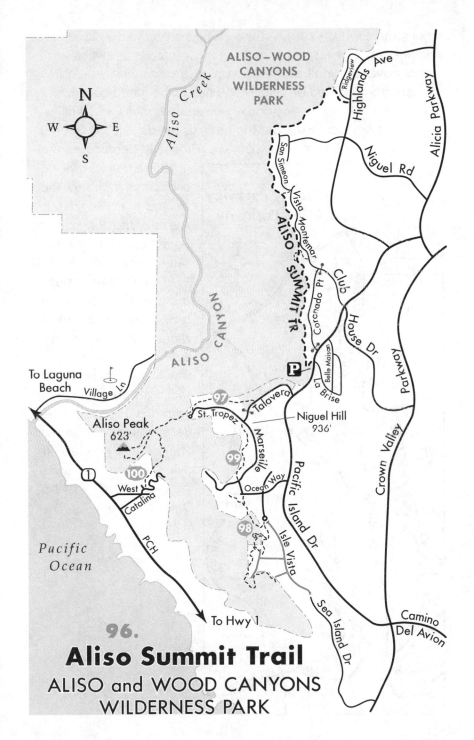

N
W   E
S

ALISO–WOOD
CANYONS
WILDERNESS
PARK

Aliso Creek

Ridgeview

Highlands Ave

Alicia Parkway

San Simeon

Niguel Rd

Vista Montemar

ALISO SUMMIT TR

Coronado Pt

Club House Dr

ALISO CANYON

ALISO

To Laguna
Beach

Village Ln

P

Belle Maison

La Brise

Parkway

Aliso Peak
623'

St. Tropez

Talavera

Niguel Hill
936'

97

99

Marseille

Crown Valley

1

100

West
Catalina

Ocean Way

98

Isle Vista

Pacific Island Dr

Pacific
Ocean

PCH

Sea Island Dr

To Hwy 1

Camino
Del Avion

96.
Aliso Summit Trail
ALISO and WOOD CANYONS
WILDERNESS PARK

along the contours of the steep cliffs just below the ridge-top homes. At 0.7 miles, a side path on the left leads through a small pine grove to a knoll, with a canyon-to-the-sea vista. Pass a trail access from the end of Vista Montemar in the gated community of Coronado Pointe (an optional turn-around point). At 1.4 miles, inland views open up across the basin to the distant San Gabriel Mountains and Santa Ana Mountains. Gradually descend to the

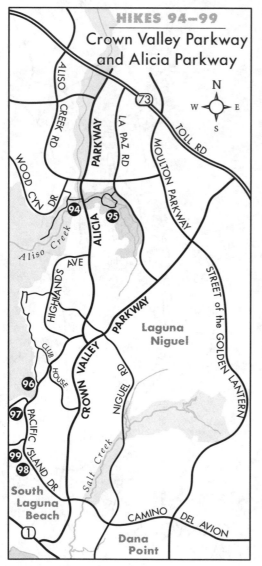

northern trailhead kiosk, and curve right to the trailhead at Highlands Avenue and Ridgeview Drive. Return along the same route.

For a loop hike through the gated residential area, return to the Vista Montemar trail access. Bear left, then follow Vista Montemar to the right to a junction with Coronado Pointe. Bear right on Coronado Pointe, and walk a half mile to the entrance gate at Pacific Island Drive. Return to the right. ■

97. Aliso Peak from Seaview Park
ALISO and WOOD CANYONS WILDERNESS PARK

Hiking distance: 0.5–2.8 miles round trip
Hiking time: 30 minutes–1.5 hours
Configuration: out-and-back
Elevation gain: level to 400 feet
Difficulty: easy
Exposure: open coastal ridge
Dogs: allowed
Maps: U.S.G.S. San Juan Capistrano
      Aliso and Wood Canyons Wilderness Park map

Seaview Park straddles the crest of 936-foot Niguel Hill on the east boundary of Aliso and Wood Canyons Wilderness Park. The ridge-top park sits on the cliffs 800 feet above Aliso Canyon and borders a residential neighborhood. At the west end of the park is the Seaview Park Overlook, a platform with displays perched on the ridge. The sweeping vistas span across the South Coast Wilderness Parks, the San Joaquin Hills, Aliso Canyon,

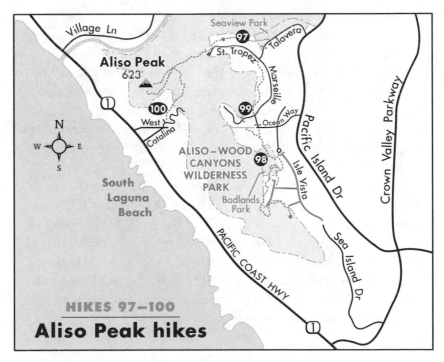

HIKES 97–100
Aliso Peak hikes

Laguna Beach, the scalloped coastline, the communities within Saddleback Valley, and the Santa Ana Mountains. The trail follows the oceanfront ridge to Aliso Peak, where the hill dramatically drops 623 feet into the sea.

To the trailhead

22729 TALAVERA DR · LAGUNA NIGUEL   33.513225, -117.732034

From I-5 (San Diego Freeway) in Laguna Niguel, take the Crown Valley Parkway exit. Head 5.7 miles south to Pacific Island Drive. Turn right (west) and drive 1.6 miles to the crest of the hill, then turn left (west) on Talavera Drive. Continue a quarter mile and park along the curb near the end of the road.

From the Pacific Coast Highway, drive 0.8 miles north on Crown Valley Parkway to Pacific Island Drive on the left (west). Turn left (west) and drive 1.6 miles to the crest of the hill, then turn left (west) on Talavera Drive. Continue a quarter mile and park along the curb near the end of the road.

The hike

Walk west along Seaview Park's grassy strip, hugging the edge of the 800-foot cliffs on the south rim of Aliso Canyon. The views extend up and down the canyon and across the valley basin to the Santa Ana Mountains. Leave the grassy parkland into the native chaparral and coastal sage scrub, topping a small rise to a view of Catalina Island. Curve west and follow the ridge past the interpretive panels to a picnic table at the Seaview Park Overlook. This is a good turn-around point for a short half-mile (route-trip) hike.

Aliso Peak Trail, a narrow footpath, continues downhill to the west, dropping to a saddle by Saint Tropez, a road in the gated Laguna Sur community. Veer away from the road, and drop down to a lower saddle. Cross the saddle, staying on the ridge to a trail split with the Valido Trail (Hike 100). Stay to the right, passing the Toovet Trail, and steadily climb to Aliso Peak. The last 40 yards to the summit are steep. From the peak are sweeping 360-degree coastal views as far as the haze allows. ▪

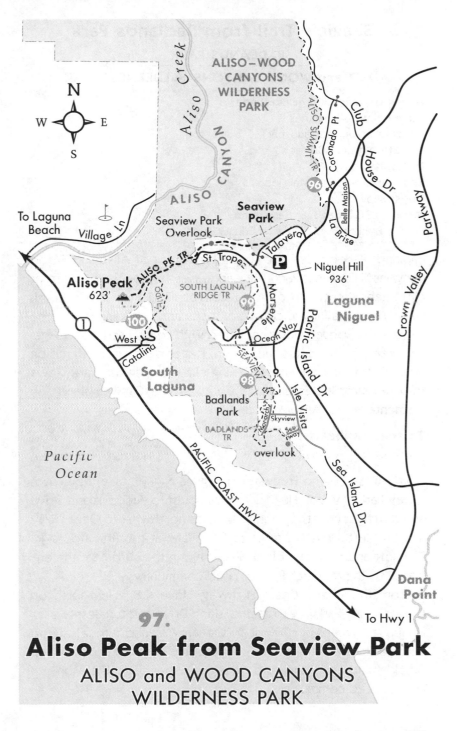

Aliso Peak from Seaview Park
ALISO and WOOD CANYONS
WILDERNESS PARK

98. Seaview Trail from Badlands Park

BADLANDS PARK

ALISO and WOOD CANYONS WILDERNESS PARK

Hiking distance: 1.5 miles round trip
Hiking time: 45 minutes
Configuration: out-and-back
Elevation gain: 100 feet
Difficulty: easy
Exposure: open coastal slopes
Dogs: allowed
Maps: U.S.G.S. San Juan Capistrano
       Franko's Map of Orange County Trails

Badlands Park borders the southeast corner of Aliso and Wood Canyons Wilderness Park. The park is perched on the oceanfront cliffs near the mouth of Aliso Canyon, 780 feet above South Laguna and the Pacific coastline. It sits amid eroding sandstone cliffs with exposed slopes covered with coastal scrub and sage. The area is on the site of an ancient beach dating back 10 million years. From the park and adjoining cliff-hugging trails are views of Dana Point, Salt Creek Beach, South Laguna, Catalina Island, San Clemente Island, Aliso Peak, and the San Joaquin Hills.

To the trailhead

31662 ISLE VISTA · LAGUNA NIGUEL   33.503904, -117.732146

From I-5 (San Diego Freeway) in Laguna Niguel, take the Crown Valley Parkway exit. Head 5.7 miles south to Pacific Island Drive and turn right (west). Continue 1.1 miles northwest to Ocean Way and turn left. Drive 0.2 miles to Isle Vista, at the first stop sign. Turn left and park one block ahead along the curb near the entrance to the Monarch Pointe gated community.

From the Pacific Coast Highway, drive 0.8 miles north on Crown Valley Parkway to Pacific Island Drive and turn left (west). Continue 1.1 miles northwest to Ocean Way and turn left. Drive 0.2 miles to Isle Vista, at the first stop sign. Turn left and park one block ahead along the curb near the entrance to the Monarch Pointe gated community.

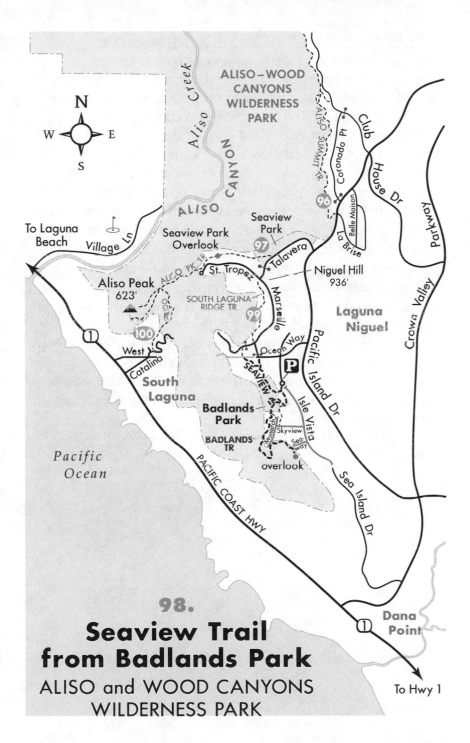

N W E S

To Laguna Beach

ALISO-WOOD CANYONS WILDERNESS PARK

Aliso Creek

Aliso

ALISO CANYON

ALISO

Village Ln

Seaview Park Overlook

Seaview Park

St. Tropez

ALISO PK. TR

Aliso Peak 623'

SOUTH LAGUNA RIDGE TR

Talavera

Niguel Hill 936'

Marseille

Laguna Niguel

Coronado Pt

Belle Maison

La Brise

Club House Dr

Parkway

Crown Valley

West Catalina

Ocean Way

SEAVIEW

Pacific Island Dr

South Laguna

Badlands Park

BADLANDS TR

Monarch

Skyview

Seaway

overlook

Isle Vista

Pacific Ocean

PACIFIC COAST HWY

Sea Island Dr

Dana Point

To Hwy 1

98.
Seaview Trail
from Badlands Park
ALISO and WOOD CANYONS
WILDERNESS PARK

The hike

Walk up the street towards the gated community. Just outside the gate, climb steps on the right to the edge of Badlands Park at a coastal overlook and a junction. Bear left a short distance to another junction. The Seaview Trail, a connector trail, continues 0.1 mile straight ahead and ends at the corner of Skyview Way and Monarch Crest. Bear right and descend the steps into Badlands Park, with a network of meandering sand paths and eroding sandstone formations. Skirt the edge of the oceanfront cliffs on the wide, graveled Badlands Trail. The path winds south, traversing the scrub-covered slopes. Curve along the south-facing cliffs, and loop around the Monarch Crest cul-de-sac. The footpath continues to the right and ends on a narrow ridge extending out towards Dana Point.

Return to the trailhead, and now take the north fork. Wind along the 780-foot cliffs toward prominent Aliso Peak. Side paths on the left cross narrow ridges between the steep-walled canyons. A short distance ahead is a trail split. The left fork ends at a concrete fire access road. The right fork leads to the Laguna Sur gated community and the trailhead for the South Laguna Ridge Trail (Hike 99). ▧

99. Aliso Peak from South Laguna Ridge Trail

ALISO and WOOD CANYONS WILDERNESS PARK

Hiking distance: 2.5 miles round trip
Hiking time: 1.5 hours
Configuration: out-and-back
Elevation gain: 200 feet
Difficulty: easy
Exposure: open coastal ridge
Dogs: allowed
Maps: U.S.G.S. San Juan Capistrano
Aliso and Wood Canyons Wilderness Park map

Aliso Peak is a 623-foot oceanfront summit with a bird's-eye view of Laguna Beach and the coastline. Three routes lead to the peak, which is located at the southern tip of Aliso and Wood Canyons Wilderness Park. This trail winds through the gated Laguna Sur residential area from the southeast, overlooking the coastal cliffs to the sea. The trail connects with the Aliso Peak Trail, following a ridge between Aliso Canyon and Valido Canyon to the Aliso Peak summit. (Hike 97 accesses Aliso Peak from the east, and Hike 100 climbs up a canyon from the south.)

To the trailhead

22631 OCEAN WAY • LAGUNA NIGUEL   33.505575, -117.733942

From I-5 (San Diego Freeway) in Laguna Niguel, take the Crown Valley Parkway exit. Head 5.7 miles south to Pacific Island Drive and turn right (west). Continue 1.1 miles northwest to Ocean Way and turn left. Drive 0.3 miles and park along the curb near the end of the road.

From the Pacific Coast Highway, drive 0.8 miles north on Crown Valley Parkway to Pacific Island Drive and turn left (west). Continue 1.1 miles northwest to Ocean Way and turn left. Drive 0.3 miles and park along the curb near the end of the road.

The hike

On the left (south) side of the road is the Seaview Trail (Hike 98). Take the trail to the right—the South Laguna Ridge Trail. It is connected by a trail easement through the Laguna Sur gated community. Walk through the entrance gate on the right. Follow the posted trail signs one block on Cannes Drive to the corner of Marseille. Cross the road and take the posted asphalt path to the corner of Marseille and Saint Tropez at Talavera Drive. Bear left and walk down Saint Tropez to the end of the road. Just before the cul-de-sac, veer right onto the dirt footpath to the Aliso Peak Trail. Bear left and descend along the ridge across the saddle, passing the Valido Trail and Toovet Trail on the left. Steadily climb west to a bench atop the 623-foot knob. The last 40 yards to the summit are steep. After enjoying the sweeping vistas, retrace your steps back to the trailhead. ∎

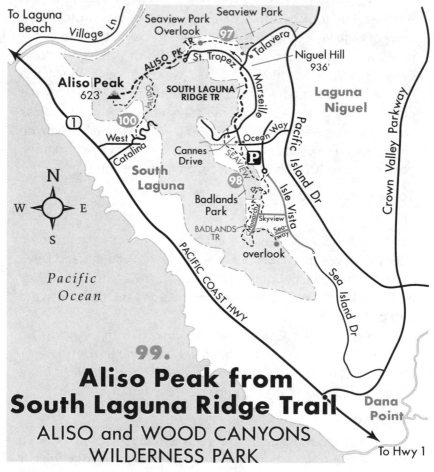

99.
Aliso Peak from
South Laguna Ridge Trail
ALISO and WOOD CANYONS
WILDERNESS PARK

100. Aliso Peak from Valido Trail

ALISO and WOOD CANYONS WILDERNESS PARK

Hiking distance: 2 miles round trip
Hiking time: 1 hour
Configuration: out-and-back
Elevation gain: 400 feet
Difficulty: easy to moderate
Exposure: open coastal slopes
Dogs: allowed
Maps: U.S.G.S. San Juan Capistrano
Aliso and Wood Canyons Wilderness Park map

Aliso Peak is located at the southern end of Aliso and Wood Canyons Wilderness Park near the Pacific coastline. Three hikes lead to the peak—the Aliso Peak Trail (Hike 97), the South Laguna Ridge Trail (Hike 99), and the Valido Trail (this route). It is the most dramatic of the three routes. The trail climbs up rugged Valido Canyon, an unspoiled stream-fed canyon, to a saddle on the ridge at the head of the canyon. From the saddle, two trail options head toward Aliso Peak. The level Toovet Trail, perched on the cliffs, loops around the south-facing cliff to the ocean side of Aliso Peak. The Aliso Peak Trail climbs directly to the 623-foot summit. From the peak are phenomenal vistas up and down the coastline.

To the trailhead

22112 PASEO DEL SUR · LAGUNA BEACH   33.506007, -117.743271

From the Pacific Coast Highway and Crown Valley Parkway at Monarch Beach, drive 1.6 miles northwest on PCH to Catalina Avenue and turn right. Continue 0.1 mile to Valido Road and veer left. Continue 50 yards to the posted trailhead on the left. Turn around and park on the north side of the street.

From the Pacific Coast Highway and Broadway in downtown Laguna Beach, drive 3.5 miles southeast on PCH to Catalina Avenue and turn left. Continue 0.1 mile to Valido Road and veer left. Continue 50 yards to the posted trailhead on the left. Turn around and park on the north side of the street.

The hike

The posted trailhead is just north (uphill) of Toto Loma Lane. Take the wide dirt path, passing a row of mature eucalyptus trees, to the south wall of Valido Canyon. The wide path narrows to a footpath and traverses the stream-fed canyon. Cross the drainage and climb up the hillside with the aid of log steps. Continue uphill to the ridge in the low spot of a saddle, 600 feet above Aliso Creek. On the ridge is a T-junction with the Aliso Peak Trail. The right fork leads to Seaview Park.

Bear left 15 yards to a junction with the Toovet Trail on the left. Detour left, skirting clockwise around the peak on a level grade. The trail ends high above the ocean and below Aliso Peak, with 180-degree vistas up and down the Orange County coast. Return to the Aliso Peak Trail on the saddle and now bear left. Steadily climb west to the 623-foot knob, with 360-degree vistas and a viewing bench. The last 40 yards to the summit are steep. After admiring the views, return along the same route. ■

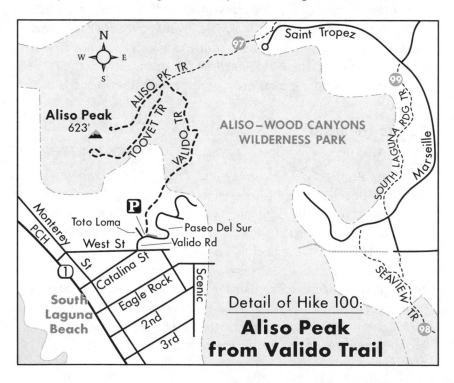

Detail of Hike 100:

**Aliso Peak
from Valido Trail**

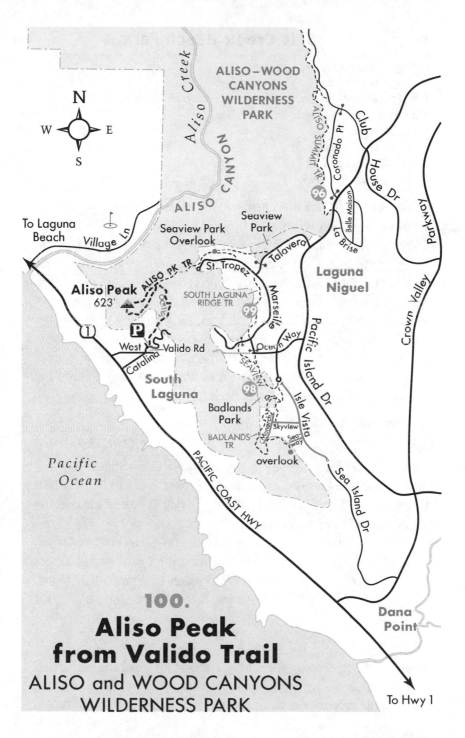

100.
Aliso Peak
from Valido Trail
ALISO and WOOD CANYONS
WILDERNESS PARK

101. Salt Creek Beach Park

Hiking distance: 2 miles round trip
Hiking time: 1 hour
Configuration: out-and-back or return loop along beach
Elevation gain: 80 feet
Difficulty: easy
Exposure: open blufftop
Dogs: allowed on trail
Maps: U.S.G.S. Dana Point

Salt Creek Beach Park is a 1.5-mile-long beach strand that stretches between Dana Point and Three Arch Cove in South Laguna. The popular surfing beach is divided by a point, on which the Ritz Carlton Hotel is perched. A paved pedestrian path leads through the Ritz Carlton Hotel grounds to Bluff Park, a seven-acre sloping grassland park with benches and picnic tables overlooking the beach. It is a great spot to view migrating gray whales and Catalina Island. A paved path follows the bluffs, with stairways and paths leading down to the beach. At the north end, the path connects with the Salt Creek Trail (Hike 102), a multi-use trail heading inland along Salt Creek.

To the trailhead

1 RITZ CARLTON DRIVE · DANA POINT   33.476653, -117.719276

From I-5 (San Diego Freeway) in San Juan Capistrano, take the Beach Cities/Highway 1 exit. Head 3.7 miles west to Ritz Carlton Drive. Turn left and drive 0.1 mile to the Salt Creek Beach parking lot on the left. A parking fee is required.

From I-5 (San Diego Freeway) in Laguna Niguel, take the Crown Valley Parkway exit, and head 6.1 miles south to the Pacific Coast Highway. Turn left and continue 0.7 miles to Ritz Carlton Drive. Turn right and drive 0.1 mile to the Salt Creek Beach parking lot on the left.

The hike

Near the west-central side of the parking lot, take the park road under Ritz Carlton Drive to the expansive, sloping parkland overlooking the ocean. As you near the bluffs, a paved path heads south (left) and climbs the bluffs through the landscaped hotel grounds to an overlook. The views extend from the Dana Point promontory to Catalina Island to the San Joaquin Hills backing South Laguna.

Return to the park road at the beachfront, and now head north on the paved blufftop path. Continue through Bluff Park towards the headland at Three Arch Cove. Just before reaching the golf course, a couple of unpaved sloping paths lead down to the beach. The Salt Creek Trail—Hike 102—continues inland along the edge of the golf course and through a tunnel under the Pacific Coast Highway. To return, curve left, leaving the bluff path to the lower path at the back edge of the sandy beach. Return on the oceanfront path to the beach access trail. The path continues south, ending at the sand. ■

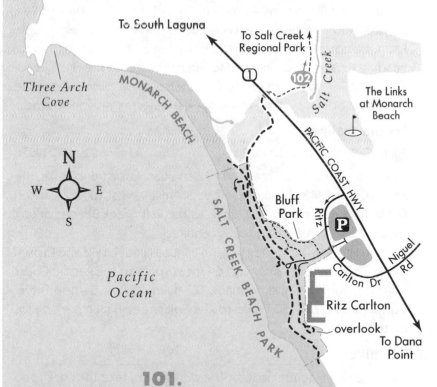

101.
Salt Creek Beach Park

102. Salt Creek Trail
FROM SALT CREEK BEACH PARK

Hiking distance: 6 miles round trip
Hiking time: 3 hours
Configuration: out-and-back
Elevation gain: 400 feet
Difficulty: easy to moderate
Exposure: open blufftop and exposed residential pathway
Dogs: allowed
Maps: U.S.G.S. Dana Point and San Juan Capistrano

The Salt Creek watershed flows through the cities of Laguna Niguel and Dana Point to the sea. A paved three-mile, multi-use trail follows Salt Creek through a wide greenbelt corridor in the heart of Laguna Niguel, connecting the beach with the coastal hills. This hike begins from Salt Creek Beach Park by the Ritz Carlton Hotel grounds, between South Laguna and Dana Point. From the north end of the beach, the paved path curves inland, heading through The Links at Monarch Beach, Salt Creek Regional Park, and San Juan Canyon to Chapparosa Community Park. The path is a popular walking route for the adjacent neighborhoods.

To the trailhead

1 RITZ CARLTON DRIVE · DANA POINT   33.476653, -117.719276

From I-5 (San Diego Freeway) in San Juan Capistrano, take the Beach Cities/Highway 1 exit. Head 3.7 miles west to Ritz Carlton Drive. Turn left and drive 0.1 mile to the Salt Creek Beach parking lot on the left. A parking fee is required.

From I-5 (San Diego Freeway) in Laguna Niguel, take the Crown Valley Parkway exit, and head 6.1 miles south to the Pacific Coast Highway. Turn left and continue 0.7 miles to Ritz Carlton Drive. Turn right and drive 0.1 mile to the Salt Creek Beach parking lot on the left.

The hike

Near the west-central side of the parking lot, take the park road under Ritz Carlton Drive to the expansive, sloping parkland overlooking the ocean. As you near the bluffs, paved paths lead in

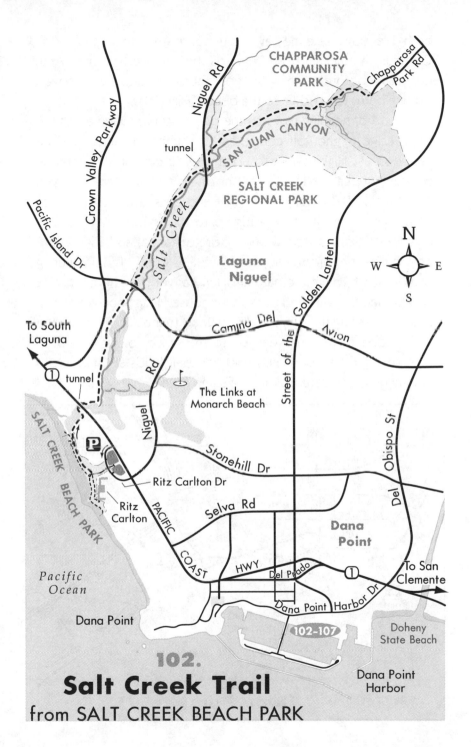

CHAPPAROSA
COMMUNITY
PARK

Chapparosa Park Rd

Niguel Rd

tunnel

SAN JUAN CANYON

SALT CREEK
REGIONAL PARK

Crown Valley Parkway

Pacific Island Dr

Salt Creek

Laguna
Niguel

N
W ⊕ E
S

Golden Lantern

Street of the

Avion

To South
Laguna

Camino Del

1 tunnel

Niguel Rd

The Links at
Monarch Beach

SALT CREEK BEACH PARK

P

Ritz Carlton Dr

Ritz
Carlton

Stonehill Dr

Obispo St

PACIFIC

Selva Rd

Del

Dana
Point

Pacific
Ocean

COAST

HWY

Del Prado

1

To San
Clemente

Dana Point

Dana Point Harbor Dr

Dana Point

102-107

Doheny
State Beach

Dana Point
Harbor

102.
Salt Creek Trail
from SALT CREEK BEACH PARK

both directions. Take the paved blufftop path to the right (north). Continue through Bluff Park towards the headland at Three Arch Cove. Just before reaching the golf course, a couple of unpaved sloping paths lead down to the beach (Hike 101).

Instead of heading towards the beach, curve inland along the north edge of the golf course and through a tunnel under the Pacific Coast Highway. Head up the wide canyon on a steady but gentle uphill grade along the north side of Salt Creek. As you near Camino Del Avion, curve right and pass under the road to a trail split. The right fork leads up to the road. Stay left, walk parallel to Camino Del Avion a short distance, and then curve right on the rim of the canyon above Salt Creek. The undulating path winds through the natural open canyon for the next mile. As you near Niguel Road at the Clubhouse Plaza Shops, make an S-curve, passing through the Niguel Road tunnel. Continue on the north slope of San Juan Canyon to the grassy picnic area with sycamore groves, rolling hills, and baseball fields at Chapparosa Community Park. Return along the same path. ▪

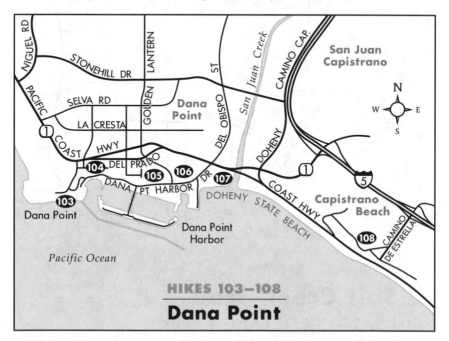

HIKES 103–108
Dana Point

103. Dana Point Harbor

Hiking distance: 2.5 miles round trip
Hiking time: 1.5 hours
Configuration: out-and-back and loop
Elevation gain: level
Difficulty: easy
Exposure: exposed coastline
Dogs: allowed on paved paths but not on beach
Maps: U.S.G.S. Dana Point

Dana Point Harbor, built in 1971, is a majestic harbor located at the base of 200-foot cliffs near the southern coastal end of Orange County. The harbor lies between the 120-acre Dana Point headland and Doheny State Beach. The Dana Point Marine Life Refuge surrounds the steep precipice from the west end of the harbor, including the offshore San Juan Rocks. Tidepools line the protected refuge, with sea urchins, anemone, starfish, and hermit crabs. Bordering the marina is a grassy waterfront park with picnic tables, a calm-water swimming beach, fishing platforms, and a paved walkway. Dana Island, a picturesque manmade island park, fronts the Dana Point Harbor. It is reached via Island Way, a vehicle/pedestrian bridge beside the boat moorings. This hike explores the harbor, Dana Island, and the shoreline beneath the Dana Point cliffs.

To the trailhead

24332 DANA POINT HARBOR DR · DANA POINT   33.463569, -117.704092

From I-5 (San Diego Freeway) in San Juan Capistrano, take the Beach Cities/Highway 1 exit. Head 1.3 miles west to Dana Point Harbor Drive. Turn left and continue 1.1 miles to the posted pier parking lot on the left.

The hike

From the grassy beachfront park, take the paved path to the right, looping around the west end of the marina. Pass a few wooden piers, the ocean institute, and a bookstore to the mile-long breakwater. At the far west end of the harbor, just past the rock jetty, steps lead down to a fenced enclosure. Pass through the open structure to the shoreline at the base of the 200-foot cliffs. Follow the base of the cliffs just above the rocky beach towards Dana Point. At low tide, the promontory can be circled, but use extreme caution.

After exploring the tidepools, return to the grassy park and beach cove by the parking lot and continue east, in the opposite direction. Pass a myriad of boat moorings, and continue to Island Way. Head south (seaward) on the walkway, crossing the 150-foot-long bridge over the water channel to Dana Island. A loop circles the narrow island that fronts the harbor channel and oceanfront. ■

104. Blufftops of Dana Point Harbor
Ken Sampson Overview Park—Hide Trail

Hiking distance: 1 mile round trip
Hiking time: 40 minutes
Configuration: out-and-back
Elevation gain: 25 feet
Difficulty: easy
Exposure: open blufftop
Dogs: allowed
Maps: U.S.G.S. Dana Point

The town of Dana Point is a small, bustling enclave with a unique history. In 1835, Richard Henry Dana, aboard the brig *Pilgrim*, helped deliver goods from Boston—around Cape Horn—in exchange for cattle hides from Mission San Juan Capistrano. In 1840, he published his experiences in *Two Years Before the Mast*. His classic memoirs describe how the hides were thrown off the 200-foot cliffs from the current site of the Ken Sampson Overview Park to the beach below, where longboats rowed them out to the ship.

This walk along the blufftop includes views across the entire harbor. The route spans from Ken Sampson Overview Park at the west end to the Hide "Blufftop" Trail at the east end. The

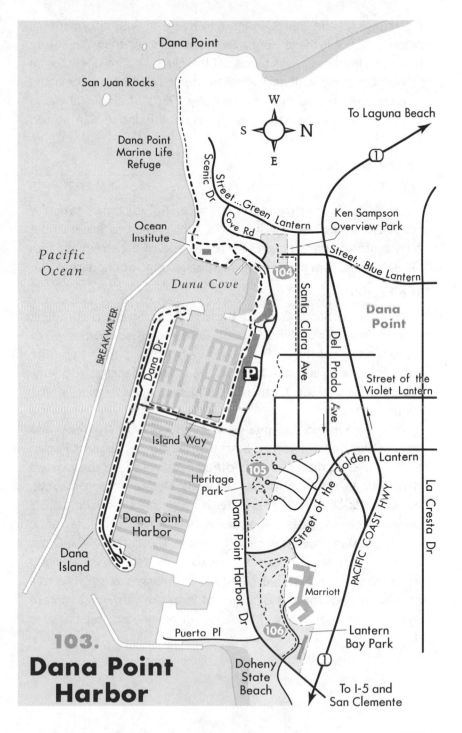

Dana Point

San Juan Rocks

Dana Point
Marine Life
Refuge

Scenic Dr

Street...Green Lantern

Cove Rd

Ocean
Institute

Pacific
Ocean

Dana Cove

BREAKWATER

Dana Dr

P

Island Way

Heritage
Park

Dana Point
Harbor

Dana
Island

Dana Point Harbor Dr

Puerto Pl

To Laguna Beach

1

Ken Sampson
Overview Park

Street... Blue Lantern

104

Santa Clara Ave

Del Prado Ave

**Dana
Point**

Street of the
Violet Lantern

105

Street of the Golden Lantern

Lantern

PACIFIC COAST HWY

La Cresta Dr

Marriott

106

Lantern
Bay Park

Doheny
State
Beach

1

To I-5 and
San Clemente

103.
Dana Point
Harbor

cliff-hugging Hide Trail is an interpretive trail with informational plaques about Richard Henry Dana and a larger-than-life statue of a hide drogher tossing hides off the cliffs. The trail includes an arched concrete wall and winding stone-lined paths, remnants of an abandoned hotel from the early 1930s. The coastal views extend across Capistrano Bay, from Dana Point to San Mateo Point.

To the trailhead

34499 RUBY LANTERN · DANA POINT   33.464510, -117.704698

From I-5 (San Diego Freeway) in San Juan Capistrano, take the Beach Cities/Highway 1 exit. Head 2.4 miles west to Street of the Ruby Lantern. Turn left and drive to the end of the street at Santa Clara Avenue. Turn either way and park alongside the street.

The hike

Walk west on Santa Clara to the corner at Street of the Blue Lantern. Bear left to Ken Sampson Overview Park and the gazebo extending off the cliffs. The views from the park include the Dana Point headland, the harbor, the point's beaches (Doheny, Capistrano, and San Clemente), and San Mateo Point at the southern county line.

Walk back inland to Santa Clara Avenue (the first street) and go one block east (right) to Street of the Amber Lantern. Return to the edge of the cliffs at another overlook. Take the posted Hide Trail east, which follows an early Native American route. Traverse the cliffs and cross a deep gorge on a footbridge to a cement archway. Notice the remnants of a rock path that once led to the Dana Point Inn, dating back to the early 1930s. Cross under the archway and climb steps to a sandstone rock wall and a nine-foot bronze statue of a hide droghing seaman. The trail ends at an overlook at the corner of Street of the Violet Lantern and El Camino Capistrano. Return by retracing your steps. ▪

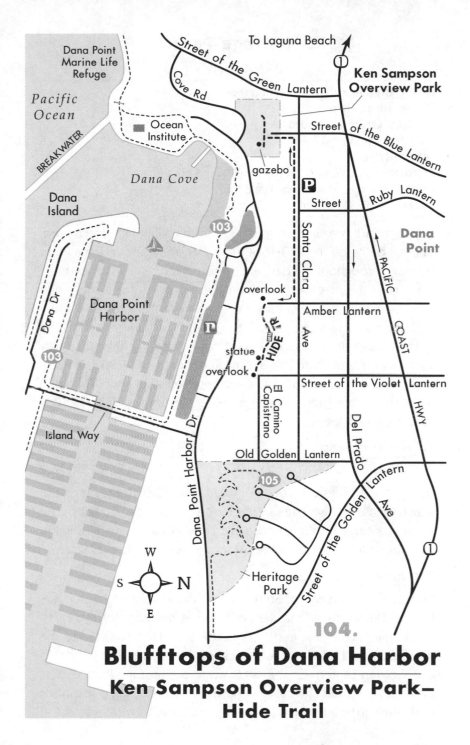

Blufftops of Dana Harbor

Ken Sampson Overview Park–
Hide Trail

104.

105. Heritage Park
DANA POINT

Hiking distance: 0.8 miles round trip
Hiking time: 1 hour
Configuration: out-and-back
Elevation gain: 120 feet
Difficulty: easy
Exposure: open coastal parkland with pockets of trees
Dogs: allowed (includes Dog Fun Zone)
Maps: U.S.G.S. Dana Point

Heritage Park is a six-acre grassland with rolling hills and paved, sinuous paths on the 120-foot marine terrace above Dana Point Harbor. Throughout the park are panoramic ocean vistas extending across the massive Dana Point Promontory, from the white sand beaches in Capistrano Bay to San Mateo Point. Walking paths and stairways lead from the bluffs to the sheltered cove at the harbor. It is a popular spot for observing migrating gray whales en route from the Bering Sea, north of Alaska, to Baja California. This park walk can be combined with Hike 104 along the bluffs—one block west—or Hike 106 through Lantern Bay Park—one block east.

To the trailhead

24601 EL CAMINO CAPISTRANO · DANA POINT   33.463474, -117.700263

From I-5 (San Diego Freeway) in San Juan Capistrano, take the Beach Cities/Highway 1 exit. Head 2.2 miles west to Street of the Violet Lantern. Turn left and drive several blocks to El Camino Capistrano and park curbside, wherever a space is available.

The hike

Walk to the south end of Street of the Violet Lantern to an overlook of Dana Harbor and the coastline at the edge of the cliffs. To the right is the east end of the Hide Trail (Hike 104). Go to the left (east), and head one block down El Camino Capistrano to Old Golden Lantern on the west edge of Heritage Park. A network of paths and staircases wind down the sloping oceanfront park through beautiful landscaped grounds with great vistas. The paths end by the harbor at Dana Point Harbor Drive near Street of the Golden Lantern. Across the street to the east is Lantern Bay County Park on the 100-foot bluffs. An access from the corner climbs the cliffs to the elevated grassy park. Across the street to the south is the harbor. ■

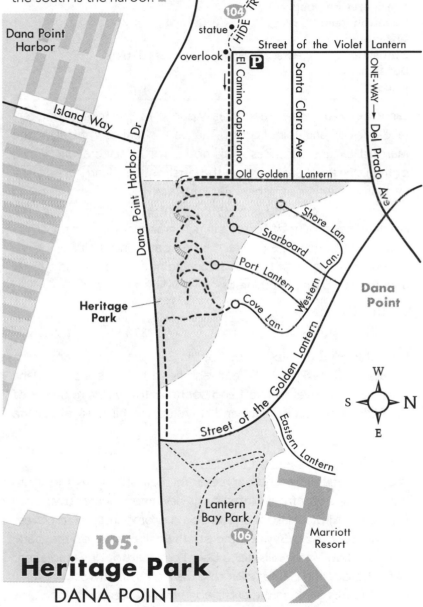

105.
Heritage Park
DANA POINT

106. Lantern Bay Park
DANA POINT

Hiking distance: 0.6-mile loop
Hiking time: 30 minutes
Configuration: loop
Elevation gain: 20 feet
Difficulty: very easy
Exposure: open coastal parkland with pockets of trees
Dogs: allowed
Maps: Dana Point

Lantern Bay Park is a 76-acre grassy park on a 120-foot marine terrace above Dana Point Harbor. The park, situated in front of the Marriott Laguna Cliffs Resort, is noted for its spectacular views of the Dana Point Promontory; the offshore San Juan Rocks; Dana Harbor; the white sand beaches of Doheny, Capistrano, and San Clemente Beaches; and San Mateo Point at the county line. The parkland has groves of Torrey pines, a grassy amphitheater, overlooks with benches, a paved walking path, and stairways connecting it to Heritage Park and Dana Point Harbor. This is a great area for observing the migrating gray whales.

To the trailhead

25111 PARK LANTERN · DANA POINT   33.464015, -117.689076

From the I-5 (San Diego Freeway) in San Juan Capistrano, take the Beach Cities/Highway 1 exit, and head 1.3 miles west to Dana Point Harbor Drive. Turn left and continue 100 yards to Street of the Park Lantern. Turn right and drive up the hill. Park along the curb.

The hike

A paved path circles the perimeter of the park. Along the south edge of the oceanfront bluffs is a grassy amphitheater overlooking the Dana Point Harbor and the bold promontory on the west end of Capistrano Bay. At the southwest corner of the park, stairs lead down the hillside to Dana Point Harbor Drive, adjacent to the harbor and Heritage Park. At the park's northwest corner, a path doubles back on the cliff's edge and descends to the steps at Dana Point Harbor Drive. The main park path returns on the inland border of the park along the resort boundary. ▪

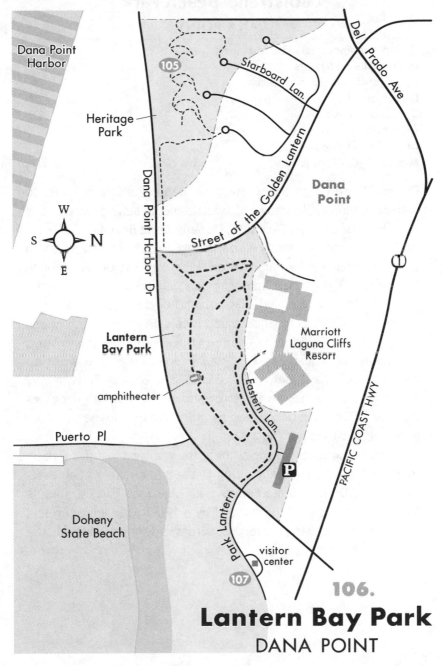

Dana Point Harbor

105

Starboard Lan.

Heritage Park

Dana Point Harbor Dr

Street of the Golden Lantern

Dana Point

Del Prado Ave

W
S ◈ N
E

Lantern Bay Park

amphitheater

Eastern Lan.

Marriott Laguna Cliffs Resort

Puerto Pl

P

PACIFIC COAST HWY

Doheny State Beach

Park Lantern

visitor center

107

106.
Lantern Bay Park
DANA POINT

343

107. Doheny State Beach to Capistrano Beach Park

DANA POINT

Hiking distance: 2.8 miles round trip
Hiking time: 1.5 hours
Configuration: out-and-back
Elevation gain: level
Difficulty: easy
Exposure: exposed beach and coastline
Dogs: not allowed on beach
Maps: U.S.G.S. Dana Point

Doheny State Beach and Capistrano Beach Park merge into an unbroken three-mile strand of white sand beach between Dana Point Harbor and San Clemente. Doheny State Beach is a 62-acre park with a mile of sandy beachfront, adjacent to the eastern end of the harbor. San Juan Creek flows into the ocean through the beach. During the summer, a sandbar restrains the creek's flow into the sea, forming a lagoon and bird sanctuary. West of the creek is a five-acre landscaped picnic area with shady trees, a rocky area with tidepools, and a visitor center with simulated tidepools and aquariums. East of San Juan Creek is a wooded campground. The Doheny Marine Life Refuge, popular with divers, is an underwater park just offshore. A bike path accesses the city of San Juan Capistrano to the north on a levee that parallels the west side of the creek.

This hike explores tidepools near the rock jetty of the harbor, then parallels the shoreline along the sandy beach. At the eastern end of Doheny State Beach, palm-lined walkway connects to Capistrano Beach Park, backed by a 120-foot marine terrace. En route, a pedestrian overpass crosses Highway 1 from the beach to the palisades.

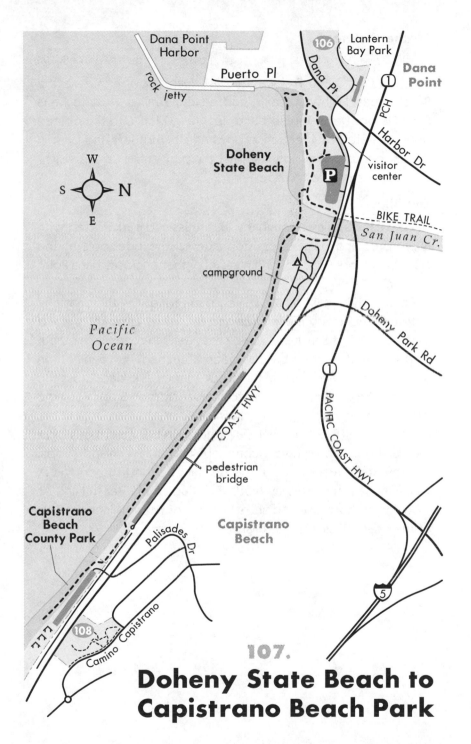

Dana Point Harbor

106

Lantern Bay Park

Puerto Pl

rock jetty

Dana Pt

PCH

Dana Point

1

Doheny State Beach

P

visitor center

Harbor Dr

W
S N
E

BIKE TRAIL

San Juan Cr.

campground

Pacific Ocean

Doheny Park Rd

1

COAST HWY

PACIFIC COAST HWY

pedestrian bridge

Capistrano Beach County Park

Palisades Dr

Capistrano Beach

5

108

Camino Capistrano

107.

Doheny State Beach to Capistrano Beach Park

To the trailhead

25300 DANA POINT HARBOR DR · DANA POINT   33.463909, -117.686271

From I-5 (San Diego Freeway) in San Juan Capistrano, take the Beach Cities/Highway 1 exit, and head 1.3 miles west to Dana Point Harbor Drive. Turn left and continue 0.1 mile to the posted Doheny State Beach entrance on the left. Turn left and park in the enormous parking lot, just past the park entrance and visitor center. An entrance fee is required.

The hike

Head west, strolling through the lush grassland park dotted with eucalyptus and palm trees. Continue to the tidepools at the state beach boundary by the rock jetty that encloses Dana Point Harbor.

Return to the east on the paved path, following the coastline between the grassy picnic area and the wide, crescent-shaped sandy beach. At San Juan Creek, cross the sandbar at the mouth of the river. If the sandbar has been breached, curve inland on the paved path and parallel the creek to the park road. Cross the creek on the bridge, and return to the beachfront. Stroll along the palm-lined beach, with views of Dana Point, the harbor, and the oceanfront cliffs. At one mile, a pedestrian bridge crosses over the Pacific Coast Highway, connecting to a few inland shops. Doheny State Beach ends a quarter mile beyond the bridge. A walkway near the highway leads into Capistrano Beach Park. At 1.4 miles, a short distance ahead, a row of houses lines the top of the beach. This is the turn-around point. ▓

108. Pines Park
DANA POINT

Hiking distance: 0.5 miles round trip
Hiking time: 30 minutes
Configuration: inter-connected pathways
Elevation gain: 100 feet
Difficulty: easy
Exposure: open parkland with several shady tree groves
Dogs: allowed
Maps: U.S.G.S. Dana Point

Pines Park is a small, tree-filled park on the Capistrano Beach Palisades. The 100-foot high blufftop park, with rolling terrain and a narrow, craggy canyon, offers beautiful views of the coastline from its picturesque, inter-twining paths. Edward "Ned" Doheny originally developed the area in the 1920s, planting an abundance of Aleppo and Canary Islands pines. Now the towering giants dominate the landscape. Paths wind through the marine terrace grasslands under the shady canopy.

To the trailhead

34941 CAMINO CAPISTRANO · DANA POINT   33.455792, -117.665161

From I-5 (San Diego Freeway) in San Clemente, take the Camino Estrella exit. Drive 0.4 miles south to Calle Hermosa. Turn right on Calle Hermosa, which curves right onto Camino Capistrano, and continue 0.3 miles to Pines Park on the left. Park along the road.

The hike

Take the winding, paved path through the lush, pine-filled park. From the south end of the park are sweeping coastal views of the Dana Point headland, Dana Point Harbor, Doheny Beach, Capistrano Beach, San Clemente Pier, and San Mateo Point at the Orange-San Diego county line. Near the center of the park is a deep gorge. The paved park path descends from both sides of the park to the gorge. An unpaved footpath drops down the gorge drainage between the steep, eroding sedimentary cliffs to the Pacific Coast Highway, across from Capistrano Beach. ∎

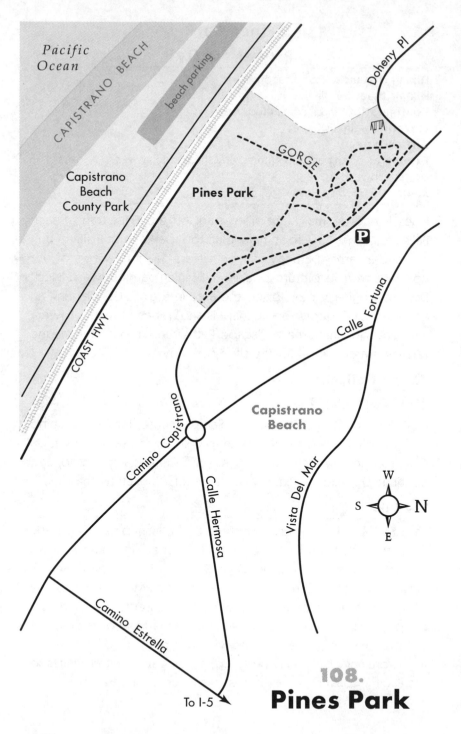

Pacific
Ocean

CAPISTRANO BEACH

beach parking

Doheny Pl

GORGE

Capistrano
Beach
County Park

Pines Park

P

Calle Fortuna

COAST HWY

Camino Capistrano

Calle Hermosa

**Capistrano
Beach**

Vista Del Mar

W
S ✦ N
E

Camino Estrella

To I-5

**108.
Pines Park**

109. Rancho San Clemente Ridgeline Trail

Hiking distance: 6 miles round trip
Hiking time: 3 hours
Configuration: out-and-back
Elevation gain: 600 feet
Difficulty: moderate
Exposure: open coastal ridge
Dogs: allowed
Maps: U.S.G.S. San Clemente

The Rancho San Clemente Ridgeline Trail is a popular neighborhood trail in the coastal hills above San Clemente. The trail follows a horseshoe-shaped ridge separating the coastal front from the inland basin, just west of the Orange–San Diego county line. The paved path stretches across the undulating ring of mountains, passing three scenic viewpoints en route to Knob Hill. Throughout the hike are sweeping coastal vistas and views across the inland valley to the Santa Ana and Santa Margarita Mountains. The trail is frequently used by dog owners.

To the trailhead

721 AVENIDA SALVADOR · SAN CLEMENTE   33.431255, -117.599050

SOUTHBOUND: From I-5 (San Diego Freeway) in San Clemente, take the El Camino Real exit. Turn right and drive 0.6 miles to Avenida Presidio. Turn right (under I-5) to the second street and turn right, staying on Avenida Presidio. Continue 0.8 miles northeast to Avenida Salvador and turn right. Drive 0.6 miles to the posted trailhead on the left, just before the crest of the hill. The trail is located at 721 Avenida Salvador, one house south of Calle Monserrat and two houses north of Calle Ameno.

NORTHBOUND: From I-5 (San Diego) Freeway in San Clemente, take the Avenida Presidio exit. Turn right, go to the second street, and turn right on Avenida Presidio. Continue 0.8 miles northeast to Avenida Salvador and turn right. Drive 0.6 miles to the posted trailhead on the left, just before the crest of the hill. The trail is located at 721 Avenida Salvador, one house south of Calle Monserrat and two houses north of Calle Ameno.

The hike

Pass the trailhead gate and walk up the paved utility access road. Curve clockwise around the water tank to an overlook of the entire horseshoe-shaped ridge, including the prominent communications towers and Knob Hill. Curve northeast and descend along the ridge to a saddle. Near the communications towers, an old road veers left up to the summit. Stay to the right, skirting around the east side of the towers to another junction at the low point of the trail. The right fork is an alternate access trail into Steed Park. Continue straight, climbing back to the tree-lined ridge on the north side of the towers to Viewpoint 2, with a picnic table and a bench. Curve right and descend to Calle De Cerro.

Cross the road and head right. Walk about 30 yards, picking up the trail on the left side of the road. Climb through a grove of eucalyptus trees. Slowly descend and cross a long saddle to the base of Knob Hill, where the pavement ends. Climb the short but steep hillside on a wide, dirt path. Just below the rounded summit, the path becomes paved again. Atop the flat, circular knoll are sweeping 360-degree vistas and two viewing benches. Return along the same route. ▪

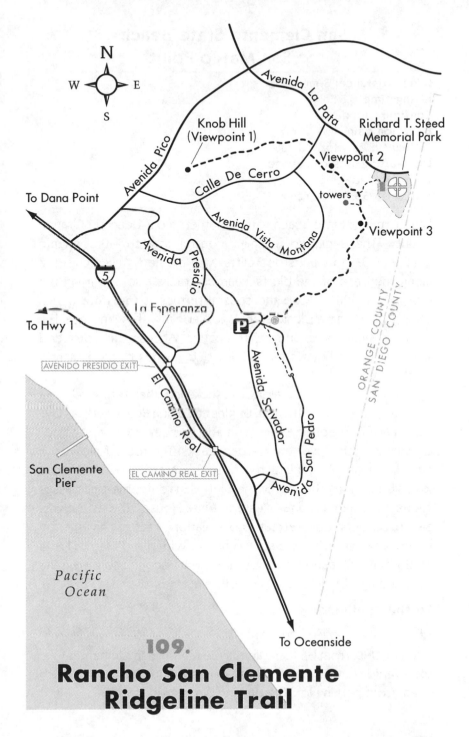

N
W E
S

Avenida La Pata

Knob Hill
(Viewpoint 1)

Richard T. Steed
Memorial Park

Avenida Pico

Calle De Cerro

Viewpoint 2

To Dana Point

towers

Avenida Vista Montana

Viewpoint 3

Avenida

Presidio

5

La Esperanza

ORANGE COUNTY
SAN DIEGO COUNTY

To Hwy 1

P

AVENIDO PRESIDIO EXIT

Avenida Salvador

Avenida San Pedro

El Camino Real

San Clemente
Pier

EL CAMINO REAL EXIT

Avenida

Pacific
Ocean

To Oceanside

109.

Rancho San Clemente
Ridgeline Trail

110. San Clemente State Beach to San Mateo Point

Hiking distance: 3-mile loop
Hiking time: 1.5 hours
Configuration: loop
Elevation gain: 100 feet
Difficulty: easy to moderate
Exposure: exposed coastline
Dogs: not allowed
Maps: U.S.G.S. San Clemente

San Clemente State Beach is the southernmost beach in Orange County. The secluded 1.5-mile coastal stretch sits beneath craggy 100-foot sandstone cliffs with eroded gullies chiseled along the base of the bluffs. Railroad tracks also run along the base of the cliffs. Atop the coastal terrace is the state beach campground and a picnic area, landscaped with palms, acacias, cypress, sycamores, and other exotics. Access trails descend from the coastal bluffs through eroded ravines to the isolated, sandy beach.

This hike makes a loop along the shoreline, then returns along a road atop the bluffs. The trail begins at Calafia Beach Park, a day-use area at the foot of Avenida Calafia. The beach provides a pedestrian crossing over the railroad tracks. The route follows the coastline from Calafia Beach Park to San Mateo Point, where it loops back along the top of the bluffs. En route, the trail passes former President Nixon's "Western White House." The estate was also used during his retreat into isolation after resigning from office. The Spanish-style stucco home, with a red tile roof, sits on 25 blufftop acres. It is obscured, but recognizable from its surroundings, by a dense cover of palm trees.

To the trailhead

243 AVENIDA CALAFIA · SAN CLEMENTE   33.405383, -117.605545

SOUTHBOUND: From I-5 (San Diego Freeway) in San Clemente, take the Avenida Calafia exit. Drive 0.4 miles west to the Calafia Beach oceanfront parking lot. The parking is metered.

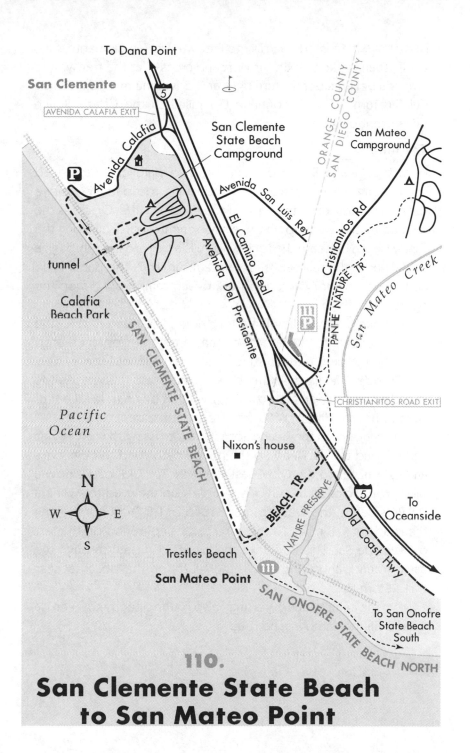

To Dana Point

San Clemente

AVENIDA CALAFIA EXIT

5

Avenida Calafia

P

San Clemente
State Beach
Campground

San Mateo
Campground

ORANGE COUNTY
SAN DIEGO COUNTY

Avenida San Luis Rey

El Camino Real

Cristianitos Rd

PANHE NATURE TR

San Mateo Creek

tunnel

Avenida Del Presidente

Calafia
Beach Park

111 P

SAN CLEMENTE STATE BEACH

Pacific
Ocean

Nixon's house

CHRISTIANITOS ROAD EXIT

5

N
W ← → E
S

BEACH TR

NATURE PRESERVE

Old Coast Hwy

To
Oceanside

Trestles Beach

San Mateo Point

111

SAN ONOFRE STATE BEACH NORTH

To San Onofre
State Beach
South

110.

San Clemente State Beach
to San Mateo Point

NORTHBOUND: From I-5 (San Diego Freeway) in San Clemente, take the Cristianitos Road exit. Turn left and cross over the freeway to Avenida Del Presidente. Turn right and drive one mile to Avenida Calafia. Turn left and continue 0.4 miles to the Calafia Beach oceanfront parking lot.

The hike

From the Calafia Beach parking lot, two parallel routes head south along the oceanfront. An undulating footpath lies above the railroad tracks, at the base of the eroding cliffs. Or, cross the railroad tracks, walk down the embankment, and stroll along the sandy beach beneath the rock wall. Pass a trail crossing through a tunnel under the railroad tracks—the return trail. This paths wind up the eroding gorges to the state beach campground atop the bluffs.

Continue south, following a low ridge. In a quarter mile, the two routes merge. Stroll past oceanfront homes perched atop the cliffs. Look for the distinctive, tropical landscape of former President Richard Nixon's home, which sets it apart. As the shoreline rounds San Mateo Point, the cliffs begin to level out at Trestles Beach (Hike 111). Surfers frequent the beach.

Curve inland on the beach access trail, crossing the low dunes and railroad tracks. Head up the paved path/road through oaks and sycamores to the Old Coast Highway. The old road is now a biking route closed to vehicles. Bear left up the road to Avenida Del Presidente, the west frontage road of I-5. Walk north along the road for 0.8 miles to the forested campground on the left by Avenida San Luis Rey. Take the pedestrian path through the campground, and wind down the bluffs on the beach access trail. Return to the right.

From the campground, you may also return directly to Avenida Calafia via the campground road. ▪

111. Trestles Beach at San Mateo Point

SAN ONOFRE STATE BEACH NORTH

Hiking distance: 2 miles round trip
Hiking time: 1 hour
Configuration: out-and-back
Elevation gain: 100 feet
Difficulty: easy
Exposure: exposed coastline
Dogs: not allowed
Maps: U.S.G.S. San Clemente

Trestles Beach straddles the Orange–San Diego county line at San Mateo Point at the north end of San Onofre State Beach. San Mateo Creek empties into the sea at the point after draining from the Santa Ana Mountains through Riverside, Orange, and San Diego Counties. The intermittent creek forms a lagoon at the mouth of the creek at the San Mateo Creek Natural Preserve. The area is a vital riparian corridor that is popular with bird-watchers.

The wide, slanted Trestles Beach is named for the old train trestle over San Mateo Creek. The beach is a well-known surfing destination. An unpaved trail begins on the south edge of San Clemente and leads about a mile to the beach. En route, the trail crosses the Old Coast Highway. (The old road is now a biking route that begins at Avenida Del Presidente and continues through the San Onofre Bluffs Campground and Camp Pendleton to Oceanside.) The beach resides within sight of the San Onofre Nuclear Power Plant just two miles south. The two ominous reactors loom over the coastal landscape. Just north of the point is former President Nixon's "Western White House." Its location can be spotted from the distinctive, tropical landscape.

To the trailhead

3967 S. EL CAMINO REAL · SAN CLEMENTE   33.396828, -117.592585

From I-5 (San Diego Freeway) in San Clemente, take the Cristianitos Road exit. Head east one block to El Camino Real. Turn left and park along the street or in the parking area on the right.

A trail also leads to the beach from the San Mateo Campground, a short distance north on Cristianitos Road.

The hike

Walk back to Cristianitos Road. Take the beach access trail across the street on the left side of the chain-link fence. Follow the wide dirt path south, overlooking the agricultural fields and the Pacific Ocean. Descend into the forested drainage and cross under I-5. Emerge on the Old Coast Highway (closed to vehicles here) by the sign for San Onofre State Beach, Trestles Beach, and San Mateo Creek Natural Preserve.

Cross the abandoned road. Continue on the beach access road/trail—now paved—winding through native grass, chaparral, oaks, and sycamores. Cross over the railroad tracks or under the trestle to the low dunes and sandy beachfront, just north of San Mateo Point. To the north are views of San Clemente, the state beach, and the pier. To the south are views of the Santa Margarita Mountains, Camp Pendleton, and the San Onofre Bluffs. Stroll a short distance north to look for President Nixon's house, where he retreated after his resignation. The Spanish-style stucco home, with a red tile roof, sits on 25 blufftop acres. Return by retracing your steps. ■

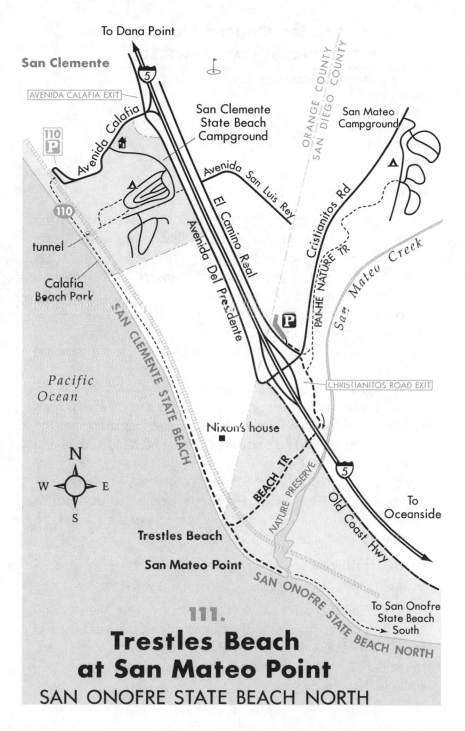

To Dana Point

San Clemente

5

AVENIDA CALAFIA EXIT

Avenida Calafia

110
P

110

tunnel

Calafia
Beach Park

San Clemente
State Beach
Campground

Avenida San Luis Rey

El Camino Real

Avenida Del Presidente

San Mateo
Campground

ORANGE COUNTY
SAN DIEGO COUNTY

Cristianitos Rd

PA-HE NATURE TR

San Mateo Creek

Sa.

P

Pacific
Ocean

SAN CLEMENTE STATE BEACH

Nixon's house

CHRISTIANITOS ROAD EXIT

5

BEACH TR.

NATURE PRESERVE

Old Coast Hwy

To
Oceanside

N
W — E
S

Trestles Beach

San Mateo Point

SAN ONOFRE STATE BEACH NORTH

To San Onofre
State Beach
South

111.
Trestles Beach
at San Mateo Point
SAN ONOFRE STATE BEACH NORTH

112. San Onofre Bluffs
SAN ONOFRE STATE BEACH SOUTH

Hiking distance: 6-mile loop
Hiking time: 3 hours
Configuration: several loop options
Elevation gain: 140 feet
Difficulty: easy to moderate
Exposure: exposed coastline
Dogs: allowed on Trails 1 and 6 only
Maps: U.S.G.S. San Onofre Bluff

The San Onofre Bluffs stretch along three miles of coastline on the south end of San Onofre State Beach. Inland, the coastal bluffs are surrounded by the Camp Pendleton Marine Base, which has restricted the area from development. There are sweeping views from atop the isolated, picturesque coastal terrace. Access to the bluffs is from the Old Coast Highway (Highway 101). The old road runs along the sheer sandstone cliffs. (The road is also a bike path that runs from San Clemente through Camp Pendleton to Oceanside.)

Located along the road are the RV and tents sites for the San Onofre Bluffs Campground, as well as six numbered access trails that cross and descend the eroding cliffs to the shoreline. The primitive, 2.6-mile strand of beach has pristine, sandy coves and quiet pockets. The long beach is shielded from civilization by the dramatic 140-foot cliffs. On the south end, at the base of Trail 6, is an unofficial clothing-optional beach. To the north lie the ever-present, surreal twin-dome reactors of the San Onofre Nuclear Power Plant.

To the trailhead

OLD PACIFIC HWY · SAN CLEMENTE   33.363739, -117.543396

From I-5 (San Diego Freeway) in San Onofre, take the Basilone Road exit. Turn southwest to the ocean side of the freeway, and drive 2.9 miles south on Old Highway 101 (the frontage road) to the San Onofre State Beach Bluffs Campground entrance. An entrance fee is required.

Parking and campsites are located along the entire stretch of the access road. There is a gate across the road at the far (south) end of the old road.

The hike

A trail parallels the entire 3-mile length of the campground and bluffs. The six numbered trails connect to the bluff path and parking lot. Each access path heads west across the bluffs and descends to the sandy beach. Every trail is different with its own distinct character. Most have a bench at the edge of the cliffs. Trail 5 descends through a gorge. Choose your own route and distance. ■

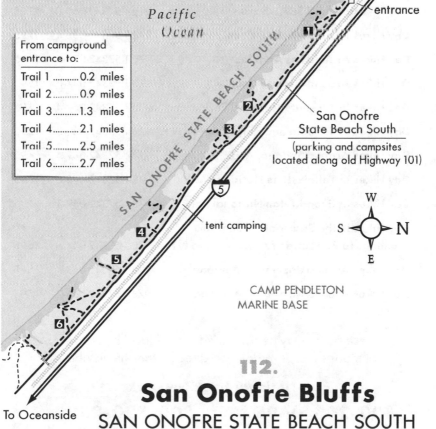

San Onofre
nuclear
power plant

To San
Clemente

Pacific
Ocean

entrance

From campground
entrance to:

Trail 1 ....0.2 miles
Trail 2 ....0.9 miles
Trail 3 ....1.3 miles
Trail 4 ....2.1 miles
Trail 5 ....2.5 miles
Trail 6 ....2.7 miles

San Onofre
State Beach South

(parking and campsites
located along old Highway 101)

SAN ONOFRE STATE BEACH SOUTH

tent camping

W
S ⊕ N
E

CAMP PENDLETON
MARINE BASE

To Oceanside

112.
San Onofre Bluffs
SAN ONOFRE STATE BEACH SOUTH

DAY HIKE BOOKS

Day Hikes On the California Central Coast.....978-1-57342-058-7 ....17.95

Day Hikes On the California Southern Coast ..978-1-57342-045-7 ...14.95

Day Hikes In the Santa Monica Mountains .....978-1-57342-065-5 ... 21.95

Day Hikes Around Sonoma County ....978-1-57342-053-2.... 16.95

Day Hikes Around Napa Valley ....978-1-57342-057-0 ... 16.95

Day Hikes Around Monterey and Carmel.......978-1-57342-067-9....19.95

Day Hikes Around Big Sur...........................978-1-57342-068-6 ... 18.95

Day Hikes Around San Luis Obispo ....978-1-57342-070-9 ... 21.95

Day Hikes Around Santa Barbara ....978-1-57342-060-0....17.95

Day Hikes Around Ventura County...............978-1-57342-062-4.....17.95

Day Hikes Around Los Angeles....................978-1-57342-071-6.... 21.95

Day Hikes Around Orange County ....978-1-57342-047-1.... 15.95

Day Hikes In Yosemite National Park ....978-1-57342-059-4 ... 13.95

Day Hikes In Sequoia and Kings Canyon N.P...978-1-57342-030-3 ... 12.95

Day Hikes Around Sedona, Arizona.............978-1-57342-049-5 ...14.95

Day Hikes In Yellowstone National Park........978-1-57342-048-8 ... 12.95

Day Hikes In Grand Teton National Park........978-1-57342-069-3....14.95

Day Hikes In the Beartooth Mountains
Billings to Red Lodge to Yellowstone N.P.....978-1-57342-064-8 ... 15.95

Day Hikes Around Bozeman, Montana ....978-1-57342-063-1.... 15.95

Day Hikes Around Missoula, Montana ....978-1-57342-066-2.... 15.95

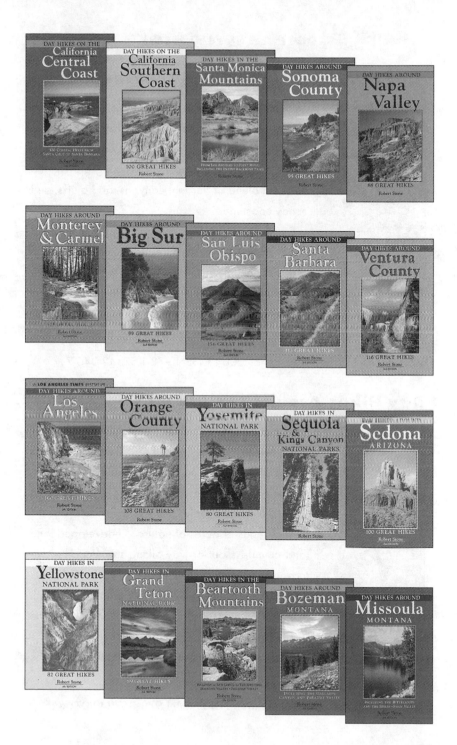

Day Hikes On the California Southern Coast

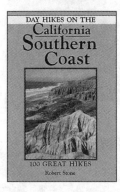

This guide is a collection of the best coastal hikes along 238 miles of southern California coastline, from Ventura County to the U.S.–Mexico border. The area has some of the most varied geography in the state...a blend of verdant canyons, arid bluffs, and sandy coastline.

Discover hundreds of miles of trails in scenic and undeveloped land, despite the expansive urban areas. Highlights include wide sand beaches, marine terraces, rocky headlands, tidal estuaries with coves and caves, sandstone cliffs, lighthouses, great locations for viewing wildlife, expansive dunes, forested canyons, waterfalls, and panoramic overlooks of the coast.

224 pages • 100 hikes • 1st Edition 2004 • ISBN 978-1-57342-045-7

Day Hikes Around Los Angeles

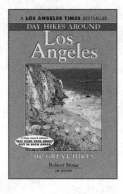

This book is an LA Times Best Seller and four-time award winner from three Outdoor Writers Associations. Now in its 6th edition, *Day Hikes Around Los Angeles* includes 160 hikes in and around a 50-mile radius of the city.

Thousands of acres of natural, undeveloped land and countless out-of-way hiking trails can be discovered tucked into the urban landscape. Highlights include year-round waterfalls, lighthouses, Griffith Park (the country's largest municipal park), the famous "HOLLYWOOD" sign, quiet canyon trails, far-reaching vistas of the city, the rugged terrain of the San Gabriel Mountains, and hikes along the entire length of the Santa Monica Mountains.

544 pages • 160 hikes • 6th Edition 2015 • ISBN 978-1-57342-071-6

INDEX

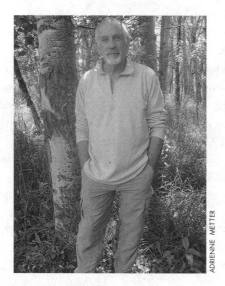

ADRIENNE METTER

About the Author

Since 1991, Robert Stone has been writer, photographer, and publisher of Day Hike Books. He is a Los Angeles Times Best Selling Author and an award-winning journalist of Rocky Mountain Outdoor Writers and Photographers, the Outdoor Writers Association of California, the Northwest Outdoor Writers Association, the Outdoor Writers Association of America, and the Bay Area Travel Writers.

Robert has hiked every trail in the Day Hike Book series. With 20 hiking guides in the series, many in their fourth and fifth editions, he has hiked thousands of miles of trails throughout the western United States. When Robert is not hiking, he researches, writes, and maps the hikes before returning to the trails. He spends summers in the Rocky Mountains of Montana and winters on the California Central Coast.